OPHTHALMIC CLINICAL ADVISOR

DIAGNOSIS AND TREATMENT

SECOND EDITION

Edited by

MYRON YANOFF, MD

Professor and Chairman
Department of Ophthalmology
Drexel University College of Medicine
Philadelphia, Pennsylvania

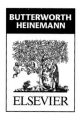

BUTTERWORTH
HEINEMANN

ELSEVIER

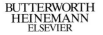

BUTTERWORTH
HEINEMANN
ELSEVIER

11830 Westline Industrial Drive
St. Louis, Missouri 63146

Library of Congress Control Number: 2007922551

Publishing Director: Linda Duncan
Acquisitions Editor: Kathryn Falk
Senior Developmental Editor: Christie M. Hart
Publishing Services Manager: Patricia Tannian
Senior Project Manager: Anne Altepeter
Cover Designer: Paula Catalano
Interior Designer: Paula Catalano

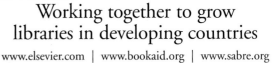

Working together to grow
libraries in developing countries

www.elsevier.com | www.bookaid.org | www.sabre.org

ELSEVIER   BOOK AID International   Sabre Foundation

Printed in China
Last digit is the print number: 9 8 7 6 5 4 3 2 1

Cataract and Systemic and Orbital Disorders

Myron Yanoff, MD
Professor and Chairman
Department of Ophthalmology
Drexel University College of Medicine
Philadelphia, Pennsylvania

Corneal and External Diseases

Parveen Nagra, MD
Drexel University College of Medicine
Philadelphia, Pennsylvania

Glaucoma

Polly Henderson, MD
Chief, Glaucoma Service
Department of Ophthalmology
Drexel University College of Medicine
Philadelphia, Pennsylvania

Neuro-ophthalmology and General Ophthalmology

Yelena Doych, MD
Instructor
Department of Ophthalmology
Drexel University College of Medicine
Philadelphia, Pennsylvania

Pediatric Ophthalmology

Gary R. Diamond, MD
Professor
Department of Ophthalmology and Pediatrics
Drexel University School of Medicine
Division of Ophthalmology
St. Christopher's Hospital for Children
Philadelphia, Pennsylvania

Retinal and Vitreous Disorders

Leo Santamaria, MD
Director, Vitreoretinal Service
Vice Chairman, Department of Ophthalmology
Drexel University College of Medicine
Philadelphia, Pennsylvania

With contributions from

Jennifer Palombi, OD
Dayton Veterans Administration Medical Center
Dayton, Ohio

Preface

Ophthalmic Clinical Advisor: Diagnosis and Treatment, Second Edition, provides expert recommendations and treatments of the conditions most often encountered by eye care providers. The design of the book (including an alphabetical listing of each entity) permits easy, rapid access of information for both the ophthalmic practitioner and the student. The layout for each entity (two-page spreads in most cases) allows for quick confirmation of the diagnosis and management of each entity. Most important, the same format is used throughout. The information given is not designed to be encyclopedic, but rather is aimed at hitting the highlights of the entities described. Full-color photographs highlight many of the conditions.

A distinctive feature of the book is the inclusion of the key coding numbers for most entities, which can be most helpful in organizing patients' medical records and in billing.

I anticipate that this book will be used by eye care providers and students as a quick reference guide of the salient points of the most commonly encountered and important entities pertaining to the eye.

Myron Yanoff

Contents

Contents

Cataract and Systemic and Orbital Disorders

Corneal and External Diseases

Glaucoma

Neuro-ophthalmology

Pediatric Ophthalmology

Contents by specialty

Retinal and Vitreous Disorders

This book provides current expert recommendations in the form of tabular summaries on the diagnosis and treatment of all major disorders throughout ophthalmology. Essential guidelines on each of the topics have been condensed into two pages of vital information, summarizing the main procedures in diagnosis and management of each disorder to provide a quick and easy reference.

Each disorder is presented on facing pages: the main procedures in diagnosis on the left and treatment options on the right.

Listed in the main column of the **Diagnosis** page is the definition; other common names; the common symptoms, signs, and complications of the disorder; pearls and considerations; and referral information, with brief notes explaining their significance and probability of occurrence, together with details of investigations that can be used to aid diagnosis.

The **left shaded side column** contains information to help readers evaluate the probability that a patient has the disorder. It may also include other information that could be useful in making a diagnosis (e.g., classification or grading systems, comparison of different diagnostic methods).

The numbers that appear in parentheses next to disease names at the top of each page and scattered throughout the text are from *The International Classification of Diseases* (New York, 1995, McGraw-Hill). These numbers are used by physicians to organize their patients' medical records and to facilitate the timely reimbursement of their services.

On the **Treatment** page, the main column contains information on lifestyle management and nonspecialist medical therapy of the disorder, with general information on specialist management when this is the main treatment.

Whenever possible under "Pharmacologic treatment," guidelines are given on the standard dosage for commonly used drugs, with details of contraindications and precautions, main drug interactions, and main side effects. In each case, however, the manufacturer's drug data sheet should be consulted before any regimen is prescribed.

The main goals of treatment (e.g., to cure, to palliate, to prevent), prognosis after treatment, precautions that the physician should take during and after treatment, and any other information that could help the clinician to make treatment decisions (e.g., other nonpharmacologic treatment options, special situations or groups of patients) are given in the **right shaded side column**. The key and general references at the end of this column provide readers with further practical information.

Acute posterior multifocal placoid pigment epitheliopathy

DIAGNOSIS

Definition
An acquired, self-limited inflammatory disorder and vasculitis of the retina, retinal pigment epithelium (RPE), and choroid in otherwise-healthy young adults.

Synonyms
None; often abbreviated AMPPE.

Symptoms
Rapid, painless loss of vision: in one or both eyes.

Signs
- Acute phase shows multiple circumscribed gray-white lesions at the level of the RPE located in the postequatorial retina (*see* Fig. 1).
- Late phase shows changes in the RPE similar to laser burns.

Associated serous detachment: uncommon.

Perivenous exudation in the retina.

Slight dilation of the retinal veins.

Papilledema, papillitis, optic neuropathy.

Episcleritis.

Iridocyclitis.

Investigations
Fluorescein angiography: in the acute phase, shows blockage of choroidal fluorescence (*see* Fig. 2), with midphase to late-phase diffuse staining of the acute lesions.

Complications
Choroidal neovascularization: rare.

Cerebritis: has been reported [1].

Pearls and Considerations
1. Spontaneous visual recovery is expected with or without systemic therapy, with most eyes achieving 20/40 or better vision in 1-6 mo from onset.
2. It is important to look for an underlying cause because the condition has been related to some antimicrobial agents, such as ampicillin and sulfonamides. If an antimicrobial agent is identified, it should be discontinued to prevent further recurrences.
3. Associated cerebral vasculitis may occur as late as 3 mo after presentation of AMPPE.

Referral Information
A computed tomography scan, magnetic resonance imaging, or cerebral arteriogram is indicated in patients with severe headache to rule out cerebral vasculitis.

Differential diagnosis
Serpiginous choroidopathy.

Cause
Unknown.

Epidemiology
- Disease affects healthy young men and women.
- One third of patients give a history of a viral prodrome.
- Recurrences are frequent.

TREATMENT

Diet and Lifestyle
- No precautions are necessary.

Pharmacologic Treatment
- Steroids should be instituted promptly if there are signs of associated cerebritis.

Nonpharmacologic Treatment
- No nonpharmacologic treatment is recommended.

Treatment aims
To observe patient.

Prognosis
- Visual prognosis is good, and there is a low incidence of recurrence after treatment.

Follow-up and management
- Based on the severity of the symptoms; patients should be followed every few weeks until they are out of the acute phase.

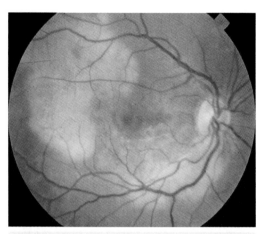

Figure 1 Acute phase of APMPPE showing multiple circumscribed gray-white lesions at the level of the retinal pigment epithelium located in the postequatorial retina.

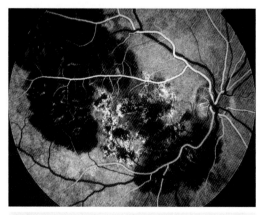

Figure 2 Fluorescein angiogram in the acute phase of the patient in Fig. 1, showing early blockage of choroidal fluorescence.

Key reference
1. Gass D: Inflammatory disease of the retina and choroid. In Gass D, editor: *Stereoscopic atlas of diseases: diagnosis and treatment*, ed 4, St Louis, 1997, Mosby.

General references
Bird AC: Acute multifocal placoid pigment epitheliopathy. In *Retina*, ed 4, E-dition, St Louis, 2006, Elsevier.
Kooragayala LM et al: Acute multifocal placoid pigment epitheliopathy, 2005, www.emedicine.com.
Pulido JS, Blake CR: Inflammatory choroiditis. In Tasman W et al, editors: *Duane's clinical ophthalmology* (CD-ROM), Philadelphia, 2004, Lippincott Williams & Wilkins.

AIDS-related ocular manifestations (042)

DIAGNOSIS

Definition
Any disease or condition of the eye or ocular adnexa that arises from a patient's underlying systemic acquired immunodeficiency syndrome (AIDS) infection or associated immuno-suppression.

Synonyms
None.

Symptoms
Decreased vision.
Eye pain.
Facial rash.
Floaters.
Red eye.
Shadow.

Signs
Human Immunodeficiency Virus (HIV) Retinopathy (Noninfectious)
Nerve fiber layer (NFL) and inner retinal hemorrhages.
Microaneurysms.
Cotton-wool spot: the most common manifestation of AIDS retinopathy.

Infectious Agents
Adnexa:
- Herpes zoster ophthalmicus (HZO).
- Molluscum contagiosum.

Cryptococcus: papilledema, multiple choroiditis, meningitis, endophthalmitis.
Cytomegalovirus (CMV) retinitis: classic intraretinal hemorrhages with white infiltrates (*see* Fig. 1).
Granular form: "brush fire" appearance.
Hemorrhagic form: "tomato ketchup fundus."
Herpes retinitis (acute retinal necrosis [ARN] or progressive outer retinal necrosis [PORN]): aggressive retinitis in which multiple white retinal infiltrates coalesce, leading to retinal detachment and visual loss (*see* Retinal necrosis, acute).
Pneumocystis **choroiditis:** multiple, deep, yellow-orange lesions at the level of the choroid (*see* Fig. 2).
Toxoplasmosis: multifocal outer retinal lesions that spread quickly; normally, little vitreous inflammation is seen in immunocompetent patients; occurs in previously diagnosed patients (*see* Fig. 3).
Microsporidia: chronic keratoconjunctivitis.
Syphilis: plaquelike serous elevations in the posterior pole.

Tumors
Kaposi's sarcoma: flat purplish lesion on the eyelid or conjunctiva similar to lesions seen on the skin; may be mistaken for subconjunctival hemorrhage.
Central nervous system (CNS) lymphoma.
Lymphomas.
Squamous cell carcinoma of the eyelid.

Neurologic Manifestations
Cranial nerve palsies.
Papilledema.
Nystagmus.
Optic neuritis.
Visual field defects.

Differential diagnosis
Cotton-wool spots: of diabetes, hypertension, ocular ischemia, and vasculitis.

Cause
- HIV infection.

Diagnosis continued on p. 6

TREATMENT

Diet and Lifestyle
- Compliance with highly active antiretroviral therapy (HAART).

Pharmacologic Treatment
For Cytomegalovirus Infection
Intravenous (IV) therapy with ganciclovir, foscarnet, or cidofovir.
Intravitreal ganciclovir implant (sustained-release device) placed in the pars plana of the eye.
Intravitreal injections of ganciclovir or foscarnet.

For *Pneumocystis* sp. Infection
Bactrim, pentamidine.

For Herpes Simplex or Zoster Infection
Aggressive treatment with IV acyclovir.

For Toxoplasmosis
Pyrimethamine, sulfa drugs, or clindamycin.

For Syphilis
High-dose IV penicillin for 10-14 days.

Cryptococcus
IV amphotericin, IV itraconazole, vitrectomy, and intravitreal amphotericin for endophthalmitis.

Microsporidia
Topical fumagillin up to every 2 hr initially, then taper slowly.

Nonpharmacologic Treatment
- Regular periodic ocular examinations (e.g., CD4+ count <50, every 3 mo).

Treatment aims
- To control the infection with appropriate antiviral and antimicrobial agents.
- To stabilize or improve vision.
- To treat secondary complications (e.g., retinal detachment) with laser or surgery.

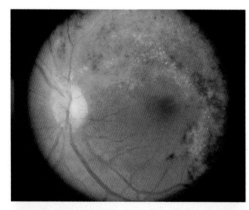

Figure 1   Cytomegalovirus (CMV) retinitis with the characteristic white perivascular retinal infiltrates and intraretinal hemorrhages, or "pizza pie fundus."

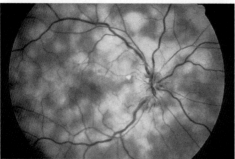

Figure 2   *Pneumocystis* choroiditis showing deep choroidal, creamy yellow-orange infiltrates throughout the posterior pole.

Treatment continued on p. 7

DIAGNOSIS—cont'd

Investigations

Careful history: reviewing the patient's past medical history often gives clues to the cause.

CD4+ count: usually <50 cells/mm^3 when patients develop CMV retinitis.

Cryptococcus: high risk of CNS infection.

PORN: CD4+ count >50 cells/mm^3 (*see* Fig. 4).

ARN: CD4+ count <50 cells/mm^3 (*see* Fig. 5).

Pneumocystis jiroveci (**previously** *P. carinii*): CD4+ count <200 cells/mm^3.

Fluorescein angiography: helpful in differentiating retinal infections.

Computed tomography and magnetic resonance imaging scans: may be necessary for patients with CNS abnormalities.

Vitreous biopsy with analysis of polymerase chain reaction: helps distinguish herpes simplex from zoster and CMV when the clinical picture is not clear-cut.

Sequential fundus photographs: help monitor patients for response to therapy and evidence of disease progression.

Complications

Visual loss.

Retinal detachment.

Medication related:

- Cidofovir: anterior uveitis and profound hypotony.
- Rifabutin (prophylaxis for atypical myobacterial infection): severe (sometimes bilateral) anterior uveitis.

Pearls and Considerations

1. Dilated fundus examination (DFE) should be performed every 3 mo in patients with a CD4+ count ≤50 cells/mm^3 because of the potential for asymptomatic CMV retinitis.
2. AIDS patients' complications should be treated cautiously with steroids because of the potential for further immunosuppression and infection.
3. Approximately 70%-80% of AIDS patients will require treatment for an ocular complication at some time in their lives.
4. CMV is the most common severe and sight-threatening ocular infection in AIDS patients.
5. Infections of the cornea and adnexa are less common than intraocular infections in AIDS patients.

Referral Information

Variable and specific to the etiology of each complication.

TREATMENT—cont'd

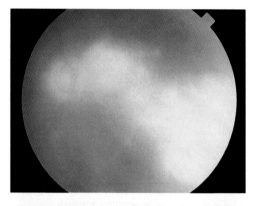

Figure 3 Outer retinal toxoplasmosis in an AIDS patient, showing the "brush fire" advancement of the infection.

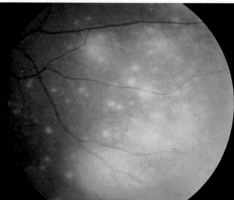

Figure 4 Progressive outer retinal necrosis (PORN). *(From Yanoff M, Duker J: Ophthalmology, ed 2, St Louis, 2003, Elsevier.)*

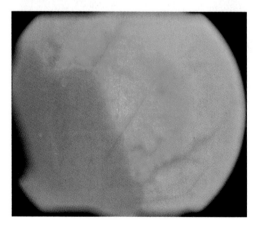

Figure 5 Acute retinal necrosis (ARN). *(From Yanoff M, Duker J: Ophthalmology, ed 2, St Louis, 2003, Elsevier.)*

General references

Copeland R et al: Ocular manifestations of HIV, 2005, www.emedicine.com.

Holland GN, Levinson RD: Ocular infections associated with acquired immunodeficiency syndrome. In Tasman W et al, editors: *Duane's clinical ophthalmology* (CD-ROM), Philadelphia, 2004, Lippincott Williams & Wilkins.

Lightman S: *HIV and the eye*, London, 2000, Imperial College Press.

Moraes HV Jr: Ocular manifestations of HIV/AIDS, *Curr Opin Ophthalmol* 13(6):397-403, 2002.

Rescigno R, Dinowitz M: Ophthalmic manifestations of immunodeficiency states, *Clin Rev Allergy Immunol* 20(2):163-181, 2001.

Rhee DJ, Pyfer MF: Acquired immunodeficiency syndrome (AIDS). In *The Wills eye manual*, Philadelphia, 1999, Lippincott Williams & Wilkins, pp 435-445.

Albinism   (270.2)

DIAGNOSIS

Definition
The classification of a group of congenital diseases that result from defective pigment production (melanogenesis); can be ocular or oculocutaneous.

Synonyms
None; associated abbreviations: OA (ocular albinism) and OCA (oculocutaneous albinism), CHS (Chédiak-Higashi syndrome), HPS (Hermansky-Pudlak syndrome), GS (Griscelli syndrome) [1].

Symptoms
Painful photophobia: in most patients.
Decreased visual acuity (worse at distance than near): in most patients.
Esthetic blemish from nystagmus: in most patients.
Poor binocular vision: because of near-total decussation of the optic nerves at the chiasm.

Signs
Horizontal nystagmus: with possible null point and head posture to maximize visual acuity.
Iris transillumination: in patients with ocular albinism.
Pink irides: in patients with oculocutaneous albinism.
Foveal hypoplasia or aplasia: with retinal vascular presence in the foveal area.
Decreased pigment in retinal pigment epithelium (RPE) and iris pigment epithelium (IPE): *see* figure.
Esotropia.
Refractive errors: often myopia.

Investigations
Skin biopsy: patients with X-linked recessive ocular albinism have macromelanosomes.
Testing for presence of tyrosinase: patients with tyrosinase-negative oculocutaneous albinism have no tyrosinase in hair bulbs; patients with tyrosinase-positive oculocutaneous albinism do.
- Patients with Chédiak-Higashi syndrome cannot opsonize certain bacteria.
- Patients with Hermansky-Pudlak syndrome have platelet adherence abnormalities and capillary fragility.

Complications
Skin disorders, including melanomas: patients with oculocutaneous albinism are at risk for skin malignancies; protection is imperative.
Photophobia: may disrupt outdoor activities.
Chronic infections, including pneumonia: in patients with Chédiak-Higashi syndrome.
Clotting abnormalities: in patients with Hermansky-Pudlak syndrome.
- Most patients with albinism and nystagmus cannot obtain a driver's license because their distance visual acuity is 20/100 to 20/200. Their near visual acuity, however, may be close to 20/20 if children are permitted to hold objects closely. Thus, children usually succeed in normal schooling environments if they are permitted to sit in the front of the classroom and walk to the blackboard when necessary. Older children may require low-vision aids for near and distant work.

Classification
Ocular albinism (X-linked recessive, rarely autosomal dominant or recessive).
Oculocutaneous albinism (autosomal recessive): tyrosinase negative, brown albinism, tyrosinase positive, rufous albinism, yellow mutant, Hermansky-Pudlak, Chédiak-Higashi.

Diagnosis continued on p. 10

Differential diagnosis
Patients have depigmented skin or adnexal structures but no increased decussation of the optic nerves at the chiasm. Various albinoid forms exist:
- *Waardenburg syndrome:* autosomal dominant association of white forelock (17%), piebald appearance, sensorineural deafness, synophrys, blepharophimosis, lateral displacement of lacrimal puncti.
- *Cross syndrome:* skin hypopigmentation with deficient melanosomes, mental retardation, microphthalmia, cataracts.
- *Åland Island disease:* believed to be a form of X-linked recessive, congenital stationary night blindness, with affected males exhibiting posterior-pole retinal depigmentation.

Cause
Congenital, hereditary, stationary.
- Oculocutaneous albinism segregates in most patients as an autosomal recessive; ocular albinism segregates in most affected patients as an X-linked recessive.

Associated features
Tyrosinase negative: white hair, pink skin.
Tyrosinase positive: white hair as children; may become blond; may develop pigmented nevi.
Yellow mutant: white hair and pink skin as infants; develop yellow hair at 6 mo and normal skin pigmentation by 3 yr.
Brown albinism: Africans with reddish brown skin, red hair, freckles, brown irides.
Autosomal dominant oculocutaneous albinism: white to cream skin, white hair, freckles, gray-blue irides.

Pathology
- Caucasian patients with ocular albinism have spotty areas of deficient melanin in the IPE melanosomes and generally no melanin in RPE melanosomes. Patients with oculocutaneous albinism have diffuse deficiency of IPE and RPE melanin; they also have varying amounts of absent dermal melanin.
- Patients with ocular and oculocutaneous albinism have absent foveal depressions, with vascular incursion into the area normally occupied by the fovea. They also have almost total decussation of the optic nerves at the chiasm.

TREATMENT

Diet and Lifestyle
- Many patients will benefit from wearing sunglasses and sunscreen protection for the skin. Low-vision aids are recommended for elderly patients.

Pharmacologic Treatment
- No pharmacologic treatment is recommended.

Treatment aims
To ensure patient comfort and safety.
To prevent bleeding diatheses in patients with Hermansky-Pudlak syndrome.
To treat infections early in patients with Chédiak-Higashi syndrome.

Other treatments
Glasses where appropriate; nystagmus prevents full benefit in many patients.

Prognosis
- Prognosis is stable in most patients; the nystagmus amplitude lessens with age, but visual acuity usually does not improve.
- Prognosis is guarded in patients with Hermansky-Pudlak or Chédiak-Higashi syndrome.

Follow-up and management
- Yearly follow-up is sufficient for most patients. Those with Hermansky-Pudlak or Chédiak-Higashi syndrome will require individualized follow-up and management of systemic problems. Many patients will want genetic counseling.

Treatment continued on p. 11

DIAGNOSIS—cont'd

Pearls and Considerations

1. Ultraviolet (UV)-protective sunglasses are recommended for patients with any variant of ocular albinism or oculocutaneous albinism.
2. Patients affected by oculocutaneous albinism should be encouraged to be screened frequently for skin cancer [1].
3. Color vision remains normal in patients with albinism [2].
4. Clinicians should be mindful of the distinction between ocular albinism (with reduced acuity of 20/70 to 20/200) and *blond fundus,* associated with lightly pigmented individuals who have normal visual acuity [2].

Referral Information

Some variations of oculocutaneous albinism are potentially fatal; therefore, medical and hematologic referral should be considered to rule out these variants [3].

TREATMENT—cont'd

Nonpharmacologic Treatment
Strabismus surgery.
Eye muscle surgery: to align the head in patients who adopt a posture resulting from the presence of a nystagmus-associated null point.

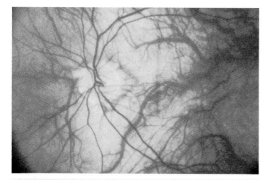

Note pale fundus caused by lack of pigment in the retinal pigment epithelium and choroid.

Key references

1. Boissy RE et al: Albinism, 2005, www.emedicine.com.
2. Seiving PA: Retinitis pigmentosa and related disorders. In Yanoff M et al, editors: *Ophthalmology*, E-dition, St Louis, 2006, Elsevier.
3. Kasier PK, Friedman NJ: Albinism. In *The Massachusetts Eye and Ear Infirmary illustrated manual of ophthalmology*, ed 2, Philadelphia, 2004, Saunders-Elsevier, pp 407-408.

General references

Carr RE, Noble KG, Siegel IM: Albinism. *Ophthalmology* 88:377, 1981.

Cortin P, Tremblay M, Lemagne JM: X-linked ocular albinism: relative value of skin biopsy, iris transillumination and funduscopy in identifying affected males and carriers, *Can J Ophthalmol* 16:121, 1981.

Creel DJ, Summers CG, King RA: Visual anomalies associated with albinism, *Ophthalmic Pediatr Genet* 11:193, 1990.

Kinnear PE, Jay B, Witkop CJ: Albinism [review], *Surv Ophthalmol* 30:75, 1985.

Mietz H, Green WR, Wolff SM, Abundo GP: Foveal hypoplasia in complete oculocutaneous albinism, *Retina* 12:254, 1992.

Amblyopia (368.0)

DIAGNOSIS

Definition
Incomplete visual development secondary to strabismus, anisometropia, or visual deprivation.

Synonym
"Lazy eye."

Symptoms
Decreased visual acuity: from lack of use of an eye.

Signs
Decreased visual acuity: during photopic acuity testing; during scotopic testing of a strabismic patient with amblyopia (see below), amblyopic eye may have equal acuity to normal eye.
Decreased accommodative ability.
Afferent pupillary defect: in severely amblyopic eyes; visual acuity less than 20/200.
Eccentric viewing: in patients with severely amblyopic eyes, may view with nonfoveal retinal areas.
Enhanced crowding phenomenon: single optotypes discerned better than linear ones.

Investigations
Visual acuity test: decreased in an eye (rarely both eyes) with normal structure; often better with isolated optotypes than with linear ones.
History of strabismus, anisometropia, media opacity.
Neutral-density filter: placing over amblyopic eye may not degrade acuity; over normal eye, acuity will be degraded.

Complications
Permanent loss of visual acuity: if amblyopia is not reversed as child.
Loss of precise stereoscopic ability.
Loss of accommodative ability.

Pearls and Considerations
1. Prolonged use of atropine may lead to systemic reactions, hypersensitivity reactions of the lids, irritation, redness, edema, and follicular conjunctivitis or dermatitis [1]. Patients treated with atropine therapy should be monitored on a regular basis for these side effects.
2. Amblyopia should be suspected in any strabismic child who appears to have a preference for one eye over the other.
3. Amblyopia should be suspected in cases of reduced visual acuity in patients with ≥2.00 diopters (D) of difference in hyperopic refractive error, or ≥4.00-D difference in myopic refractive error [2].
4. Because of crowding phenomenon, patients with amblyopia often read better when presented with single letters rather than a whole line of letters [3].
5. Although vision loss from amblyopia may be profound, light perception is always maintained.
6. Patients with profound amblyopia are at increased risk for accidents because as much as one fourth of their binocular visual field may be obscured or lost secondary to their reduced vision.
7. Microstrabismic amblyopia (or monofixation syndrome) is often detected later than other strabismic amblyopias because the small-angle esotropia is not obvious. Careful cover test analysis should be undertaken in all children to facilitate early detection.

Referral Information
All children with suspected amblyopia should undergo a complete sensorimotor examination; children with strabismic amblyopia may be referred for extraocular muscle (EOM) realignment surgery. Consider referring other children to appropriate pediatric specialists for the implementation and monitoring of patching, orthoptic devices, and medical therapy.

Differential diagnosis
Decreased visual acuity from another cause with subtle structural eye pathology, including:
- Central nervous system lesions.
- Optic nerve dystrophies.
- Keratoconus.
- High refractive errors and dishabituation to clear retinal image.
- Subtle foveal lesions.

Cause
Strabismus: from foveal suppression in non-fixing eye.
Anisometropia: from persistently blurred image in eye with greater refractive error.
Deprivation: from media opacity (e.g., cataract, corneal lesion).
Isometropic (refractive): from persistent binocular image blurring caused by high refractive errors; controversial (many will respond to refractive correction alone).

Epidemiology
- Incidence: 2.0%-2.5% in the general population.
- No de novo condition develops after 5.5 yr of age. The earlier the onset, the more rapidly amblyopia develops and the deeper it is; conversely, the earlier it is detected, the easier it is to reverse.

Associated features
Strabismus, anisometropia, media opacities; perhaps bilateral highly refractive errors.

Pathology
- Deprivation amblyopia: axon bodies in lateral geniculate layers 2, 3, 5 (ipsilateral) decreased 18%-25% in size; deprived-eye receptive bands in cortical layer IVc narrower than normal-eye receptive bands.
- Anisometropic amblyopia: no human specimens available; in monkeys, pathology is similar to deprivation amblyopia but at a slightly smaller effect.
- Strabismic amblyopia: as with deprivation amblyopia, but in the lateral geniculate; body axons receiving input from the central 10 degrees of fixation are affected.

TREATMENT

Diet and Lifestyle
• No special precautions are necessary.

Pharmacologic Treatment
• Recent trials of oral levodopa and carbidopa suggest efficacy in temporarily improving acuity from an average of 20/121 to 20/96 in older amblyopic children and teenagers.
• **Penalization** (atropinization of a highly hyperopic patient's better-sighted eye to switch fixation to the amblyopic eye) is recommended in some patients.

Nonpharmacologic Treatment
Occlusion of the better-sighted eye: either all waking hours or some fraction, followed by 1-2 hr/day occlusion until the patient's ninth birthday; this can be accomplished by a patch or occluding contact lens.

Pleoptics: dazzling of extrafoveal retina with bright light, followed by foveal stimulation; attempted in Europe on older patients with amblyopia.

Game-format devices: often used together with occlusion to stimulate amblyopic fovea.

Red-glass treatment: red filter placed over amblyopic eye to stimulate central fixation in patients with deep amblyopia having eccentric viewing; rarely used today.

Complications of Occlusion Treatment
Decrease in acuity of better-sighted eye.
Disruption of binocular vision, leading to emergence of strabismus.

Treatment aims
To equalize and maintain acuity between the eyes without creating amblyopia in the sound eye.

Other treatments
Anisometropic amblyopia patients will require refractive correction.
Patients who have media opacities will require surgery for these.

Prognosis
• Most children who have strabismic amblyopia will respond to treatment if initiated before 7 or 8 yr of age; children as old as ~15 yr deserve an attempt at treatment, and many will respond.
• Children who have anisometropic amblyopia are less responsive to treatment; those with media opacities are least responsive.

Follow-up and management
• Patients who have aligned eyes and peripheral fusion should be patched no more than 5 hr/day. Patients who have constant strabismus can be patched all waking hours. Patients undergoing full-time occlusion should be reexamined weekly per year of age (e.g., q 3 wk in a 3-year-old) until the acuity is equal.
• Successfully treated patients with amblyopia should be patched 1 hr/day to maintain visual acuity in the previously amblyopic eye.

Key references
1. Hom MM. Atropine. In *Mosby's ocular drug consult*, St Louis, 2005, Mosby-Elsevier, p 50.
2. Diamond JR. Amblyopia. In Yanoff M et al, editors: *Ophthalmology*, E-dition, St Louis, 2006, Elsevier.
3. Yen KG: Amblyopia, 2006, www.emedicine.com.

General references
Eggers HM, Blakemore C: Physiologic basis of anisometropic amblyopia, *Science* 201:264-272, 1978.
Helveston EM: Relationship between degree of anisometropia and depth of amblyopia, *Am J Ophthalmol* 62:757-765, 1966.
Leguire LE, Rogers GL, Bremer DL, et al: Levodopa/carbidopa for childhood amblyopia, *Invest Ophthalmol Vis Sci* 34:3090, 1993.
Leske MC, Hawkins BS: Screening: relationship to diagnosis and therapy. In Tasman W et al, editors: *Duane's clinical ophthalmology* (CD-ROM), Philadelphia, 2004, Lippincott Williams & Wilkins.
Levi DM, Klein SA, Aitsebaomo AP: Vernier acuity, crowding and cortical magnification, *Vision Res* 25:963-972, 1985.
Von Noorden GK, Crawford MLJ, Levacy RA: The lateral geniculate nucleus in human anisometropic amblyopia, *Invest Ophthalmol Vis Sci* 24: 788-796, 1983.

Anatomically narrow angle   (365.02)

DIAGNOSIS

Definition
A condition in which the anterior chamber angle is narrow or partially closed with an associated shallow anterior chamber, putting the patient at increased risk for angle-closure glaucoma.

Synonyms
None; associated abbreviations include ACG (angle-closure glaucoma) and CACG (chronic angle-closure glaucoma).

Symptoms
- Patients are asymptomatic.

Signs
Hyperopia: because these patients usually have smaller-than-average eyes, they will be hyperopic.

Shallow peripheral anterior chamber: generally with a van Herick grading of ≤2 when examined with the slit lamp (*see* figure).

Narrow angle on gonioscopy: the anterior-chamber angle will appear quite narrow on gonioscopy, usually ≤20 degrees; by definition, these patients do not have a closed angle or elevated intraocular pressure (IOP). However, the angle may appear optically closed, meaning that no angle structures are visible on gonioscopy, and the iris appears to be in contact with the peripheral cornea. An asymptomatic, anatomically narrow angle should open past the trabecular meshwork with pressure gonioscopy.

Investigations
Complete eye examination, including gonioscopy: in patients with critically narrow or optically closed angles, pupil dilation for funduscopy may provoke an attack of angle-closure glaucoma; such patients may be candidates for prophylactic peripheral iridectomy (*see* Nonpharmacologic treatment).

A-scan ultrasound biometry: measurement of the anterior-chamber depth and axial length of the eye gives some indication of the risk of angle closure; an anterior-chamber depth of <2 mm is associated with a high risk of subsequent angle closure.

B-scan ultrasound biomicroscopy: this recently introduced imaging technique allows a precise measurement of the width of the anterior-chamber angle and the relative positions of the iris root, angle structures, and ciliary body.

Complications
Angle-closure glaucoma: estimated lifetime risk is ~30% in patients with critically narrow angles.

Pearls and Considerations
1. Anterior-chamber depth can be measured by ultrasound. A normal finding is generally ~3.5 mm. Anterior chambers ≤2.5 mm are considered at risk for angle closure.
2. Gonioscopy is contraindicated in patients with hyphema, compromised cornea, or laceration of the globe.
3. Pilocarpine may result in severely blurred vision in patients with central lenticular opacities [1]. A full ophthalmic examination should be performed to rule out such opacities before initiating pilocarpine therapy.
4. Pilocarpine should be used with caution in patients with cholelithiasis, biliary tract disease, cardiovascular disease, and pulmonary disease [1].

Referral Information
Referral should be considered for prophylactic peripheral iridotomy. Appropriate glaucoma workup should be obtained in patients with suspected acute or chronic angle-closure events; and in those with high IOP, referral for trabeculectomy or filtering surgery should be considered to lower pressure adequately [2].

Differential diagnosis
Other conditions that may produce a narrow anterior-chamber angle on gonioscopy without elevated IOP or other signs of glaucoma include:
- Plateau iris configuration.
- Phacomorphic angle narrowing: caused by a large lens.
- Nanophthalmos.
- Retinopathy of prematurity.
- Subluxation of the lens.
- Spherophakia.

Cause
Anatomically narrow angles result from the anatomy and configuration of the structures of the anterior segment of the eye. The eyes are smaller than average with a short axial length, shallow anterior chamber, small corneal diameter, anteriorly inserted iris root, and a normal or larger-than-normal crystalline lens. The result is an increase in the normal physiologic resistance to aqueous flow at the pupillary margin and a forward bowing and displacement of the peripheral iris toward the angle and peripheral cornea. The forward bowing of the iris may become great enough to cause the iris to adhere to the trabecular meshwork, obstruct the outflow of the aqueous, and cause angle-closure glaucoma (365.2).

Epidemiology
Population studies have found that anatomically narrow angles occur in 0.5%-1.0% of the white and black American population. In some other ethnic groups (e.g., Koreans, North American Inuit), narrow angles are much more common.

Associated features
- Hyperopia.
- Small optic discs with very small or absent physiologic cups.

TREATMENT

Diet and Lifestyle

- Avoid drugs and activities that may dilate the pupil; such agents may provoke an attack of angle closure.
- Many antihistamines and sympathomimetics found in proprietary cold and allergy medications should be avoided.
- Phenothiazine and many other psychotropic drugs should be avoided.
- Certain activities that cause the pupils to dilate, such as being in low-light situations (e.g., movie theater) or sexual intercourse, may cause pupillary dilation and angle-closure glaucoma in susceptible individuals.

Pharmacologic Treatment
Miotics

- The use of miotics (e.g., pilocarpine) may reduce the risk of angle closure for a time. Studies have shown, however, that long-term use of pilocarpine does not prevent angle closure in high-risk individuals. With long-term use, miotics actually increase the likelihood of developing angle closure.

Nonpharmacologic Treatment
Laser Iridectomy

- Laser iridectomy is definitive treatment. By creating an alternative route for the aqueous from the posterior chamber to the anterior chamber, the relative pupil block and the forward bowing of the iris are eliminated. This allows the angle to widen and removes the risk of future angle closure. The treatment is almost 100% effective and very safe. Serious complications following laser iridectomy are extremely rare.

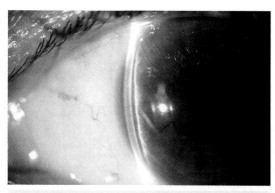

Anatomically narrow angle. Van Herick test demonstrating shallow peripheral anterior chamber with the slit-lamp beam.

Treatment aims

To widen the angle and eliminate the risk of angle closure.

Prognosis

Studies have shown that the risk of angle closure in subjects with asymptomatic but very critically narrow angles is between 15% and 30%, a fairly high risk for a serious and potentially blinding disease. Many clinicians therefore advocate the use of prophylactic laser iridectomy in such patients, especially if pupil dilation is required regularly (e.g., diabetic patient at risk for retinopathy).

Follow-up and management

Patients with critically narrowed angles should be advised of the risks and offered a laser iridectomy. Once an iridectomy has been done, the patient is no longer at risk for angle closure and may be followed as would any otherwise-normal individual. Patients who decline iridectomy should be advised of the symptoms of angle closure and instructed to seek medical attention immediately if any symptoms develop. In the absence of symptoms, patients declining iridectomy should be followed once or twice a year with gonioscopy and IOP measurements.

Key references

1. Hom MM: Pilocarpine. In *Mosby's ocular drug consult*, St Louis, 2005, Mosby-Elsevier, pp 444-446.
2. Kasier PK, Friedman NJ: Angle closure glaucoma. In *The Massachusetts Eye and Ear Infirmary illustrated manual of ophthalmology*, ed 2, Philadelphia, 2004, Saunders-Elsevier, pp 203-207.

General references

Alward WL: *Color atlas of gonioscopy*, London, 1994, Mosby–Year Book Europe.

Palmberg P: Gonioscopy. In Ritch R, Shields MB, Krupin T, editors: *The glaucomas*, ed 2, St Louis, 1996, Mosby, pp 455-469.

Panek WC, Christensen RE, Lee DA, et al: Biometric variables in patients with occludable anterior chamber angles, *Am J Ophthalmol* 110:185-188, 1990.

Sawada A, Sakuma T, Yamamoto T, et al: Appositional angle closure in eyes with narrow angles: comparison between fellow eyes of acute angle-closure glaucoma and normotensive cases, *J Glaucoma* 6:288-292, 1997.

Wilensky JT, Kaufman PL, Frohlichstein D, et al: Follow-up of angle-closure glaucoma suspects, *Am J Ophthalmol* 115:338-346, 1993.

Wilensky JT, Ritch R, Kolker AE: Should patients with anatomically narrow angles have prophylactic iridectomy? *Surv Ophthalmol* 41:31-36, 1996.

Angioid streaks   (363.43)

DIAGNOSIS

Definition
Full-thickness breaks in calcified, thickened Bruch's membrane with disruption of overlying retinal pigment epithelium (RPE) [1].

Synonyms
None.

Symptoms
- Patients are usually asymptomatic in the early course.

Gradual decrease in vision: common with increase in age.

Loss of vision to legal blindness: seen in ~50% of patients.

- Scotoma.
- Metamorphosia.

Signs
Radially oriented cracks in the pigment layer emanating from the optic nerve: *see* Fig. 1.

"Peau d'orange" or mottled appearance of the RPE: *see* Fig. 2.

Peripheral atrophic spots.

Disc drusen.

Subretinal crystalline deposits.

Subretinal hemorrhage: if associated with trauma or choroidal neovascularization.

Choroidal neovascular membrane (CNVM).

Investigations
Physical examination: to rule out systemic disorders, such as pseudoxanthoma elasticum (PXE), Ehlers-Danlos syndrome, Paget's disease, and sickle cell disease.

Fluorescein angiogram: if choroidal neovascularization is suspected.

Serum alkaline phosphatase and urine calcium: if considering Paget's disease.

Sickle cell prep and hemoglobin electrophoresis: if considering sickle cell disease.

Complications
High risk of subretinal bleeding secondary to blunt trauma.

RPE detachment.

Choroidal neovascularization.

Disciform scarring.

Pearls and Considerations
1. In patients with angioid streaks, minor trauma can result in rupture of Bruch's membrane with resultant hemorrhage or choroidal neovascularization [1,2].
2. Patients with angioid streaks benefit from regular Amsler grid testing to monitor for visual changes associated with formation of subretinal neovascular membrane (SRNVM).
3. The color of angioid streaks depends on natural fundus coloration and the amount of overlying RPE atrophy. Streaks appear red in blond fundi or medium to dark brown in more pigmented fundi [3].

Referral Information
1. Patients who present with associated choroidal neovascularization should be referred for laser photocoagulation, submacular surgery, or photodynamic therapy (PDT) as appropriate.
2. Patients identified with angioid streaks should have an appropriate medical referral to rule out underlying systemic disease. Evaluation should include skin biopsy and photographs.

Differential diagnosis
Senile angioid streaks.
Choroidal rupture secondary to trauma.
Senile macular degeneration.
Idiopathic choroidal neovascularization.
Myopia with lacquer cracks.
Presumed ocular histoplasmosis.
Choroidal folds.
Toxoplasmosis.

Cause
Idiopathic, 50%.
PXE, 34%.
Paget's disease, 10%.
Sickle cell hemoglobinopathies, 6%.
Ehlers-Danlos syndrome.
Greenblad-Strandberg syndrome.

Epidemiology
- 50% of patients with angioid streaks will have systemic associations.
- 85% of patients with PXE have evidence of angioid streaks.
- 8%-15% of patients with Paget's disease have angioid streaks.

Associated features
- Peau d'orange appearance.
- PXE: "plucked-chicken skin," gastrointestinal tract bleeding, cardiac abnormalities.

Pathology
- Thickening, elastic degeneration, and calcification of Bruch's membrane.
- Breaks in the elastic and collagenous layers of Bruch's membrane.
- Fibrovascular ingrowth.
- Secondary RPE atrophy, choriocapillaris damage, photoreceptor loss, RPE hypertrophy, serous retinal detachment, disciform scarring.

TREATMENT

Diet and Lifestyle
Safety glasses should be worn, because trauma precipitates hemorrhage.

Pharmacologic Treatment
- No pharmacologic treatment is recommended.

Nonpharmacologic Treatment
Amsler grid testing: for early detection of choroidal neovascularization.
Laser photocoagulation: of choroidal neovascularization.
- Despite laser intervention, there is a high incidence of recurrence.
- Prophylactic laser treatment should not be performed because it may induce choroidal neovascularization.
- PDT may be an option in certain cases.

Treatment aims
To educate patients and detect secondary choroidal neovascularization early.
- Low-vision aids may be useful.
- Genetic counseling should be considered for hereditary conditions.

Prognosis
- Long-term prognosis is guarded. Patients can lose vision to the level of legal blindness if the streaks involve the fovea or if secondary choroidal neovascularization in the fovea occurs.

Follow-up and management
- Amsler grid testing daily.
- Dilated fundus examination every 6 mo.

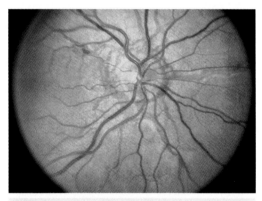

Figure 1 Note the radially oriented cracks in the pigment layer emanating from the optic nerve.

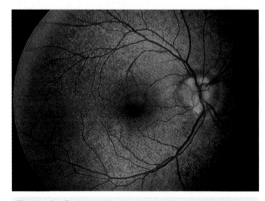

Figure 2 Patient with pseudoxanthoma elasticum and "peau d'orange" appearance to the retinal pigment epithelium.

Key references
1. Kasier PK, Friedman NJ: Angioid streaks. In *The Massachusetts Eye and Ear Infirmary illustrated manual of ophthalmology*, ed 2, Philadelphia, 2004, Saunders-Elsevier, pp 333-335.
2. Abusamak M: Angioid streaks, 2005, www.emedicine.com.
3. Atebara NH: Miscellaneous abnormalities of the fundus. In Tasman W et al, editors: *Duane's clinical ophthalmology* (CD-ROM), Philadelphia, 2004, Lippincott Williams & Wilkins.

General references
Aessopos A, Farmakis D, Loukopoulos D: Elastic tissue abnormalities resembling pseudoxanthoma elasticum in beta thalassemia and the sickling syndromes, *Blood* 99(1):30-35, 2002.
Landy J, Brown GC: Update on photodynamic therapy, *Curr Opin Ophthalmol* 14(3):163-168, 2003.

DIAGNOSIS

Definition
Ischemia of the anterior optic nerve head secondary to underlying systemic granulomatous vasculitis of the large and medium-sized blood vessels; a sight-threatening medical emergency [1].

Synonyms
Giant cell arteritis (GCA), temporal arteritis; abbreviated AAION.

Symptoms
Acute unilateral or bilateral blindness: 2-9 wk after onset of headaches.
Premonitory amaurosis fugax: may present in 10% of patients.
Amaurosis: induced by bright light.
Painful diplopia: may present in 6% of patients.

Systemic Symptoms
Recent headache in temple, occipital region, neck, eye, or ear; jaw claudication; tongue pain and numbness; toothache; intermittent fevers; night sweats; anorexia, weight loss; malaise; depression.
Proximal muscle pain, myelopathy, polymyalgia rheumatica.
- *Note:* Many patients may have no constitutional complaints and will present only with the eye sign (occult GCA).

Headache
- Headache is the initial manifestation of GCA in 50%-90% of patients.
- Head pain is a "different kind of headache" that can be severe and boring.
- Headache is worse at night and with exposure to cold.
- There is tenderness of the scalp overlying the greater superficial temporal arteries. These arteries may appear enlarged, nodular, and erythematous. Patients may complain of sensitivity when brushing hair or placing head on pillow because of scalp and temple tenderness.
- Pain may involve neck, face, jaw, tongue, ear, or throat. Jaw claudication and neck pain have a high specificity.

Signs
Afferent pupillary defect (APD), if unilateral.
Anterior ischemic optic neuropathy (AION) with pallid disc swelling, **bilateral AION, central retinal artery occlusion (CRAO), branch retinal artery occlusion** (rare), **combined CRAO and AION, cilioretinal artery occlusion** (combined with any of the above).
Choroidal ischemia, infarcts of the nerve fiber layer, pupil-sparing third-nerve paresis, sixth- and seventh-nerve palsies, ischemic ocular syndrome.

Investigations
Westergren erythrocyte age-adjusted sedimentation rate (ESR) of 47-107 mm/hr: in about 9% of patients, ESR will be normal.
C-reactive protein: >2.45 mg/dL.
Complete blood count: normochromic, normocytic anemia.
Reactive thrombocytosis.
Fluorescein angiography: with an abnormal choroidal filling time >18 sec that carries a 93% sensitivity and a 94% specificity for GCA.
Biopsy of greater superficial temporal artery (GSTA): bilateral GSTA biopsies increase yield by 5%-14%.
Ocular pneumopthysmography.

Complications
Permanent bilateral visual loss (in 40% of patients), **myocardial infarction, transient ischemic attacks, stroke.**

Differential diagnosis
Idiopathic anterior ischemic optic neuropathy.
Acute angle-closure glaucoma.
Herpes zoster sine eruptione.
Aneurysm.
Temporomandibular joint syndrome.
Pituitary apoplexy.
Carotid artery dissection.
Wegener's granulomatosis.
Systemic cholesterol microembolization syndrome.
Carotid-cavernous fistula.

Cause
Autoimmune vasculitis of the elderly of unknown cause.

Epidemiology
Overall incidence, 2.9:100,000; 50-59 yr of age, 1.7:100,000; >80 yr of age, 55.5:100,000.
- Mean age of presentation is 75 yr with lower limit of 50 yr.
- More common in white women; less common in black and Asian populations.

Associated features
Polymyalgia rheumatica. (Ret. 4)
- GCA may be the cause of death (myocardial infarction, dissecting aortic aneurysm, cerebral infarction).

Immunology
- An autoimmune syndrome develops from the immunologic response directed toward antigens residing in the wall of medium-sized arteries.
- Genetic risk is supported by a sequence motif in the HLA-DRBI gene.
- T lymphocytes undergoing clonal expansion have been demonstrated infiltrating the temporal artery wall.
- A small number of tissue-infiltrating T cells produce interferon-γ, an important cytokine governing the disease process.
- Circulating macrophages secrete interleukin-6, the major inducer of acute-phase reactants.

Pathology
- Active disease is characterized by fragmentation and destruction of the internal elastic lamina and inflammatory infiltrate in the vessel wall.
- Healed vasculitis shows a diffuse intimal thickening, intimal and medial fibrosis, and fragmentation or loss of internal elastic lamina.

Diagnosis continued on p. 20

Anterior ischemic optic neuropathy, arteritic (giant cell arteritis, temporal arteritis) (377.30)

TREATMENT

Diet and Lifestyle
- No special precautions are necessary.

Pharmacologic Treatment
- Protect the unaffected eye.
- Patient should be hospitalized immediately and pulse steroids administered.

Standard dosage Solu-Medrol, 250 mg IV every 6 hr for 3 days, then oral prednisone, maximum of 60-80 mg/day.

Special points After 1 mo, taper by 5 mg/wk using the patient's symptoms and ESR as a guide (<20 mm/hr).

Slow reduction to about 20 mg by 8th wk is typical.

A maintenance dose of 10-15 mg may be needed for up to 2 yr!

Other Drugs
Immunosuppressive drugs, including cyclophosphamide, methotrexate, and azathioprine.
- *Note:* There are no data to support a therapeutic advantage to immunosuppressive drugs.

Treatment aims

To preserve the vision in the remaining eye.
To prevent systemic complications of the disease, such as stroke.

Prognosis
- If left untreated, 30%-40% of patients may go bilaterally blind, with the highest risk of vision loss within 10 days.
- Despite treatment, 5%-10% go blind.
- Risk of vision loss remains high up to 2 mo.
- Vision loss after 4 mo is unlikely.
- A slight improvement with treatment occurs in 15%-34%.

Follow-up and management
- Because there is a 26% relapse rate in patients under age 2 yr, these patients must be meticulously monitored.
- ESR and symptoms should decline with effective treatment.

Treatment continued on p. 21

DIAGNOSIS—cont'd

Classification
1990 criteria for the classification of giant cell (temporal) arteritis [2]:

1. Age at disease onset ≥50 yr.
2. New headache.
3. Temporal artery abnormality.
4. Elevated ESR.
5. Abnormal artery biopsy.

- If three of the five criteria are present, patient is said to have GCA.

Pearls and Considerations

1. Temporal artery biopsy (TAB) remains the only confirmatory test for AAION.
2. On confirmation of AAION, high-dose corticosteroid treatment is mandatory.
3. High-dose corticosteroid therapy has a high incidence of undesirable side effects in this patient population because of advanced age and comorbidity. Complications of high-dose corticosteroid therapy include diabetes mellitus, hypertension, Cushing's syndrome, osteoporosis, muscle wasting, gastrointestinal disturbance, avascular necrosis of the femoral head, and mental disturbances. Patients must be monitored for these side effects, and the beneficial effects of treatment must be balanced against the side effects [1].
4. In general, the life expectancy of patients with GCA is reportedly similar to that of the general population; however, the risk for death from cardiovascular disease in the first year after diagnosis, if patient is inadequately treated, is significantly higher than in the general population [1].

Referral Information

1. On presentation, refer to laboratory for complete blood workup and TAB.
2. On confirmation, refer for hospitalization and systemic treatment.

TREATMENT—cont'd

Nonpharmacologic Treatment

Trendelenburg's position: patient is supine on the bed with the head tilted downward 30-40 degrees, and the bed is angulated beneath the knees.

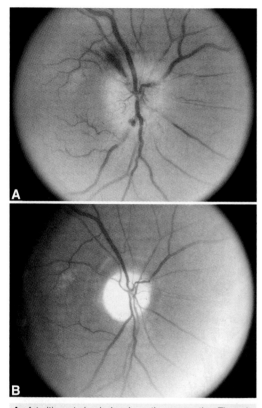

A, Arteritic anterior ischemic optic neuropathy. There is pallid swelling of a right optic disc with a flame-shaped hemorrhage. This 76-yr-old patient had no constitutional signs or symptoms but had an ESR of 110 and a positive temporal artery biopsy. **B**, Optic atrophy 2 mo later.

Key references

1. Rahman W, Rahman FZ: Giant cell (temporal) arteritis: an overview and update, *Surv Ophthalmol* 50:415-428, 2005.
2. Hunder GG, Bloch DA, Michel BA, et al: The American College of Rheumatology 1990 criteria for the classification of giant cell arteritis, *Arthritis Rheum* 33:1122-1128, 1990.

General references

Diaz VA, DeBroff BM, Sinard J: Comparison of histopathologic features, clinical symptoms, and erythrocyte sedimentation rates in biopsy-positive temporal arteritis, *Ophthalmology* 112(7):1293-1298, 2005.

Niederkohr RD, Levin LA: Management of the patient with suspected temporal arteritis: a decision-analytic approach, *Ophthalmology* 112(5):744-56, 2005.

Nordborg E, Nordborg C: Giant cell arteritis: strategies in diagnosis and treatment, *Curr Opin Rheumatol* 16(1):25-30, 2004.

Salvarani C, Cantini F, Boiardi L, Hunder GG: Polymyalgia rheumatica, *Best Pract Res Clin Rheumatol* 18(5):705-722, 2004.

DIAGNOSIS

Definition
Ischemia of the anterior optic nerve head caused by underlying vasculopathy or disruption of blood flow within the optic nerve head and often associated with hypertension and diabetes.

Synonyms
None; abbreviated NAION.

Symptoms
Acute (hours) and subacute (days) monocular visual loss: may worsen over weeks; visual nadir is ~3-4 days.

Bilateral NAION: extremely unusual and suggests an alternative diagnosis.

- The patient usually has no pain and often notices the condition on awakening in the morning.

Signs
Hyperemic, edematous optic nerve head: with segmental infarction, flame-shaped hemorrhages, and luxury perfusion (*see* Fig. 1).

Small optic disc without a physiologic cup ("disc at risk"; *see* Fig. 2).

Relative afferent pupillary defect.

Inferior altitudinal, inferior nasal, or central scotoma.

Vision better than 20/200: in ~50% of patients.

Investigations
Blood pressure measurement.

Westergren erythrocyte sedimentation rate (ESR).

C-reactive protein.

Complete blood count.

Fluorescein angiography.

Biopsy of greater superficial temporal artery (GSTA).

Pearls and Considerations
1. Clinical features that help differentiate NAION from AAION include a relatively younger age at onset, less severe vision loss, and relatively little or no reported pain with NAION.
2. Full clinical workup is still indicated to rule out the arteritic form of the disease.

Referral Information
Referral to laboratory for full clinical workup, including blood tests and temporal artery biopsy.

Differential diagnosis
Giant cell arteritis.
Papillitis.

Cause
Unknown, but thought to result from the occlusion of posterior ciliary arteries providing the laminar, prelaminar, and retrolaminar blood supply to the optic nerve.
Risk factors include hypertension; diabetes mellitus; cigarette smoking; and elevated fibrinogen, cholesterol, and triglyceride levels.

Associated features
Systemic hypertension (35%-50% of patients).
Nocturnal arterial hypotension (10%-25% of patients).
Favism.
Diabetes mellitus.
Systemic vasculitis.
Migraine.
After cataract extraction (within 2 wk).
Elevated intraocular pressure.
Coagulopathies (e.g., anticardiolipin antibody syndrome, protein S and protein C deficiencies).
Acute blood loss, anemia, hypotension.

Pathology
Unknown.

TREATMENT

Diet and Lifestyle
- Patients should stop smoking.
- If patient takes blood pressure medication at bedtime, consider different medication schedule.

Pharmacologic Treatment
- Although controversial, aspirin may offer a short-term benefit (1-2 yr) in reducing the incidence of second-eye NAION. Long-term benefit (5 yr) has not been established.

Nonpharmacologic Treatment
- No nonpharmacologic treatment is recommended.

Other Treatments
- Optic nerve fenestration has been shown ineffective in treating patients and produces a poorer visual outcome than the natural course of the disease.

Treatment aims
To treat the underlying vasculopathy; if none present, no treatment will be effective.

Prognosis
- Approximately 24% of patients will have a significant improvement in visual acuity and visual field.
- There is <5% chance of recurrence in the same eye.
- There is a 25%-50% chance that the fellow eye will be involved within 5 yr.
- No concrete relationship has been established between NAION and cerebrovascular disease.

Follow-up and management
- Serial testing of visual fields should be performed over 12 mo to monitor improvement.

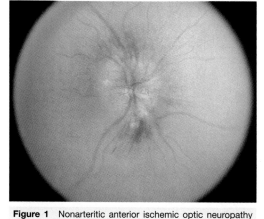

Figure 1 Nonarteritic anterior ischemic optic neuropathy (NAION) of right eye in 60-yr-old woman with hypertension. There is diffuse disc edema and flame-shaped hemorrhages at the 6 and 12 o'clock positions. Note the absence of a physiologic cup.

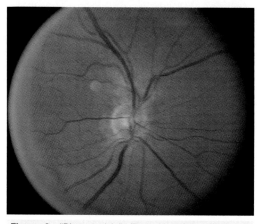

Figure 2 "Disc at risk." *(From Yanoff M, Ducker J: Ophthalmology, ed 2, St Louis, 2003, Elsevier.)*

General references
Hayreh SS: Posterior ischaemic optic neuropathy: clinical features, pathogenesis, and management, *Eye* 18(11):1188-1206, 2004.
Rucker JC, Biousse V, Newman NJ: Ischemic optic neuropathies, *Curr Opin Neurol* 17(1):27-35, 2004.
Yanoff M, Duker J: *Ophthalmology*, ed 2, St Louis, 2003, Elsevier.

DIAGNOSIS

Definition
Inflammation of the uveal tract.

Synonyms
Iritis, uveitis, pars planitis.

Symptoms
Pain.
Redness.
Photophobia.
Increased lacrimation.
Blurry vision.
- Pain, decreased vision, and redness may be minimal in subacute cases.

Signs
Acute
Ciliary injection of conjunctiva (hyperemia around limbus), **posterior synechiae, iris bombé; shallow anterior chamber.**
Fine to large keratic precipitates (granulomatous) and fibrin dusting of corneal endothelium.
Anterior chamber shows many cells, variable flare, and in rare cases, a hypopyon.
Dilated iris vessels and rarely a hyphema.
Posterior synechiae (adhesion of pupillary iris to lens).
Iris nodules.
Anterior vitreous cells.
Cystoid macular edema and rarely a disc edema; **peripheral anterior synechiae** on gonioscopy.
Low intraocular pressure (IOP) (low aqueous production): with cyclitis.
High IOP: trabeculitis or obstruction of trabecular meshwork by inflammatory debris; partial or complete pupillary block caused by posterior synechiae.

Chronic
Variable conjunctival redness as well as anterior-chamber reaction.
Secluded/occluded pupil.

Investigations
Histories: onset and duration of symptoms, systems review (especially of arthritic, gastrointestinal, and genitourinary disorders), insect bite, rash, sexual, drug, family back disorders (e.g., ankylosing spondylitis).
Visual acuity testing.
Slit-lamp examination (SLE).
IOP.
Dilated fundus examination.
- If uveitis is bilateral, granulomatous, associated with positive review of systems, poorly responsive to usual dose of topical steroids, significant flare, or recurrent: **complete blood count, erythrocyte sedimentation rate (ESR), antinuclear antibody (ANA), rapid plasma reagin, Lyme disease titers, angiotensin-converting enzyme (ACE), fluorescent treponemal antibody (FTA) absorption, purified protein derivative (PPD, tuberculin) with anergy panel.** Obtain a **chest radiograph** and **HLA-B27.**

Complications
Cataract.
Glaucoma.
Corneal edema.
Cystoid macular edema.

Differential diagnosis
Rhegmatogenous retinal detachment (pigment cells in the anterior chamber).
Leukemia.
Retinoblastoma: in children.
Intraocular foreign body.
Malignant melanoma.
Juvenile xanthogranuloma.

Cause
Idiopathic: most common.
HLA-B27–positive iridocyclitis.
Juvenile rheumatoid arthritis (most cases pauciarticular or oligoarticular arthritis, rheumatoid factor (–), ANA (+), young girls).
Fuchs' heterochromic iridocyclitis.
Herpes simplex keratouveitis.
Syphilis.
Traumatic, sarcoid, and tuberculosis iridocyclitis.

Associated features
Iris heterochromia, corneal band keratopathy.

Immunology
Mostly type III hypersensitivity reaction, but also type II.

Pathology
Neutrophils, eosinophils, and lymphocytes in anterior chamber and on corneal endothelial and iris surfaces: large keratic precipitates and iris nodules are granulomas.

Diagnosis continued on p. 26

TREATMENT

Diet and Lifestyle
- No special precautions are necessary.

Pharmacologic Treatment
Cycloplegia

Standard dosage   Cyclopentolate 1%-2%, 3 times daily for mild to moderate inflammation. Atropine 1%, 2 or 3 times daily for moderate to severe inflammation. Prednisolone acetate 1%, every 1-6 hr.

Special points   Consider subtenons injection of steroid or systemic steroid if patient unresponsive to topical therapy.
Treat secondary glaucoma with topical antiglaucoma medication.
If an infectious cause is determined, the specific management should be added to the above regimen.
Consider a rheumatology consult.

Treatment aims
To lessen or obviate inflammatory response in anterior chamber and anterior vitreous.

Other treatments
- Other immunosuppressive therapy may be necessary to control inflammation.

Prognosis
- Prognosis is usually good with therapy.
- There is a high complication rate with cataract surgery in patients with juvenile rheumatoid arthritis but *not* with Fuchs' heterochromic iridocyclitis.
- Patients with sarcoid, tuberculosis (TB), and syphilis do well with appropriate therapy.
- Make sure anti-TB systemic treatment is addressed before initiating prednisone.

Follow-up and management
- Patients should be followed every 1-7 days in the acute phase and every 1-6 mo when stable. Complete ocular examination should be performed at each visit.
- If the anterior-chamber reaction is improving, the steroid should be tapered slowly. In some patients, chronic low-dose steroids may be needed to prevent recurrence.

Treatment continued on p. 27

DIAGNOSIS—cont'd

Classification

Acute: signs and symptoms appear suddenly and last for up to 6 wk.

Chronic: onset is gradual, and inflammation lasts longer than 6 wk.

Granulomatous: insidious onset; chronic course; eye almost white; iris nodules and large keratic precipitates ("mutton fat") present; posterior segment often involved.

Nongranulomatous: acute onset; shorter course; red eye and intense flare present; no iris nodules.

Infectious: viruses, bacteria, rickettsiae, fungi, protozoa, parasites.

Noninfectious: exogenous (trauma, chemical injury), endogenous (immunologic types 1-4 hypersensitivities).

Pearls and Considerations

1. On second presentation of idiopathic iridocyclitis, patients should be referred for full systemic workup.
2. Anterior-chamber cells and flare are best observed at SLE, with a bright conic section and room lights very dim.

Referral Information

See Pearls and Considerations.

TREATMENT—cont'd

Nonpharmacologic Treatment
Glaucoma surgery (e.g., tube-shunt devices): to control IOP.

Cataract surgery: usually not undertaken until the eye is quiet for at least 6 mo.

Laser peripheral iridectomy: for posterior synechiae with iris bombé to prevent acute angle-closure glaucoma (AACG). Multiple iridectomies may be needed because they can close by inflammation.

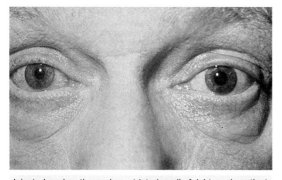

Injected conjunctiva and constricted pupil of right eye in patient with acute iritis.

General references

Albert DM, Jakobiec FA, editors: *Principles and practice of ophthalmology*, vol I, Philadelphia, 1994, Saunders.

American Academy of Ophthalmology: *Basic and clinical science*, section 8, San Francisco, 1994-1995, American Academy of Ophthalmology.

Menezo V, Lightman S: The development of complications in patients with chronic anterior uveitis, *Am J Ophthalmol* 139(6):988-992, 2005.

Monnet D, Breban M, Hudry C, et al: Ophthalmic findings and frequency of extraocular manifestations in patients with HLA-B27 uveitis: a study of 175 cases, *Ophthalmology* 111(4):802-809, 2004.

Smith JR: HLA-B27–associated uveitis, *Ophthalmol Clin North Am* 15(3):297-307, 2002.

Wright K: *Textbook of ophthalmology*, Baltimore, 1997, Lippincott Williams & Wilkins.

Asteroid hyalosis and synchysis scintillans (379.22)

DIAGNOSIS

Definition
Asteroid Hyalosis

White refractile crystals composed of calcium soaps that float in the vitreous and *do not* settle with gravity [2].

Synchysis Scintillans

Brown refractile crystals composed of cholesterol that float in the vitreous and *do* settle with gravity [1].

Synonyms
None.

Symptoms
- Patients are usually asymptomatic.

Floaters.

Signs
Asteroid Hyalosis

Small, white refractile particles: made of calcium soap; float in the vitreous; do not settle with gravity (*see* Fig. 1).

Monocularity: in 75% of cases.

- Asteroid hyalosis occurs more often in diabetic patients [2].

Synchysis Scintillans

Numerous yellow-white or gold particles: made up of cholesterol; located in the vitreous and anterior chamber; settle to the bottom of the eye with gravity (*see* Fig. 2).

Investigations
Asteroid Hyalosis

Fluorescein angiogram: can be performed to view the macula clearly if patients present with decreased vision and if the view of the posterior pole is obscured by the asteroid.

Synchysis Scintillans

Careful history: to determine if there was previous surgery or trauma to the eye.

Pearls and Considerations
Asteroid hyalosis has no clinical association, whereas synchysis scintillans is often found after vitreous hemorrhage, uveitis, or trauma [3].

Referral Information
None.

Differential diagnosis

Past vitreous hemorrhage.
Uveitis.
Pigment floating in the vitreous.

Cause

Asteroid hyalosis
An innocuous degenerative disease of unknown origin.
Usually diagnosed in patients >60 yr of age [4].

Synchysis scintillans
History of severe, accidental, or surgical trauma associated with a large intraocular hemorrhage [3].

Epidemiology

Asteroid hyalosis
- More common in older individuals.
- Overall incidence, 1:200.

Associated features

Synchysis scintillans
Posterior vitreous detachment; this often allows the crystals to settle interiorly.

Pathology

Asteroid hyalosis
Calcium and lipid particles ranging from 0.01-0.10 mm in diameter [5].

Synchysis scintillans
Cholesterol particles.

TREATMENT

Diet and Lifestyle
Asteroid Hyalosis
- No special precautions are necessary.

Synchysis Scintillans
- Safety glasses should be worn to protect the better eye.

Pharmacologic Treatment
- No pharmacologic treatment is recommended.

Nonpharmacologic Treatment
- Treatment is generally not indicated unless an unrelated cause of decreased vision must be treated, in which case a pars plana vitrectomy should be performed to clear out the vitreous cavity.
- Conditions often associated with the need for vitrectomy include diabetic macular edema and choroidal neovascularization.

Prognosis
Asteroid hyalosis
Good, because it is asymptomatic and does not affect vision.
Synchysis scintillans
Good, but often associated with trauma or inflammation; in such patients, vision may be decreased from structural changes to the eye caused by the trauma or inflammation, in addition to the cholesterol found in the vitreous cavity.

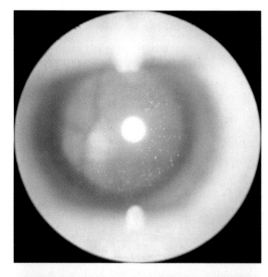

Figure 1 Fundus reflex of a patient with asteroid hyalosis.

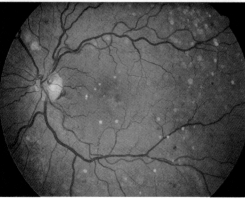

Figure 2 Small, round, yellow dots floating in the vitreous in a patient with diabetic retinopathy.

Key references
1. Kasier PK, Friedman NJ: Synchysis scintillans. In *The Massachusetts Eye and Ear Infirmary illustrated manual of ophthalmology*, ed 2, Philadelphia, 2004, Saunders, p 287.
2. Yazar Z, Hanioglu S, Karakoc G, Gursel E: Asteroid hyalosis, *Eur J Ophthalmol* 11(1): 57-61, 2001.
3. Spraul CW, Grossniklaus HE: Vitreous hemorrhage, *Surv Ophthalmol* 42(1):3-39, 1997.
4. Mitchell P, Wang MY, Wang JJ: Asteroid hyalosis in an older population: the Blue Mountain Eye Study, *Ophthalmic Epidemiol* 10(5):331-335, 2003.
5. Komatsu H, Kamura Y, Ishi K, Kashima Y: Fine structure and morphogenesis of asteroid hyalosis, *Med Electron Microscopy* 36(2): 112-119, 2003.

Bacterial endophthalmitis (360.0)

DIAGNOSIS

Definition
An intraocular infection caused by microbial organisms.

Synonyms
None.

Symptoms
Rapid visual loss.
Pain.
Redness.
Tearing.

Signs
Conjunctival injection.
Chemosis.
Hypopyon.
Severe vitritis.

Investigations
Careful measurement of visual acuity.
Full slit-lamp and dilated eye examinations.
Gonioscopy: to look for a microhypopyon.
B-scan ultrasound: if the view of the vitreous and retina is obscured by the anterior-chamber inflammation. (Check for vitreous opacities.)
Gram stain, culture, and sensitivity: both the anterior-chamber fluid and the vitreous fluid.

Complications
Loss of vision.
Secondary retinal detachment.
Loss of the eye: if severe pain or phthisis develops.

Classification
Endogenous bacterial endophthalmitis (usually acute or subacute).
Exogenous bacterial endophthalmitis (usually acute or subacute).
Fungal endophthalmitis (usually chronic).

Pearls and Considerations
1. Endophthalmitis is considered a sight-threatening ophthalmic emergency.
2. Infection rarely spreads outside the confines of the sclera to surrounding tissue [1].
3. The Endophthalmitis Vitrectomy Study (EVS) determined that up to one quarter of patients did not initially report pain with endopthalmitis. Rather, the nearly universal presenting symptom was *blurred vision*. This should therefore be considered a critical symptom when triaging postcataract patients [2].

Referral Information
A patient with endophthalmitis should be referred immediately to a vitreoretinal surgeon [2].

Differential diagnosis
Sterile endophthalmitis.
Panuveitis.
Viral retinitis (e.g., acute retinal necrosis).

Cause
Exogenous after intraocular surgery
Occurs after any type of eye surgery; patients usually present 48-72 hr after initial surgery with complaints of pain and decreased vision; common organisms include *Staphylococcus epidermidis* and *S. aureus*. *Streptococcus pneumoniae* and *Haemophilus influenzae* occur more often after filtering blebs; *Propionibacterium acnes* infection presents as a persistent low-grade anterior uveitis with white plaques on the posterior capsule (*see* figure).

Endogenous endophthalmitis
Systemic infection seeds the eye; patient workup for endocarditis; can also occur in patients with indwelling catheters; immunocompromised patients are at higher risk.

Posttraumatic endophthalmitis
Can follow penetrating eye injuries; it is important to rule out retained intraocular foreign bodies; more serious pathogens, such as *Bacillus cereus* or a polymicrobial inoculum, can occur in rural settings.

Endogenous fungal endophthalmitis [6]
Usually secondary to indwelling catheters and long-term parenteral nutrition; patients are often immunocompromised and usually present with gradual decrease in vision and increasing floater formation; most common organism is *Candida albicans*. Less common forms (e.g., *Aspergillus*, *Cryptococcus*, and *Fusarium* spp.) are seen in severely immunosuppressed patients.

Epidemiology
- Postoperative exogenous endophthalmitis occurs in 0.04% of patients after cataract extraction [3].
- A reported 10.7% of patients with intraocular foreign bodies will develop endophthalmitis [4].
- The incidence of *Candida* endophthalmitis in association with documented candidemia is reported at 9% [5].

Pathology
- Polymorphonuclear leukocytic infiltration into the involved tissues.

TREATMENT

Diet and Lifestyle
- No precautions are necessary.

Pharmacologic Treatment
For Endogenous Endophthalmitis
- Systemic antibiotic therapy will usually be sufficient treatment for bacterial and fungal organisms.

For Exogenous Endophthalmitis
Topical fortified antibiotics (e.g., ancef, vancomycin, aminoglycoside); once response to antibiotics evident, administer steroids and cycloplegics (e.g., atropine).
- Inject intravitreal antibiotics tailored to the organism involved. Most patients receive combination therapy (e.g., vancomycin and amikacin with or without steroids) at the time of diagnosis to cover both gram-positive and gram-negative organisms until the Gram stain and cultures are available. Additional intravitreal injections may be necessary for more virulent strains or fungi. One exception is the treatment for *Propionibacterium acnes*. Patients require clindamycin intravitreally, and often the capsular bag must be removed to eradicate the infection.

Nonpharmacologic Treatment
Pars plana vitrectomy may be necessary if (1) the patient presents with vision worse than hand motions (HM) [3], (2) there is evidence of retinal detachment, or (3) if the patient is getting worse after initial intravitreal antibiotic therapy.
Follow EVS guidelines:
- If visual acuity (VA) light perception (LP) or worse: vitrectomy + intravitreal antibiotics.
- If VA HM or better: vitreous tap + intravitreal antibiotics.

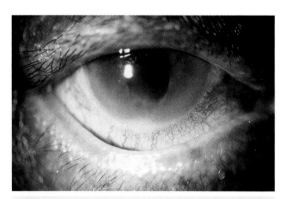

Patient who developed endophthalmitis after glaucoma filtering surgery. Note the conjunctival injection and the layered hypopyon in the anterior chamber.

Treatment aims
To eradicate the infection.
To decrease inflammation.
To restore vision.

Prognosis
- Visual prognosis is poor even with prompt treatment.

Follow-up and management
- Once the diagnosis of endophthalmitis has been made and treatment instituted, patients need to be followed daily, looking for improvement, a poor response to the chosen antibiotics, or a secondary complication of retinal detachment.
- Once culture results have provided sensitivity information on which antibiotics are effective in treating the offending organism, the antibiotic therapy may have to be augmented or changed.
- Virulent gram-negative organisms may need repeated intravitreal antibiotic injections within 48 hr of the initial therapy.
- Subjectively, a decrease in pain usually correlates with response to treatment, even though ocular examination may not change initially.

Key references
1. Graham RH, Wong DT, Lakosha H: Bacterial endophthalmitis, 2006, www.emedicine.com.
2. Endophthalmitis Vitrectomy Study Group: Results of the Endophthalmitis Vitrectomy Study: a randomized trial of immediate vitrectomy and of intravenous antibiotics for the treatment of postoperative bacterial endophthalmitis, *Arch Ophthalmol* 113:1479-1496, 1995.
3. Miller JJ, Scott IU, Flynn HW Jr, et al: Acute-onset endophthalmitis following cataract surgery (2000-2004): incidence, clinical settings, and visual acuity outcomes after treatment, *Am J Ophthalmol* 139(6):983-987, 2005.
4. Flynn HW Jr, Scott IU, Brod RD, Han DP: Current management of endophthalmitis, *Int Ophthalmol Clin* 44(4):115-137, 2004.
5. Donahue SP, Greven CM, Zuravleff JJ, et al: Intraocular candidiasis in patients with candidemia: clinical implications derived from a prospective multicentered study, *Ophthalmology* 1994, 101:1302-1309.
6. Jackson TL, Eykyn SJ, Graham EM, Stanford MR: Endogenous bacterial endophthalmitis: a 17-year prospective series and review of 267 reported cases, *Surv Ophthalmol* 48(4):403-423, 2003.

General references
Bialasiewicz AA: Therapeutic indications for local anti-infectives: bacterial infections of the eye, *Dev Ophthalmol* 33:243-249, 2002.
Das T, Sharma S: Current management strategies of acute post-operative endophthalmitis, *Semin Ophthalmol* 18(3):109-115, 2003.
Kowalski RP, Dhaliwal DK: Ocular bacterial infections: current and future treatment options, *Expert Rev Antiinfect Ther* 3(1):131-139, 2005.

DIAGNOSIS

Definition
Failure of the eyes to work together efficiently for any reason, including extraocular muscle imbalance, accommodative dysfunction, and anisometropia.

Synonyms
Varied and related to the specific disorder; include "lazy eye," "crossed eyes," "walleyes," and "double vision."

Symptoms
- On onset of strabismus, patients may develop:

Diplopia: perception of one object as being located in two different positions in space.

Visual confusion: perception of two objects being located in the same position in space.

Asthenopia (visual discomfort): caused by diplopia and visual confusion.

- To obviate diplopia and visual confusion, children <7 yr of age may develop:

Suppression: absolute scotoma under binocular viewing conditions that prevents diplopia for the object of regard of the fixing eye.

Anomalous retinal correspondence (ARC): reordering of visual cortical directional values to prevent sensations of diplopia and visual confusion for peripheral objects.

Signs
Squinting and rubbing of eyes: signs of asthenopia.

Visual comfort in a patient with obvious strabismus: signs of suppression and ARC.

Investigations
Sensory test: to determine the presence or absence of sensory adaptations to strabismus in patients who developed strabismus before age 7 yr.

Motor test: to determine alignment of the eyes.

Complications
- Patients with suppression and ARC have no stereoptic ability, and if the suppression scotoma is large, they may have little monocular input from the strabismic eye.
- Patients with diplopia and visual confusion have difficulty locating objects in space, especially if the acuity is equal in each eye. They may have difficulty walking, driving, or reading.

Pearls and Considerations
Topic too broad for specific recommendations.

Referral Information
Varied; specific to the underlying etiology of binocular vision disorder.

Differential diagnosis
Monocular diplopia may occur in patients with cataracts, corneal lesions, or other media anomalies. These patients do not have strabismus, and the diplopia persists when the other eye is covered. Monocular diplopia may be obviated by viewing through a pinhole or by bringing a card up from below until it covers one of the images.

Cause
- Diplopia and visual confusion are caused by sensory inputs from seeing eyes that do not have the same visual directions.

The sensory adaptations of suppression and ARC occur spontaneously in patients who initially develop strabismus before age 7 yr. Suppression is a cortical phenomenon in which the retinal locus (on which falls the foveated image in the other [straight] eye) is not viewed. The suppression scotoma is absolute and facultative (it exists only under binocular viewing conditions). ARC is a cortical phenomenon in which peripheral directional values arising in the strabismic eye are altered. This obviates peripheral diplopia and visual confusion.

Epidemiology
- Sensory adaptations of suppression and ARC occur in children who initially develop strabismus before 7-9 yr of age.
- Diplopia and visual confusion occur in older children and adults who initially develop strabismus after 7-9 yr of age.

Associated features
- Strabismus is associated with disorders of binocular vision, but the eye misalignment may be so small as to be undetectable except by careful sensory and motor tests.

TREATMENT

Diet and Lifestyle
- No special precautions are necessary.

Pharmacologic Treatment
- No pharmacologic treatment is recommended.

Nonpharmacologic Treatment
- Alignment of the visual axes in strabismic eyes will treat diplopia and visual confusion. Children will revert to normal retinal correspondence, and suppression will disappear over time.
- Treatment may require glasses, fusional training exercises, prisms, or surgery.

Treatment aims
In adults
To ensure disappearance of diplopia and visual confusion.
To recover peripheral fusion and stereopsis.
In children
To achieve normal retinal correspondence.
To recover peripheral fusion and stereopsis.

Prognosis
- The prognosis for a sensory cure is better in younger children and poor in older adults. It is probably better in patients not neurologically impaired. The prognosis also depends on the length of time the eyes were strabismic and whether the strabismus was intermittent (better prognosis) or constant.
- Adults with diplopia and visual confusion may learn over time to ignore the displaced image. It is often less distinct than the image seen by the fixing eye.

Follow-up and management
- Management options are listed under Nonpharmacologic treatment.

General references
Burian HM: The sensorial retinal relationships in comitant strabismus, *Arch Ophthalmol* 37: 336-340, 1947.

Diamond G: *Textbook of ophthalmology*, vol 5. Yanoff M, Podos S, editors: *Strabismus and pediatric ophthalmology*, London, 1993, Mosby-Wolfe.

Jampolsky A: Characteristics of suppression in strabismus, *Arch Ophthalmol* 37:336-340, 1947.

Parks MM: Stereoacuity as an indicator of bifixation. In Knapp P, editor: *Strabismus Symposium*, New York, 1968, Karger, pp 361-364.

Travers T: Suppression of vision in squint and its association with retinal correspondence and amblyopia, *Br J Ophthalmol* 22:557-604, 1938.

Blepharitis   (373.0) and blepharoconjunctivitis   (372.2)

DIAGNOSIS

Definition
Blepharitis: a family of inflammatory processes of the eyelids.
Blepharoconjunctivitis: inflammation of the conjunctiva secondary to blepharitis.

Synonyms
None.

Symptoms
Itching, burning, tearing.
Mild pain.
Foreign body sensation.
Crusting around the eyes on awakening.

Signs
Crusty, red, thickened eyelid margins with prominent blood vessels.
Inspissated oil gland at the eyelid margins (meibomianitis).
Conjunctival injection with papillary reaction and/or papillofollicular reaction.
Swollen eyelids.
Mild mucus discharge.
Superficial punctate keratitis (SPK), marginal infiltrates.
Phylectenules: elevated milky whitish nodules on the conjunctiva or rarely the cornea.

Investigations
History: chronic history of eye irritation, often worse in the morning.
Complete external examination: noting health of the periorbital region and facial skin (e.g., telangiectasia and rhinophyma [acne rosacea], scaling [seborrhea], vesicles [herpes simplex or zoster], umbilicated nodules [molluscum contagiosum]).
Visual acuity test: may be decreased because of tear-film abnormalities and SPK.
Intraocular pressure (IOP).
Slit-lamp examination: eyelash debris and collerates (flat crusted rings surrounding the eyelash base) may be seen in infectious blepharitis.
Dilated fundus examination: usually normal.
- For persistent inflammation despite therapy, consider swab culture of the eyelids and conjunctiva.

Complications
Corneal pannus and scarring.
Peripheral keratitis: occurs more often with bacterial infection.
Phylectenule: often related to *Staphylococcus aureus.*

Pearls and Considerations
Long-term use of topical steroid may result in steroid-related complications such as cataract or elevated IOP because of the potential for corneal penetration. Patients should be closely monitored for such complications.

Referral Information
Referral not required in most cases. Consider referral to dermatologist for underlying rosacea or other skin disease.

Differential diagnosis
Preseptal cellulitis.
Sebaceous gland carcinoma.
Discoid lupus.

Cause and classification
Infectious
Bacterial (*Staphylococcus aureus, S. epidermidis, Streptococcus pneumoniae, Haemophilus influenzae, Moraxella lacunata*). Viral (herpes simplex, herpes zoster, molluscum contagiosum).
Noninfectious
Acne rosacea.
Eczema.
Seborrhea.
Meibomian gland dysfunction.

TREATMENT

Diet and Lifestyle
- Lid hygiene is crucial in the treatment and prevention of blepharitis and blepharoconjunctivitis.
- Scrub the eyelid margins twice daily with mild shampoo on a cotton-tipped applicator.
- Apply warm compresses for 15 min 2-4 times daily; most effective when used before eyelid scrubs.

Pharmacologic Treatment
For Bacterial and Seborrheic Blepharitis
- Administer artificial tears 4-8 times daily.
- Apply topical antibiotic ointment (erythromycin, bacitracin, gentamicin, or sulfacetamide) to the eyelids 2 or 3 times daily. Seborrheic blepharitis may have an infectious component.
- If significant inflammatory component, consider topical corticosteroid (loteprednol or fluorometholone) 3 or 4 times daily with rapid taper, and/or topical cyclosporine 0.05% twice daily.
- Consider systemic treatment (especially when seen with rosacea) with doxycycline, 100-200 mg daily.

For Herpetic Blepharitis and Conjunctivitis
Standard dosage	Trifluridine 1% solution, 5 times daily.
Special points	Chronic trifluridine therapy may produce a toxic superficial keratitis and conjunctivitis. May apply topical antibiotic ointment on the skin lesions to prevent bacterial superinfection (erythromycin or bacitracin ophthalmic ointment).

For Recurrent Meibomianitis
Standard dosage	Doxycycline, 100 mg PO daily or twice daily.
	Tetracycline, 250 mg PO 4 times daily.
Contraindications	Pregnancy; can be deposited in a fetus's growing teeth, discoloring them.
Special points	Patients taking doxycycline or tetracycline may develop skin photosensitivity and should avoid skin sun exposure.

Nonpharmacologic Treatment
- No nonpharmacologic treatment is recommended.

Treatment aims
To reduce bacterial count.
To prevent corneal complications (pannus, scarring).

Prognosis
- Patients do well with appropriate therapy.
- Lid hygiene and chronic therapy are often necessary to maintain ocular health.

Follow-up and management
- Every 3-4 wk as needed; if steroid is being used, need to follow up every 2 wk to monitor IOP.

General references
Albert DM, Jakobiec FA, editors: *Principles and practice of ophthalmology*, vol I, Philadelphia, 2000, Saunders.
American Academy of Ophthalmology: *Basic and clinical science*, section 8, San Francisco, 2006-2007, The Academy.
Wright K: *Textbook of ophthalmology*, Baltimore, 1997, Williams & Wilkins.

Blepharophimosis   (374.46)

DIAGNOSIS

Definition
Genetically inherited, severe, bilateral ptosis with poor levator function in which the palpebral fissures are horizontally shortened [1].

Synonyms
None.

Symptoms
Chin-up head posture with severe ptosis.

Signs
Bilateral telecanthus, ptosis, variable epicanthus inversus: leads to greatly reduced horizontal fissure size; partial syndrome if one feature missing (*see* figure).

Flattened supraorbital ridges with eyebrow arching: important finding seen in virtually all patients with full syndrome (*see* figure).

Variable vertical lid shortening: leads to ectropion of lateral half of lower lids.

Variable antimongoloid lid-fissure slant.

Investigations
- Ptosis and epicanthus inversus are variable; each patient should be carefully studied before surgery is performed.

Complications
Amblyopia: may occur in patients with severe ptosis and anisometropia.

Puncturing of lacrimal sac: may occur during surgical repair of telecanthus; transnasal wiring through nasal bones for correction of telecanthus puts sac at risk.

Pearls and Considerations
Blepharophimosis is associated with primary amenorrhea in some families.

Referral Information
Oculoplastics referral for repair with medial canthal tendon and local skin flaps, bilateral frontalis suspension, and skin grafting as appropriate [1].

Differential diagnosis
- Each feature of the syndrome may occur without the others.

Cause
- Unknown.

Epidemiology
- No known racial predilection, but tends to segregate in families.
- Males predominantly affected.

Associated features
- Flattened supraorbital ridges with eyebrow arching.
- Vertical lid shortening.
- Antimongoloid lid-fissure slant.

TREATMENT

Diet and Lifestyle
- No special precautions are necessary.

Pharmacologic Treatment
- No pharmacologic treatment is recommended.

Nonpharmacologic Treatment
- Surgery is often deferred until after 18 mo of age. Epicanthus and telecanthus are repaired first, then ptosis. Transnasal wiring is usually required to repair telecanthus because of the strong tension on medial canthal tendons. Levator resections are often initially effective, but lids fall with time, and most patients will eventually require sling procedures. Many surgeons wait 1 yr after telecanthus repair to perform ptosis surgery.

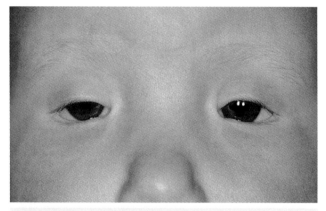

Note symmetric bilateral ptosis, telecanthus, and epicantal folds.

Treatment aims
To obviate telecanthus and epicanthal folds. To provide normally positioned lids with normal function.

Prognosis
- Prognosis is excellent for stable result of telecanthus and epicanthal folds.
- Ptosis tends to recur after levator surgery, and many patients ultimately require sling procedures.

Follow-up and management
- The uncommon patient with amblyopia and anisometropia should be managed in the usual manner with typical surgical postoperative care.

Key reference
1. Custer PL: Blepharoptosis. In Yanoff M, Duker JS, editors: *Ophthalmology*, E-dition, St Louis, 2006, Elsevier.

General references
Callahan A: Ptosis. In Troutman RC, Converse JM, Smith B, editors: *Plastic and reconstructive surgery of eye and adnexae*, London, 1962, Butterworth, pp 361-385.
Mustarde JC: Ptosis. In *Repair and reconstruction in the orbital region*, ed 2, Edinburgh, 1980, Churchill Livingstone, pp 952-962.
Roveda JM: Epicanthus et blepharophimosis: notre, technique de correction, *Ann D'oculist* 200:551-562, 1967.

DIAGNOSIS

Definition

A late complication of **extracapsular cataract extraction** (ECCE) in which the capsular epithelium proliferates and opacifies the posterior lens capsule.

Synonyms

Secondary cataract; **posterior capsular opacification** (PCO).

Symptoms

• Symptoms follow ECCE, either nuclear expression or phacoemulsification.

Obscuration of vision: (366.53; if vision is not obscured. 366.52) may occur as early as a few weeks after ECCE, but usually occurs months to years later.

Blurred vision.

Dim vision: patients often complain of a combination of dim vision ("vision used to be brighter") and blurred vision.

Hazy vision.

Haloes at night.

• *Note:* Some patients may be asymptomatic. Reduced vision may first be detected during a routine eye examination, because if the vision is normal in the other eye, patients generally do not notice reduced vision in the eye with increased PCO.

Signs

Opacification of posterior lens capsule: the posterior lens capsule initially appears mildly translucent (rather than transparent); with progression, the translucency advances to a watery, milky color and finally, in the end stage, to white and opaque; generally the loss of transparency is diffuse, but the posterior lens capsule usually contains islands of differing density.

Cellular reaction on anterior surface of intraocular lens implant: the reaction is one of large foreign body giant cells that are often admixed with pigment; this usually occurs weeks to months after an ECCE.

Fibrinous reaction on anterior surface of intraocular lens implant: generally the fibrinous reaction is seen in the early postoperative period. Rarely the anterior capsular opacification can become so severe as to interfere with vision.

Elschnig's pearls: remaining lens epithelial cells form new lens "fibers"; Elschnig's pearls are seen on slit-lamp examination as tiny balls of new lens fibers resembling fish eggs.

Soemmerring's ring (366.51): lens cortex trapped in equatorial part of "lens capsular bag"; because Soemmerring's ring cataract occurs in the equatorial (peripheral) portion of the "lens bag," it may not be observed until the pupil is dilated widely and does not interfere with vision.

Investigations

Visual acuity testing: usually the best visual acuity is reduced over the last visit; however, sometimes the patient sees the same as the last visit but notes that the visual acuity screen is less bright.

Refraction: reduced vision may be secondary to a refractive change rather than to PCO.

Intraocular pressure (IOP).

Undilated and dilated slit-lamp examination.

Dilated fundus examination: with the use of a high plus in the direct ophthalmoscope, the red reflex is less bright than normal and also uneven; when focused on the retina, the image is blurred.

Differential diagnosis

• Other causes of decreased vision after cataract surgery include:

Refractive change: probably most common cause of postoperative change in visual acuity.

Cystoid macular edema: occurs in ≤5% of post-ECCE patients.

Age-related macular degeneration: usually predates cataract surgery but may not have been visualized because of the cataract.

Corneal edema: occurs in ≤1% of post-ECCE patients.

Intraocular inflammation: extremely rare and may be sterile or infectious.

Retinal detachment: occurs in <1% of patients after ECCE.

Cause

• Proliferation of residual anterior lens capsular epithelium onto the posterior lens capsule.

Epidemiology

• Occurs in ~25% of patients after ECCE and lens implantation.

Classification

Grade I: diaphanous haze.

Grade II: mild haze (has a watery, milky appearance).

Grade III: moderate haze (often has geographic areas of differing densities).

Grade IV: white, capsular haze.

Pathology

• The proliferated lens epithelium undergoes fibrous metaplasia, which results in the formation of scar tissue over the posterior lens capsule. The proliferated metaplastic cells are both fibroblasts and myofibroblasts and therefore have the potential for contraction.

Diagnosis continued on p. 40

TREATMENT

Pharmacologic Treatment

- No medical treatment is available to prevent, stabilize, or reverse posterior capsular lens opacities.
- An early fibrinous inflammatory reaction on the anterior surface of the lens implant usually responds well to 1% corticosteroid solutions given topically, 1 drop every 2-4 hr daily.

Nonpharmacologic Treatment
Neodymium:Yttrium-Aluminum-Garnet (Nd:YAG) Laser (668.21)

- Inflammatory membranes on the anterior surface of the lens implant that do not respond to corticosteroid therapy can be removed easily by the use of the Nd:YAG laser, using an energy level of 0.8-1.0 millijoule (mJ).
- Before treatment, the undilated pupil is examined to make certain that it is centered or, if not, to see where the pupil is in relation to the lens opacity so that an opening in the posterior lens opacity can be made in the appropriate location. The pupil is dilated. One drop of apraclonidine 1% sterile ophthalmic solution (Iopidine; Alcon Laboratories, Randburg, South Africa) is instilled in the eye. YAG laser capsulectomy (either direct or with special posterior capsulectomy contact lens) is performed at the minimum energy level that can be used to dissolve the posterior lens opacity (start at 0.8 mJ and increase energy in increments of 0.1-0.2 mJ). After an adequate opening in the proper anatomic location is obtained, another drop of Iopidine is instilled. The patient is asked to wait for a few hours to make certain that the IOP does not rise above normal (if a persistent IOP rise occurs, it should be treated appropriately with antiglaucoma medications). The patient is then discharged with no medication or perhaps a mild corticosteroid eyedrop to be used four times daily. Follow up with patient in about a week.
- Because the YAG energy is propagated anteriorly, when performing the YAG laser capsulectomy on the posterior lens capsule, the helium-neon (HeNe) aiming beam should be focused slightly posterior to the posterior lens capsule to avoid "pinging" the lens implant. If no dissolution of the posterior capsule occurs, the aiming beam can be moved cautiously, by tiny increments, anteriorly until capsular dissolution results. Conversely, when performing the YAG laser on a membrane on the anterior lens capsule (YAG laser membranectomy), again because the YAG energy is propagated anteriorly, the focusing of the HeNe aiming beam is not nearly as critical as when focusing on the posterior capsule.

Treatment aims

To provide an adequate opening in the opacified posterior lens capsule for clear vision within the visual axis.

To avoid placing energy anterior to the posterior lens capsule by carefully aligning and aiming the HeNe beam so as not to "ping" the lens implant (fortunately, if this happens, it is rarely clinically significant).

To avoid post-Nd:YAG complications, which include glaucoma (use preoperative and postoperative pressure-lowering drops); cystoid macular edema (wait at least 4-6 wk after cataract surgery before performing another Nd:YAG surgical treatment).

Prognosis

After Nd:YAG laser treatment, ~100% of patients are cured (meaning that the opening created in the posterior lens capsule is permanent). In extremely rare cases the opening may close (usually in an eye that has an anterior uveitis).

Follow-up and management

Patients should be checked a few days to a few weeks after Nd:YAG laser treatment to make certain that (1) visual acuity has improved, (2) an adequate opening is present in the posterior lens capsule, (3) IOP is normal, (4) cystoid macular edema has not developed, and (5) a retinal tear or detachment is not present.

Treatment continued on p. 41

DIAGNOSIS—cont'd

Complications
Decreased vision: patient may note the decreased vision as an actual decrease in clarity of vision, a darkening of vision, or a combination of both.

Subluxation or dislocation of intraocular lens implant (secondary to capsular contraction).

Delayed infection: usually caused by *Staphylococcus epidermidis* or *Propionibacterium acnes* trapped in the lens capsule at cataract surgery; this infection tends to be indolent and may not appear until many months after surgery.

Pearls and Considerations
Frequency of "after cataract" is age related, with almost all children developing PCO and the incidence decreasing in adults [1].

Referral Information
Referral for yttrium-aluminum-garnet (YAG) laser capsulotomy is indicated.

TREATMENT—cont'd

Other Treatments
- Surgical incision of posterior capsule: rarely performed since the advent of Nd:YAG laser treatment.

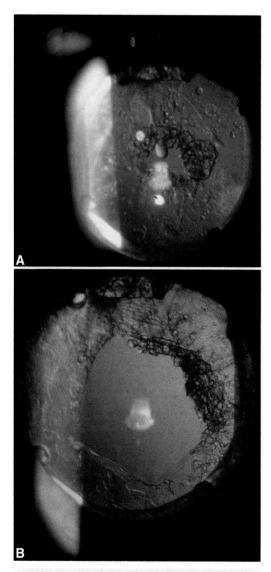

Figure 1 **A,** Posterior lens capsule has become opaque a few years after cataract extraction and lens implantation. **B,** Large opening has been made in the posterior lens capsule with a YAG laser.

Key reference
1. Boulton M, Saxby LA: Secondary cataract. In Yanoff M, Duker JS, editors: *Ophthalmology*, E-dition, St Louis, 2006, Elsevier.

General references
Caballero A, Garcia-Elskamp C, Losada M, et al: Natural evolution of Elschnig pearl posterior capsule opacification after posterior capsulotomy, *J Cataract Refract Surg* 27(12): 1979-1986, 2001.

Schaumberg DA, Dana MR, Christen WG, et al: A systemic overview of the incidence of posterior capsule opacification, *Ophthalmology* 105(7):1213-1221, 1998.

Shirai K, Saika S, Okada Y, et al: Histology and immunochemistry of fibrous posterior capsule opacification in an infant, *J Cataract Refract Surg* 30(2):523-526, 2004.

Tetz MR, Nimsgern C: Posterior capsule opacification. Part 2. Clinical findings, *J Cataract Refract Surg* 25(12):1662-1674, 1999.

DIAGNOSIS

Definition
"Senescent lens changes related, in part, to ultraviolet B radiation" [1].

Synonym
Senile cataract.

Symptoms
Obscuration of vision: the onset of decreased vision tends to be insidious, usually over many years; occasionally, however, the onset may be rapid (perception of rapidity may be brought on when, for the first time in a long time, patient covers the good eye and notes decreased vision in the cataractous eye, which may have been present for some time; true rapidity of decreased vision occurs rarely, with some rapidly developing posterior subcapsular cataracts and mature cataracts); patient may describe obscuration of vision as blurred, dim, or hazy vision.

Haloes at night: in low light when the pupils are semidilated or fully dilated; nuclear cataracts can cause haloes to appear around lights; it is important to differentiate this phenomenon from the same symptom that occurs with angle-closure glaucoma (with nuclear cataract, the eye is white, painless, and has a normally reactive pupil, whereas with angle-closure glaucoma, the eye is red, painful, and the pupil is dilated and fixed).

- *Note:* Many patients may be asymptomatic, and cataract may first be detected during a routine eye examination.

Signs
Opacification within the lens cortex (*cortical cataract* [366.15]) **and/or nucleus** (*nuclear cataract* [366.16]): *see* Fig. 1.

Opacification just posterior to the anterior lens capsule (*anterior subcapsular cataract* [366.13]) **or just anterior to the posterior lens capsule** (*posterior subcapsular cataract* [366.14]): *see* Fig. 2.

Completely white (mature) cataract (366.17): as the cortex undergoes cataractous change, it becomes liquefied (morgagnian degeneration; seen with the slit lamp as cortical spokes); the cortex then becomes more and more milky until finally it becomes opaque (mature cataract); the liquefied cortex can escape through the intact lens capsule, causing capsular folds (*hypermature cataract* [366.18]); *see* Fig. 3.

Investigations
Visual acuity testing: in moderate or advanced cataracts, testing visual acuity with the Snellen chart gives a reasonable estimate of the patient's vision.

- *Note:* Some patients with normal or near-normal visual acuity can be quite symptomatic. For example, a posterior subcapsular cataract may be small, dense, and centrally located, but with the pupil at a normal size, the patient can see around the cataract, and the vision may be normal. However, when the patient goes outside into bright sunlight and the pupil constricts, the patient's vision may fall precipitously because the cataract now occupies the entire pupil. Special testing for brightness (brightness acuity tester) and glare is often indicated in the evaluation of a patient who has a cataract.

Refraction; intraocular pressure; undilated and dilated slit-lamp examination; dilated fundus examination.

Differential diagnosis
- Cataracts may not be primary ("senile") and may be related to a secondary process (e.g., neoplasm).
- Other causes of decreased vision include:
Cystoid macular edema.
Age-related macular degeneration.
Diabetic retinopathy.
Glaucoma.
Retinal detachment.
Vitreous hemorrhage.
Corneal edema.

Cause
- Risk factors include heredity, age, diabetes mellitus, oral or inhaled corticosteroid therapy, exposure to ultraviolet B (UVB) radiation, poor nutrition, and smoking.

Epidemiology
- Cataracts are common, and cataract surgery is the most frequently performed surgery in the elderly patient.
- Cataracts can occur at any age. The two peaks are in patients <10 yr (congenital cataracts) and those >65 yr, but cataracts occur in every decade of life.

Classification
- Cataracts can be classified as *cortical* (366.15), *nuclear* (366.16), *anterior subcapsular* (366.13), *posterior subcapsular* (366.14), or *mature* (366.17).

Pathology
- The pathology depends on the type of cataract. In general, degenerative changes are found in the nucleus, cortex, or anterior or posterior subcapsular areas.
- Early cataractous changes in the cortex appear as tiny areas of liquefaction called *morgagnian degeneration,* seen clinically as cortical spokes. The liquefaction can progress to involve the entire cortex, which then appears milky white. The cataractous nucleus loses its artifactitious clefts and appears homogeneous in microscopic sections.

Diagnosis continued on p. 44

TREATMENT

Diet and Lifestyle
- Diet and lifestyle have no effect on most cataracts. Avoidance of excess UVB radiation exposure may be helpful.

Pharmacologic Treatment
- No pharmacologic treatment is recommended.

Nonpharmacologic Treatment
- If visual potential exists in the eye, surgical treatment may be indicated.
- Even if the vision is reduced significantly and testing shows an excellent chance for good vision after cataract surgery, the patient may not want surgery. The benefits and risks of cataract surgery and lens implantation and the patient's lifestyle and expectations must be discussed thoroughly with the patient. For example, a taxi driver who has a posterior sub-capsular cataract and a visual acuity of 20/30 may choose cataract surgery before a retired individual who mainly reads and watches television and has a nuclear cataract that reduces visual acuity to 20/60. Only through a comprehensive discussion with the patient and other involved family members or friends can a mutual decision for cataract surgery be reached.
- Some patients who have a nuclear cataract note that they are able to read for the first time in years without glasses. This increased ability for near vision, known as *second sight*, is caused by the increased index of refraction of the nuclear cataract, which induces nearsight-edness. Despite that the nuclear cataract may reduce distance vision, patients who spend most of their time using near vision (reading, watching television) will be most unhappy with cataract surgery if they now need glasses to read. Again, a full discussion, including the patient's expectations, is mandatory.

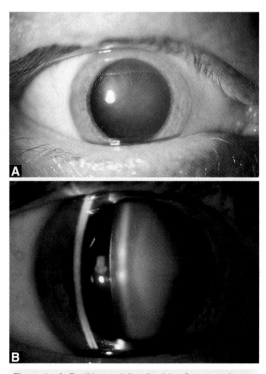

Figure 1   A, Pupil has a dull, yellowish reflex secondary to a nuclear cataract (nuclear sclerosis). **B,** Slit beam demonstrates the yellow nuclear cataract and white cortical cataract.

Treatment aims
To improve vision.
To rehabilitate the patient as rapidly as possible.
- With modern small-incision, no-stitch, outpatient phacoemulsification ECCE surgery, wound stability is rapid and rehabilitation is minimal. The patient generally can resume normal activities the day after surgery. Glasses, if needed, may be prescribed in 2-8 wk.
- With the larger incision needed for nuclear expression ECCE, the time course is somewhat delayed. Glasses, if needed, generally are not prescribed for 4-10 wk after surgery.

Other treatments
- In the rare instances of phacolytic glaucoma or secondary angle-closure glaucoma, cataract removal usually alleviates the problem.

Prognosis
- Cataract surgery results in about 95% visual improvement to a visual acuity of 20/40 or better.

Follow-up and management
- Long-term follow-up is needed to ensure proper visual rehabilitation and to check for postoperative complications, such as corneal edema, opacification of the posterior lens capsule ("after cataract"), glaucoma, intraocular inflammation, cystoid macular edema, and retinal detachment.

Treatment continued on p. 45

DIAGNOSIS—cont'd

Complications

Decreased vision: infrequently a swollen, mature cataract can cause a secondary angle-closure glaucoma; rarely a hypermature cataract can "leak" fluid, leading to a secondary open-angle glaucoma called *phacolytic glaucoma*.

Pearls and Considerations

1. A diagnosis of exclusion; secondary causes should be ruled out [1].
2. Potential acuity meter (PAM) is a useful tool in predicting postextraction visual acuity.
3. Success rate for routine cataract surgery is >95% [1].

Referral Information

Refer for cataract extraction and intraocular lens implantation once the cataract becomes visually significant.

TREATMENT—cont'd

Extracapsular Cataract Extraction

- An extracapsular cataract extraction (ECCE), either by nuclear expression or phacoemulsification, usually with intraocular lens implantation, can be performed. The decision of whether to perform nuclear expression ECCE or phacoemulsification ECCE depends on several factors. First and foremost is the skill of the individual surgeon and the type of procedure with which the surgeon is most comfortable. In general the type of surgery depends on the hardness of the nuclear component of the cataract (all cortical cataracts are soft). If the nuclear cataract is soft to moderately hard, most surgeons will perform phacoemulsification ECCE. If the nuclear cataract is very hard, some surgeons will perform nuclear expression ECCE. Most surgeons perform phacoemulsification ECCE on almost all cataracts.

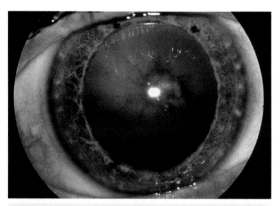

Figure 2   A density can be seen toward the back of the lens in this posterior subcapsular cataract.

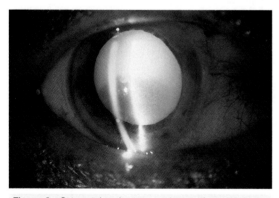

Figure 3   Cataract has become mature and appears as a milky reflex in the pupil. Note yellow-brown nucleus has been displaced inferiorly in milky, liquid cortex.

Key reference
1. Kasier PK, Friedman NJ: Lens. In *The Massachusetts Eye and Ear Infirmary illustrated manual of ophthalmology*, ed 2, Philadelphia, 2004, Saunders, p 268.

General references
Hiller R, Sperduto RD, Podgor MJ, et al: Cigarette smoking and the risk of development of lens opacities: the Framingham Studies, *Ophthalmology* 104:1113, 1997.

Italian-American Cataract Study Group: Incidence and progression of cortical, nuclear, and posterior subcapsular cataracts, *Am J Ophthalmol* 118(5):623-631, 1994.

Klein BEK, Klein R, Lee KE, et al: Socioeconomic and lifestyle factors and the 10-year incidence of age-related cataracts, *Am J Ophthalmol* 136(3):506-512, 2003.

Sachdev NH, Di Girolamo N, Nolan TM, et al: Matrix metalloproteinases and tissue inhibitors of matrix metalloproteinases in the human lens: implications for cortical cataract formation, *Invest Ophthalmol Vis Sci* 45(11):4075-4082, 2004.

Vrensen G, Willekens B: Biomicroscopy and scanning electron microscopy of early opacities in the aging human lens, *Invest Ophthalmol Vis Sci* 31(8):1582-1591, 1990.

DIAGNOSIS

Definition
Opacity of the lens that is present from birth.

Synonyms
None.

Symptoms
Decreased visual acuity.
Glare.

Signs
Leukokoria (white pupillary reflex).
Nystagmus: in untreated cases or in patients not responding to treatment.
Squinting in sunlight.
Strabismus.
Amblyopia.
Microphthalmos: common.

Investigations
Evaluation of red reflex: in every newborn; preferably before discharge from nursery.
Pupil dilation and evaluation of retina and other internal structures.
Evaluation of serum glucose, urea nitrogen, galactose enzymes, TORCH (toxoplasmosis, other infections, rubella, cytomegalovirus infection, and herpes simplex) **titers, or urine glucose and protein:** in some bilateral congenital cases.

Complications
Nystagmus: untreated cases usually develop irreversible nystagmus at ~2-3 mo of age; best corrected visual acuity after surgery is then <20/200.
Glaucoma: ~40% of children undergoing uncomplicated lensectomy will develop glaucoma at a later age, usually of uncertain cause; all aphakic children must be followed carefully because of this risk.
Infection, hemorrhage: after surgery.
Infection, corneal abrasion, lost lenses: after contact lens treatment.
Intraocular inflammation, cyclitic membrane formation, glaucoma, lens slippage: after intraocular lens placement.

Associated Features
• Microphthalmia is often associated with congenital cataract. Cataracts are found in patients with the following syndromes:
Renal diseases: Lowe syndrome, Alport syndrome.
Central nervous system diseases: Marinesco-Sjögren syndrome, Sjögren syndrome.
Mandibulofacial syndromes: Hallermann-Streiff syndrome, Pierre Robin syndrome, Treacher Collins syndrome.
Dermal syndromes: incontinentia pigmenti, congenital ectodermal dysplasia, Werner syndrome, Rothmund-Thomson syndrome.
Chromosomal disorders: trisomies 13, 18, 21.
Metabolic syndromes: galactosemia, galactose-kinase deficiency, Wilson syndrome, Fabry syndrome, Refsum syndrome, homocystinuria, myotonic dystrophy, pseudohypoparathyroidism.
Other ocular abnormalities: Norrie disease, aniridia, pigmentary retinopathy.

Pearls and Considerations
1. Congenital cataract is of particular concern because of the potential for deprivation amblyopia and secondary glaucoma. Early detection and intervention are key to a desirable visual outcome.
2. Not all cataracts are visually significant. Cataracts not visually significant should be monitored regularly because of the potential for progression [1].

Referral Information
Refer to pediatric ophthalmologist for cataract extraction.

Differential diagnosis
• All causes of leukokoria, including:
Retinoblastoma.
Toxocariasis.
Coats' disease.
Persistent hyperplastic primary vitreous.
TORCH diseases.
Myelinated nerve fibers.
Others.

Causes
• 33% of cases are sporadic, 25% are familial (usually autosomal dominant).
• Must consider galactosemia, Lowe syndrome, and TORCH diseases in bilateral congenital cases.

Epidemiology
• Most frequent form of remediable childhood blindness.
• Found in 0.4% of live births, but many cataracts are not visually significant. Rubella was a major cause of bilateral congenital cataracts in the past (*see* figure).

Pathology
• Pathology of nuclear, cortical, and posterior subcapsular cataracts is similar to that in adults.
• Posterior lenticonus opacities show a thin posterior lens capsule with posteriorly bulging cortex with abnormal lens epithelial cells.

TREATMENT

Diet and Lifestyle
- Patients with galactosemia and galactose-kinase deficiency should be placed on a galactose-free diet. The cataracts may improve.

Pharmacologic Treatment
- No pharmacologic treatment is recommended.

Nonpharmacologic Treatment
- Lensectomy should be performed as soon as possible in all children with visually significant congenital cataracts (axial opacities >3.0 mm in diameter).
- Unilateral congenital cataracts should be removed when discovered, preferably before 3 wk of age.
- Bilateral congenital cataracts should be removed before 8 wk of age, either simultaneously or within 3 days of one another.
- After lensectomy, the refractive power of the lens must be replaced with either an intraocular lens (reserved for children >2 or 3 yr of age), contact lens, or glasses (generally, bilateral aphakes with contraindications to intraocular lens or contact lens treatment).

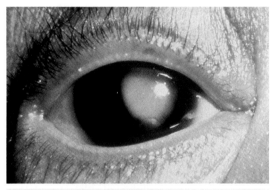

Cataract caused by rubella in 4-wk-old child.

Treatment aims
To clear visual axes and achieve excellent visual acuity in each eye.

Other treatments
- Patching one eye for treatment of amblyopia is often required.

Prognosis
Monocular congenital cataracts: if surgery is performed very early in life and compliance with patching and refractive treatment is good, the patient may develop 20/20 visual acuity, straight eyes, binocular vision, and stereopsis; compliance is often less than adequate, however, or surgery is delayed, and poor acuity, nystagmus, and strabismus result.
Bilateral congenital cataracts: often symmetric, and amblyopia is less threatening; the outcome in each eye is generally better than in unilateral cases.

Follow-up and management
- Immediately after surgery, patients should be seen approximately twice weekly; a few days after surgery, patients should be fitted with contact lenses. Frequent refraction and acuity evaluations are necessary because amblyopia in infancy can occur, reversing quickly with treatment. Patching regimens and refractive corrections are altered as necessary.
- Intraocular pressure, refractions, and optic nerve appearance are monitored because glaucoma occurs frequently in the aphakic population.

Key reference
1. Bashour M, Menassa J, Gerontis CC: Congenital cataract, 2006, www.emedicine.com.

General references
Haargaard B, Wohlfahrt J, Fledelius HC, et al: A nationwide Danish study of 1027 cases of congenital/infantile cataracts: etiological and clinical classifications, *Ophthalmology* 111(12): 2292-2298, 2004.

Junk AK, Stefani FH, Ludwig K: Bilateral anterior lenticonus: Scheimpflug imaging system documentation and ultrastructural confirmation of Alport syndrome in the lens capsule, *Arch Ophthalmol* 118(7):895-897, 2000.

Kramer PL, LaMorticella D, Schilling K, et al: A new locus for autosomal dominant congenital cataracts maps to chromosome 3, *Invest Ophthalmol Vis Sci* 41(1):36-39, 2000.

Lambert SR, Drack AV: Infantile cataracts, *Surv Ophthalmol* 40(6):427-458, 1996.

Cataract, infantile, juvenile, and presenile   (366.0)

DIAGNOSIS

Definition
Acquired opacity of the lens found in children and young adults.

Synonyms
None.

Symptoms
Decreased vision: in infants or very young children, decreased vision is difficult to evaluate; the parent often will notice that the infant or child is not focusing on objects or that the eyes are wandering aimlessly.

Strabismus: often an infant or young child who has a unilateral cataract will develop strabismus to remove the blurred image caused by the cataractous eye from the macular portion of the retina.

Leukokoria (white pupil): noted by parent; this type of presentation is rare and occurs when the cataract becomes "mature" and has a white, milky appearance; the leukokoria (cat's eye reflex) may mimic that which is seen with retinoblastoma.

- *Note:* Some patients may be asymptomatic, and cataract may first be detected during a routine eye examination.

Signs
Opacification within the lens cortex (366.03) **and/or nucleus** (366.04) **or at the junction of nucleus and cortex** (*zonular cataract* [366.03]) (*see* Fig. 1).

Opacification just posterior to the anterior lens capsule (*anterior subcapsular or polar cataract* [366.01]) **or just anterior to the posterior lens capsule** (*posterior subcapsular or polar cataract* [366.02]): an opacification caused by an abnormal anterior (anterior polar or anterior pyramidal cataract) or posterior (posterior polar cataract) curvature of the lens; an "oil globule" reflex is seen within the pupillary red reflex (*see* Fig. 2).

Completely white (mature) cataract (366.17).

Investigations
History: important because congenital and infantile cataracts may be autosomal dominant (most common), autosomal recessive, X-linked, or a chromosomal abnormality; the cataract may arise secondarily to an intrauterine infection (e.g., rubella).

Visual acuity testing.

Refraction.

Intraocular pressure.

Undilated and dilated slit-lamp examination: other ocular congenital anomalies may occur along with the congenital cataract, such as colobomata of the iris.

Dilated fundus examination: especially in infants and young children; other ocular congenital anomalies may occur along with the congenital cataract, such as colobomata of the choroid.

Appropriate evaluation of any underlying cause as indicated.

Differential diagnosis
- Cataracts in children can be secondary to:
Tumor (e.g., retinoblastoma).
Trauma.
Intraocular inflammation.
Metabolic (e.g., galactosemia) or systemic (e.g., diabetes mellitus) diseases.

Cause
Congenital (accounts for ~50% of all childhood cataracts).
Genetic without systemic abnormalities (e.g., autosomal dominant cataract).
Genetic with systemic abnormalities (e.g., oculocerebral syndrome of Lowe, incontinentia pigmenti).
Metabolic (e.g., galactosemia, diabetes mellitus).
Chromosomal abnormalities (e.g., trisomies 13 [Patau syndrome] and 21 [Down syndrome]).
Intrauterine (e.g., rubella), or postpartum intraocular infection.
Therapeutic drugs (e.g., steroids).

Epidemiology
- Cataracts occur in ~0.3% of all children; most have no known cause or associated systemic conditions.

Classification
- Infantile cataracts occur from 0-10 yr.
- Juvenile cataracts occur from 11-20 yr.
- Presenile cataracts occur ≤45 yr.

Associated features
- Approximately 50% of patients have no associated systemic features, but some may have other ocular abnormalities (e.g., amblyopia, strabismus, intraocular structural abnormalities).
- In the other 50%, associated features depend on the underlying cause (e.g., chromosomal or metabolic disorders, systemic syndromes with ocular manifestations, trauma, infections).

Pathology
- The pathology depends on the type of cataract, with degenerative changes found in the nucleus, cortex, and anterior or posterior subcapsular areas.

Diagnosis continued on p. 50

TREATMENT

Diet and Lifestyle

- In the vast majority of patients, diet and lifestyle have no effect on the cataracts. However, in patients with metabolic cataracts (e.g., galactosomia), appropriate diet can have a dramatic effect on the cataract.
- Galactosemia is an autosomal recessive disease resulting from a deficiency of galactose-1-phosphate uridyl transferase. The cataract usually is noted a few days to a few months after birth.

Pharmacologic Treatment

- In the vast majority of patients, pharmacologic treatment has no effect on the cataracts. However, in metabolic cataracts (e.g., diabetes mellitus), appropriate therapy can impede or even reverse the cataract.

Nonpharmacologic Treatment

- If visual potential exists in the eye, surgical treatment is indicated. Extracapsular cataract extraction (ECCE), usually by the irrigation-and-aspiration (I&A) technique in patients ≤30 yr of age and by I&A or phacoemulsification in older patients. Depending on the patient's age, intraocular lens implantation may or may not be indicated.
- Special care must be taken if congenital ectopic cataracts are present, such as Marfan syndrome (autosomal dominant; excessive hydroxyproline urinary excretion) and homocystinuria (autosomal recessive; deficiency of cystathionine synthetase). In these patients the cataractous lens generally is subluxated (in posterior chamber but not in normal position) or dislocated (out of posterior chamber into vitreous or anterior chamber).
- The residual lens epithelium in children is quite reactive, and opacification of the posterior capsule after ECCE is almost inevitable. Most surgeons therefore will perform a posterior capsulotomy (opening) or capsulectomy (removal) at the time of ECCE.
- Because the eye does not reach adult size until the middle to late teens, the decision on whether or not to implant an intraocular lens at the time of cataract surgery in a child is controversial. Although some advocate postoperative contact lenses, posterior-chamber lens implantation is generally desirable. The strength of the lens must be estimated because the eye is still growing.

Treatment aims

To improve vision.
To prevent or treat amblyopia and strabismus.

Prognosis

- Prognosis depends on many factors, such as age at onset, other associated intraocular abnormalities, and presence of amblyopia.

  In young children <10 yr of age, special attention must be paid to visual rehabilitation and the prevention or treatment of amblyopia. Children <10 yr of age who have blurred vision in one eye (e.g., from unilateral congenital cataract) tend to rotate that eye internally or externally so that the image does not fall on the macula. Although these children are able to suppress the image in the deviating eye, thereby avoiding the debilitating symptom of double vision (diplopia), the deviating eye itself becomes "lazy," and amblyopia develops. After good vision is restored by cataract surgery, this type of amblyopia often can be treated successfully by patching the nonamblyopic eye. Once the amblyopic child passes the age of ~10-12 yr, however, the amblyopia becomes so deep seated that it cannot be reversed by patching or any other means.

Follow-up and management

- Long-term follow-up is needed to ensure proper visual rehabilitation and treatment of such postoperative complications as glaucoma and retinal detachment.

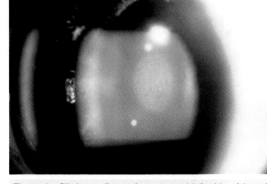

Figure 1   Slit beam (front of eye toward left side of beam) shows central granular opacity in the center of the lens, characteristic of a congenital nuclear cataract.

Treatment continued on p. 51

DIAGNOSIS—cont'd

Complications

Amblyopia

If strabismus develops (usually with unilateral congenital cataract and in patients <10 yr of age), the child will not properly use the macula. This disuse of the macula in one eye causes the image to be suppressed. The advantage of this is that the child does not have to deal with double vision (diplopia). The disadvantage is that a "lazy eye" (amblyopia) develops.

Phacolytic Glaucoma

A mature cataract can "leak" fluid and cause a secondary glaucoma called *phacolytic glaucoma*. The liquefied cortex leaks out through an intact capsule, gaining access to the anterior chamber, where it acts as a weak antigen. Macrophages engulf the cortex, become swollen, and occlude the open anterior-chamber angle. Blockage of aqueous outflow causes acute open-angle glaucoma.

Pearls and Considerations

Same as for congenital cataracts.

Referral Information

Same as for congenital cataracts.

TREATMENT—cont'd

- If strabismus and amblyopia existed before surgery, immediate attention to these conditions must be given postoperatively. The amblyopic eye needs to be patched and carefully followed. Strabismus surgery may be needed if conservative therapy fails.
- If phacolytic glaucoma (*see* Complications) develops, cataract extraction and lens implantation usually are curative unless irreversible damage to the optic nerve has been caused by the glaucoma.

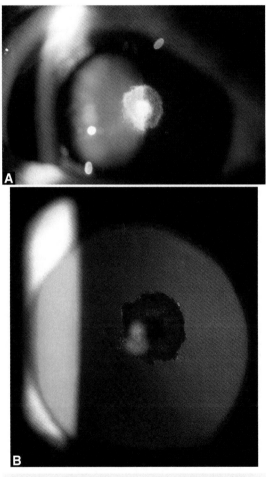

Figure 2 A, Slit beam (front of eye toward left side of beam) shows an opaque plaque on the back part of the lens in a young adult, characteristic of a congenital posterior polar cataract. **B,** Red reflex clearly demonstrates the posterior polar cataract.

General references

Bateman JB, Johannes M, Flodman P, et al: A new locus for autosomal dominant cataract on chromosome 12q13, *Invest Ophthalmol Vis Sci* 41(9):2665-2670, 2000.

Haargaard B, Wohlfahrt J, Fledelius HC, et al: A nationwide Danish study of 1027 cases of congenital/infantile cataracts: etiological and clinical classifications, *Ophthalmology* 111(12): 2292-2298, 2004.

Junk AK, Stefani FH, Ludwig K: Bilateral anterior lenticonus: Scheimpflug imaging system documentation and ultrastructural confirmation of Alport syndrome in the lens capsule, *Arch Ophthalmol* 118(7):895-897, 2000.

Kramer PL, LaMorticella D, Schilling K, et al: A new locus for autosomal dominant congenital cataracts maps to chromosome 3, *Invest Ophthalmol Vis Sci* 41(1):36-39, 2000.

Lambert SR, Drack AV: Infantile cataracts, *Surv Ophthalmol* 40(6):427-458, 1996.

Cataract, secondary to ocular and other complications   (366.3)

DIAGNOSIS

Definition
Opacity of the lens secondary to other ocular inflammation or disease process.

Synonyms
None.

Symptoms
Obscuration of vision: depending on the underlying condition, the onset of decreased vision may be *rapid* (e.g., sudden, usually reversible osmotic cataract of juvenile diabetes) or *insidious* (e.g., posterior subcapsular cataract of retinitis pigmentosa); the patient may perceive obscuration of vision as blurred, dim, or hazy vision.

Haloes at night: in low light when the pupils are semidilated or fully dilated, nuclear cataracts can cause haloes to appear around lights; it is important to differentiate this phenomenon from the same symptom that occurs with angle-closure glaucoma (with nuclear cataract, the eye is white, painless, and has a normally reactive pupil, whereas with angle-closure glaucoma, the eye is red and painful and the pupil is dilated and fixed).

Red eye: depending on the underlying cause of the cataract (e.g., uveitis, acute angle-closure glaucoma, Stevens-Johnson syndrome), the eye may be red secondary to ciliary injection.

Painful eye: depending on the underlying cause of the cataract, the eye may be painful; usually associated with those entities that cause ciliary injection.

- *Note:* Some patients may be asymptomatic, and cataract may first be detected during a routine eye examination.

Signs
Opacification within the lens cortex (*cortical cataract* [366.15]) **and/or nucleus** (*nuclear cataract* [366.16]).

Opacification just posterior to the anterior lens capsule (*anterior subcapsular cataract* [366.13]) **or just anterior to the posterior lens capsule** (*posterior subcapsular cataract* [366.14]).

Completely white (mature) cataract (366.17): as the cortex undergoes cataractous change, it becomes liquefied (*morgagnian degeneration;* seen with the slit lamp as cortical spokes); the cortex then becomes more and more milky until finally it becomes opaque (mature cataract); the liquefied cortex can escape through the intact lens capsule, causing capsular folds (*hypermature cataract* [366.18]).

Elschnig's pearls: remaining lens epithelial cells form new lens "fibers" (*see* Cataract, after).

Soemmerring's ring (366.51): lens cortex trapped in equatorial part of "lens capsular bag" (*see* Cataract, after).

Subluxation (within posterior chamber but not in normal position) **or dislocation** (in anterior chamber or vitreous compartment).

Ciliary injection: if eye inflamed.

Differential diagnosis
Primary cataracts unrelated to a secondary process.
Other causes of decreased vision (e.g., diabetic retinopathy).

Cause
See Boxes 1 and 2.

Epidemiology
- Although all the entities listed in Boxes 1 and 2 may be associated with cataracts, the exact frequency is not known.
- Cataracts often complicate chronic intraocular inflammation.
- Degenerative disorders (especially retinitis pigmentosa and Wilson's disease) have a high frequency of associated cataracts.

Classification
- Cataracts can be classified as:
  Cortical (366.15).
  Nuclear (366.16).
  Anterior subcapsular (366.13).
  Posterior subcapsular (366.14).
  Mature (366.17).

Pathology
- The pathology depends on the type of cataract.

Complications
Decreased vision.
Retinal detachment.
Uveitis.
- Infrequently, a swollen mature cataract can cause a secondary angle-closure glaucoma.
- Rarely, a hypermature cataract can "leak" fluid, leading to a secondary open-angle glaucoma called *phacolytic glaucoma* (*see* Cataract, infantile, juvenile, and presenile).

Diagnosis continued on p. 54

TREATMENT

Diet and Lifestyle
- In the vast majority of patients, no special precautions are necessary.

Pharmacologic Treatment
For Cataracts Secondary to Ocular Complications
- Appropriate pharmacologic treatment is indicated for the relevant underlying conditions.
- In most of these cases, however (although the underlying condition may be brought under control), the cataract is not reversible, and cataract surgery must be performed.

Box 1. Causes of cataracts secondary to ocular complications

Cataract complicata (366.30)

Acute angle-closure glaucoma

   Glaukomflecken (366.31)

Intraocular inflammation

   Chronic choroiditis (363.0)

   Iridocyclitis (364.1)

Degenerative disorders

   Retinitis pigmentosa (362.74)

Box 2. Cataracts secondary to systemic and other entities

Diabetic (366.41)

   Secondary to diabetes mellitus (250.5)

   Sunflower cataract of Wilson's disease (366.34)

Tetanic (366.42)

   Secondary to calcinosis (275.4)

   Hypoparathyroidism (252.1)

Myotonic (366.43)

   Secondary to myotonic dystrophy (359.2)

Other systemic syndromes

   Craniofacial dysostosis (756.0)

   Galactosemia (271.1)

Toxic or drug induced (366.45)

   Posterior subcapsular cataract secondary to corticosteroids or radiation induced (366.46)

Other entities

   Acquired immunodeficiency syndrome (AIDS)

   Stevens-Johnson syndrome

   Vitamin A deficiency

Treatment aims
To improve vision.
- Patients who have cataracts secondary to ocular and systemic problems often do not achieve 20/20 vision. Many of these patients, however, usually appreciate any improvement in vision. For example, removing a cataract from an incapacitated patient with hand-motions vision can give the patient 20/200 or 20/400 vision, which can increase mobility and independence.

Other treatments
- Other treatments are aimed at the underlying conditions. Unfortunately, this generally does not reverse the cataractous lens changes, and if visual incapacity results from the cataract, surgery is required.

Prognosis
- The prognosis depends on the underlying ocular or systemic condition; by the time the underlying condition is controlled, however, irreversible cataractous changes may have occurred in the lens.

Follow-up and management
- Long-term follow-up is needed to ensure proper visual rehabilitation and treatment of the underlying ocular or systemic condition.
- Cataract extraction and lens implantation in this group of patients is fraught with complications. The patient must be followed to diagnose the early stages of glaucoma, recurrence of intraocular inflammation, retinal tear and detachment, and other conditions.

Treatment continued on p. 55

DIAGNOSIS—cont'd

Investigations

History: a meticulous history of past episodes of red eye (e.g., previous iridocyclitis), metabolic defects (e.g., secondary to hypoparathyroidism), and inherited conditions (e.g., retinitis pigmentosa) is extremely important in establishing the cause of the cataract.

Visual acuity testing.

Refraction.

Intraocular pressure.

Undilated and dilated slit-lamp examination.

Dilated fundus examination.

Appropriate evaluation of any underlying cause: as indicated.

Pearls and Considerations

If vision worsens, refer to an eye care physician.

Referral Information

Varied and dependent on the suspected etiology of the disease.

TREATMENT—cont'd

For Cataracts Secondary to Systemic Diseases

- Appropriate pharmacologic treatment is indicated for the relevant underlying conditions.
- In rare cases (e.g., osmotic cataract of juvenile diabetes, tetanic cataract of calcinosis secondary to hypoparathyroidism), cataracts may be reversible when the underlying condition can be brought under control. In most of these patients, however (although the underlying condition may be managed), the cataract is not reversible, and cataract surgery must be performed.

Nonpharmacologic Treatment

- If visual potential exists in the eye, surgical treatment is indicated. Extracapsular cataract extraction (ECCE), either by nuclear expression or phacoemulsification (usually with intraocular lens implantation), is performed.
- Some conditions have surprisingly better results than would be expected from the clinical data. For example, patients with advanced retinitis pigmentosa who are legally blind because of their restricted visual field become even more disabled by the characteristic subcapsular cataract that develops in this condition. Cataract extraction and lens implantation often greatly benefit these patients. Another example is heterochromic iridocyclitis (Fuchs'), which might indicate cataract surgery on an inflamed eye. Experience, however, shows that these patients tolerate intraocular surgery quite well, and active inflammation here is not a contraindication to surgery.

General references

Cumming RG: Use of inhaled corticosteroids and the risk of cataracts, *N Engl J Med* 337(1): 8-14, 1997.

Garbe E, Suissa S, LeLorier J: Exposure to allopurinol and the risk of cataract extraction in elderly patients, *Arch Ophthalmol* 116(12):1652-1656, 1998.

Stambolian D, Scarpino-Myers V, Eagle RC Jr, et al: Cataracts in patients heterozygous for galactokinase deficiency, *Invest Ophthalmol Vis Sci* 27(3):429-433, 1986.

Toogood JH, Markov AE, Baskerville J, et al: Association of ocular cataracts with inhaled and oral steroid therapy during long-term treatment of asthma, *J Allergy Clin Immunol* 91(2): 571-579, 1993.

Cataract, traumatic   (366.22)

DIAGNOSIS

Definition
Opacity of the lens secondary to blunt trauma or penetrating injury.

Synonyms
None.

Symptoms
Obscuration of vision: the onset of decreased vision depends on the underlying cause; for example, following blunt trauma, a typical petal-shaped cataract (*see* Figs. 1 and 2) may take years to progress to the point where vision is decreased; on the other hand, perforating trauma may injure the lens and cause instant loss of vision; the patient may describe obscuration of vision as blurred, dim, or hazy vision.

Haloes at night: blunt trauma may cause nuclear cataracts, which, when the pupils are semi-dilated or fully dilated, can cause haloes to appear around lights; it is important to differentiate this phenomenon from the same symptom that occurs with angle-closure glaucoma (with nuclear cataract, the eye is white, painless, and has a normally reactive pupil, whereas with angle-closure glaucoma, the eye is red and painful and the pupil is dilated and fixed).

Red and/or painful eye: depending on the underlying cause of the cataract (e.g., traumatic uveitis, endophthalmitis, secondary angle-closure glaucoma), the eye may be red secondary to ciliary injection, which often also causes pain.

- *Note:* Some patients may be asymptomatic, and cataract may first be detected during a routine eye examination.
- A traumatic cataract, usually following blunt trauma, may take years to develop to the point at which vision is affected.

Signs
Opacification within the lens cortex (*cortical cataract* [366.15]) **and/or nucleus** (*nuclear cataract* [366.16]).

Opacification just posterior to the anterior lens capsule (*anterior subcapsular cataract* [366.13]) **or just anterior to the posterior lens capsule** (*posterior subcapsular cataract* [366.14]).

Completely white (mature) cataract (366.17).

Completely white but shrunken (hypermature) cataract (366.18).

Investigations
Visual acuity testing: it is extremely important to test visual acuity after ocular trauma, especially after penetrating ocular trauma in which uveal prolapse occurs; if after 1 wk to 10 days no useful vision is present, the eye should be enucleated to avoid the development of *sympathetic uveitis* (*see* Uveitis, sympathetic).

Refraction.

Intraocular pressure: a clue to an occult rupture of the globe may be a reduced pressure in the injured eye, especially when accompanied by a deeper-than-normal anterior chamber or a vitreous hemorrhage.

Undilated and dilated slit-lamp examination.

Dilated fundus examination.

Differential diagnosis
Primary (presenile or "senile") or secondary cataracts unrelated to trauma.
- Other causes of decreased vision include:
Cystoid macular edema.
Age-related macular degeneration.
Diabetic retinopathy.
Glaucoma.
Retinal detachment.
Vitreous hemorrhage.
Corneal edema.

Cause
Most often caused by blunt trauma to the eye; also, can be secondary to penetrating trauma to the eye; may not become apparent or symptomatic for months to years after blunt trauma.

Epidemiology
- Although the majority of cataracts are caused by the aging process, a significant percentage are traumatic.

Classification
- Traumatic cataracts (366.2) also can be classified as:
Cortical (366.15).
Nuclear (366.16).
Anterior subcapsular (366.13).
Posterior subcapsular (366.14).
Mature (366.17).
Completely white but shrunken, i.e., hypermature (366.18).

Associated features
- The trauma that caused the cataract can also cause corneal problems, glaucoma, Berlin's edema, retinal detachment, vitreous hemorrhage, intraocular foreign bodies, endophthalmitis, and traumatic chorioretinopathy.

Pathology
- The pathology depends on the type of cataract. In general, degenerative changes are found in the nucleus, cortex, or anterior or posterior subcapsular areas. Globe pathology depends on the associated injury and its consequences.

Diagnosis continued on p. 58

TREATMENT

Diet and Lifestyle
- In the vast majority of patients, no special precautions are necessary.

Pharmacologic Treatment
- Pharmacologic treatment has no effect on the cataracts but may be extremely important in some of the consequences of the trauma. For example, perforating trauma may introduce into the eye pathogenic organisms that must be treated vigorously (usually by topical and intravenous antibiotics and often along with vitrectomy and intraocular antibiotics). The type and dosage of the antibiotic depend on the particular protocol in use by the surgeon.

Nonpharmacologic Treatment
- If visual potential exists in the eye, surgical treatment may be indicated. Visual acuity potential can be measured by a variety of methods (e.g., potential acuity measurement instrument, laser interferometry, color discrimination).
- Extracapsular cataract extraction (ECCE), either by nuclear expression or phacoemulsification (usually with intraocular lens implantation), is performed. Often, with perforating trauma, a vitrectomy is combined with a lensectomy and intraocular lens insertion. Other problems, such as traumatic retinal detachment, can be repaired at the same time.
- If a cataractous lens is *subluxated* (i.e., in posterior chamber but not in its normal location) or *dislocated* (i.e., not in posterior chamber but in vitreous or anterior chamber), special precautions need to be taken during surgery. An intracapsular cataract extraction or a pars plana lensectomy may be warranted.

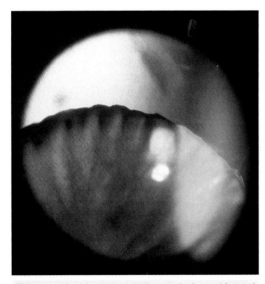

Figure 1   After blunt trauma to the eye, the lens subluxated inferiorly.

Treatment aims
To improve vision.

Other treatments
- Other ocular problems secondary to the trauma should be dealt with as indicated. Often the traumatic cataract is the least of the vision-threatening complications that can occur after ocular trauma (e.g., secondary glaucoma, anterior-chamber hemorrhage, retinal tears or detachment, vitreous hemorrhage, endophthalmitis).

Prognosis
- Prognosis depends on other associated ocular injuries. If no other vision-threatening ocular injuries are present, cataract extraction and intraocular lens implantation result in ~95% visual improvement to a visual acuity of 20/40 or better.

Follow-up and management
- Long-term follow-up is needed to ensure proper visual rehabilitation and to check for postoperative complications, such as corneal edema, opacification of the posterior lens capsule ("after cataract"), glaucoma, intraocular inflammation, cystoid macular edema, and retinal detachment. Also, any other ocular injuries resulting from the trauma need to be appropriately managed.
- A delayed type of glaucoma can result from blunt injury, especially when the injury causes an anterior-chamber hemorrhage.

Treatment continued on p. 59

DIAGNOSIS—cont'd

Complications
Decreased vision.

Glaucoma, secondary open-angle: e.g., contusion deformity of the anterior-chamber angle (angle-recession glaucoma).

Glaucoma, secondary angle-closure: e.g., iris neovascularization (neovascular glaucoma); infrequently, a mature cataract can cause a secondary angle-closure glaucoma.

Ocular complications caused by the trauma: e.g., vitreous hemorrhage, retinal tears and detachment, choroidal rupture, perforation of the globe, intraocular foreign bodies.

• Rarely, a swollen, hypermature cataract can "leak" fluid, leading to a secondary open-angle glaucoma called *phacolytic glaucoma*.

Pearls and Considerations
Infrared energy, electric shock, and ionizing radiation are other, less common causes of traumatic cataract [1].

Referral Information
Surgical referral for cataract extraction as appropriate.

TREATMENT—cont'd

- With a subluxated or dislocated lens, vitreous usually is present in the anterior chamber. ECCE by nuclear expression or phacoemulsification may be extremely difficult. Sometimes the safest method is a pars plana lensectomy or an intracapsular cataract extraction with an anterior-chamber lens implant or a scleral, fixated, sewn-in posterior-chamber lens implant.
- When the eye cannot be salvaged by surgical or medical means, enucleation may be necessary. This needs to be carefully explained to the patient before surgery; however, the patient may not be alert enough to comprehend the impact of enucleation. In such cases, therefore, surgical and medical care should be performed. Postoperatively, when the patient is aware that no useful vision is present, enucleation can be discussed. In any event, if no useful vision is present and if ocular perforation with uveal prolapse occurred at the time of the injury, the eye should be enucleated within 5-10 days after the trauma to prevent sympathetic uveitis.

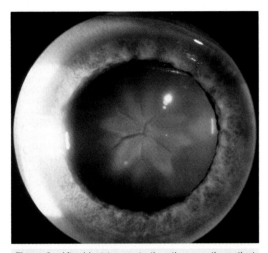

Figure 2 After blunt trauma to the other eye, the patient developed a typical petal-shaped cataract.

Key reference
1. Mulrooney BC, Allinson RW, et al: Traumatic cataract, 2006, www.emedicine.com.

General references
Charles NC, Rabin S: Calcific phacolysis: salvageable vision following treatment, *Arch Ophthalmol* 113(6):786-788, 1995.

Finkelstein M, Legmann A, Rubin PAD: Projectile metallic foreign bodies in the orbit: a retrospective study of epidemiologic factors, management, and outcomes, *Ophthalmology* 104(1):96-103, 1997.

Giovinazzo VJ, Yannuzzi LA, Sorenson JA, et al: The ocular complications of boxing, *Ophthalmology* 94(6):587-596, 1987.

Portellos M, Orlin SE, Kozart DM: Electric cataracts, *Arch Ophthalmol* 114(8):1022-1023, 1996.

Wong TY, Seet B, Ang CL: Eye injuries in twentieth century warfare: a historical perspective, *Surv Ophthalmol* 41(6):433-459, 1997.

Cavernous sinus syndrome   (Cavernositis 607.2)

DIAGNOSIS

Definition
Refers to a myriad of disease processes occurring within the cavernous sinus with resultant signs and symptoms of ophthalmoplegia, chemosis, proptosis, Horner's syndrome, or trigeminal sensory loss [1].

Synonyms
None.

Symptoms
Diplopia.
Ptosis.
Painful or painless.

Signs
Ptosis.
Ophthalmoparesis.
Third-, fourth-, and sixth-nerve palsies.
Oculosympathetic paresis (Horner's syndrome: postganglionic third-order neuron affected).
Proptosis: up to 4 mm.
Loss of sensation along V1, V2.

Investigations
Anisocoria: check in bright and dim illumination.
Cocaine ophthalmic solution (4%-10%) **or Paredrine** (hydroxyamphetamine; Pharmics, Salt Lake City, Utah) **pupil testing:** no dilation to both in Horner's syndrome.
Forced ductions.
Magnetic resonance imaging.
Lumbar puncture.
Indirect pharyngoscopy.
Biopsy of nasopharynx.
Laboratory studies (e.g., MMA-TP, RPR, ANA, ESR, CXR).

Pearls and Considerations
Varied and dependent on the etiology of the disease.

Referral Information
A full medical workup and imaging are required to determine the nature of the disease.

Differential diagnosis
Myasthenia gravis.
Giant cell arteritis.
Ischemic ocular syndrome.
Chronic progressive external ophthalmoplegia (bilateral).
Miller-Fisher variant of Guillain-Barré syndrome.
Botulism.

Cause
Trauma.
Intracavernous carotid artery aneurysm.
Carotid cavernous fistula or thrombosis.
Neoplasm.
Metastases.
Inflammation/infection (e.g., herpes zoster, mucormycosis, *Treponema pallidum, Mycobacterium tuberculosis*).
Sarcoidosis.
Wegener's granulomatous disease.
Tolosa-Hunt syndrome (THS): diagnosis of exclusion; inflammatory, painful idiopathic ophthalmoplegia.

Classification
- Retrocavernous sinus involvement is suggested by involvement of V1, V2, and V3.
- Inferior cavernous sinus involvement is indicated by parasympathetic paresis of the pupil and loss of sensation in V1.
- Involvement of the anterior cavernous sinus/superior orbital fissure is implied by proptosis and involvement of the optic nerve.

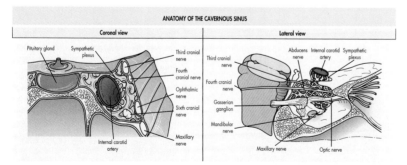

Figure 1   Cross section of cavernous sinus. It contains cranial nerves (CN) III, IV, VI, V1 (anteriorly), and V2 (posteriorly); internal carotid artery (ICA); and sympathetics. *(From Yanoff M, Duker J, editors: Ophthalmology, ed 2, St Louis, 2003, Elsevier.)*

TREATMENT

Diet and Lifestyle
- No special precautions are necessary.

Pharmacologic Treatment
- Treatment directed toward underlying cause.
- Tolosa-Hunt syndrome: oral prednisone, 1-1.5 mg/kg/day; possible initial IV steroids; exclude infection before initial steroid therapy.

Nonpharmacologic Treatment
- No nonpharmacologic treatment is recommended.

Treatment aims
Depends on cause.

Prognosis
Depends on cause.

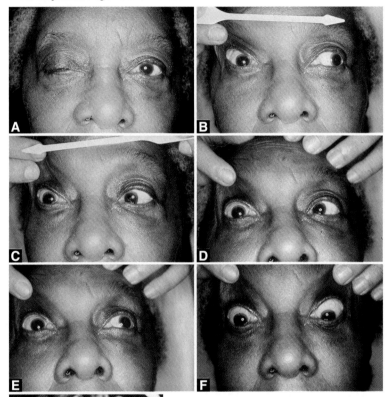

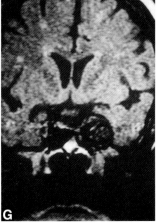

Figure 2   A, Woman age 55 yr has acute onset of right ophthalmoparesis. **B,** While lifting her eyelid, she is unable to adduct her right eye. **C** to **E,** She is also unable to abduct her right eye **(C)** and cannot elevate it up and in **(D)** or up and out **(E). F,** She is equally unable to depress her right eye, which is consistent with third-, fourth-, and sixth-nerve palsies. Furthermore, the right pupil is miotic and implicates the oculosympathetic fibers. **G,** This constellation of signs localized a lesion to the cavernous sinus. This coronal T1-weighted magnetic resonance image shows an aneurysm involving the right cavernous sinus.

Key reference
1. Kattah J, Pula J: Cavernous sinus syndromes, 2006, www.emedicine.com.

General references
Keane JR: Cavernous sinus syndrome: analysis of 151 cases, *Arch Neurol* 53(10):967-971, 1996.
Levin A: *Neuro-ophthalmology*, New York, 2005, Thieme Medical Publishers.
Zarei M, Anderson JR, Higgins JN, Manford MR: Cavernous sinus syndrome as the only manifestation of sarcoidosis, *J Postgrad Med* 48(2):119-121, 2002.

Chemical burns   (941.02)

DIAGNOSIS

Definition
Traumatic injury to the eye or adnexa resulting from contact with any chemical agent.

Synonyms
None.

Symptoms
Pain.
Photophobia.
Burning.
Foreign body sensation.
Decreased vision.
Epiphora.

Signs
Mild to Moderate Burns
Corneal epithelial defects: from superficial punctate keratitis to focal epithelia loss to sloughing of the entire epithelium (*see* figure).
Conjunctival hyperemia/injection.
- No signs of absent blood vessels, conjunctival chemosis, hyperemia, or hemorrhage.

Moderate to Severe Burns
Corneal edema and opacification.
Significant chemosis and perilimbal blanching.
High intraocular pressure.
Poor fluorescein stain despite complete epithelial loss.
Conjunctival ischemia/absent blood vessels.

Investigations
History: time of injury, type of chemical, duration of exposure, duration of irrigation.
Visual acuity test.
Slit-lamp examination and eyelid eversion: to look for foreign body.
Intraocular pressure.
Dilated fundus examination.

Complications
Corneal ulceration and infection.
Corneal opacity and vascularization.
Corneal melt and perforation.
Symblepharon formation.
Anterior-segment ischemia.
Cataract.
Local necrotic retinopathy.

Pearls and Considerations
Treatment with copious irrigation should be instituted immediately, even before testing vision or undertaking any other testing, and should be continued until a neutral pH is achieved [1].

Referral Information
Depends on severity of disease; referral for hospitalization, palliative care, or corneal graft surgery may be required depending on the severity of the burn.

Differential diagnosis
Traumatic corneal abrasion.
Dry eyes.
Episcleritis.
Scleritis.
Stevens-Johnson syndrome.
Ocular cicatricial pemphigoid.

Cause
Alkali (lye, cements, plasters), acids, solvents, detergents, mace.

Classification
Alkali burns: penetrate ocular surface easily.
Acid burns: coagulate surface tissue.

Pathology
- Acids denature and precipitate proteins in tissue. Tissue damage is mainly at the surface, and the coagulated surface forms a barrier against penetration of the agent.
- Alkylating agents raise the pH of tissue and cause saponification of fatty acids in cell membranes, subsequently disrupting them. The agent is then able to penetrate the ocular tissue rapidly, entering the anterior chamber, where it causes intense inflammation.

TREATMENT

Diet and Lifestyle
Protective eyewear around chemicals.

Pharmacologic Treatment
- Emergency treatment is mandatory. Copious irrigation of the eyes with saline or with nonsterile water if it is the only liquid available. This might take up to 4-6 L to neutralize the pH. Place a lid speculum and topical anesthesia in the eye before irrigation. Inspect the upper and lower fornices well, sweep with moistened cotton swab, and irrigate thoroughly. Use IV tubing connected to an irrigating solution to facilitate irrigation.

For Mild Burns
- After the eye is irrigated and the pH is neutral, instill cycloplegia.

Standard dosage   Homatropine 5%, 2 times daily.
- Place topical antibiotic ointment.

Standard dosage   Erythromycin, 4 times daily.
- Consider pressure patch for 24 hours.

For Moderate to Severe Burns
- Debride necrotic tissue, instill cycloplegia (*see* For mild burns), place topical antibiotic ointment up to 8 times daily (*see* For mild burns), and apply topical steroid.

Standard dosage   Prednisolone acetate 1%, 4-8 times daily for 1-2 wk, then rapid taper.
Special points   Consider pessure patch between drops.

- If the intraocular pressure is elevated, administer antiglaucoma medication. Destroy conjunctival adhesions using a glass rod with antibiotic ointment.
- If corneal melt occurs, may use collagenase inhibitors (e.g., Mucomyst every 4 hr), and if melting progresses, consider cyanoacrylate adhesive.
- Consider doxycycline (100 mg twice daily) for its collagenase inhibitor effect and vitamin C, 2 g daily (1 g twice daily or 500 mg 4 times daily), to promote collagen synthesis.
- Frequent lubrication with preservative-free tears, every 1-2 hr, essential in promoting reepithelialization.
- Consider topical citrate 10%, 4-8 times daily, for its anticollagenase effect and topical ascorbate 10%, 4-8 times daily, to promote collagen synthesis.

Nonpharmacologic Treatment
- Soft/bandage contact lenses, patching, tarsorrhaphy, and amniotic membrane transplantation may be required to promote reepithelialization.
- Corneal transplant may be performed either as an emergency procedure for corneal melt or perforation or later because of corneal scarring.
- Limbal stem cell transplant may be necessary to replace damaged limbal stem cells, alone or before corneal transplantation.

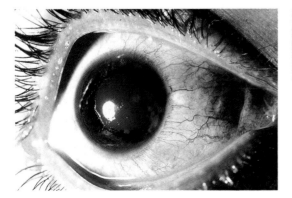

Corneal and conjunctival abrasion after chemical burn caused by car battery explosion (HNO_3). There is no limbal ischemia.

Prognosis
- Poor for severe burns, especially those caused by alkylating agents.

Follow-up and management
Mild burns
- Recheck daily, consider patching, until corneal abrasion heals.

Moderate to severe burns
- Daily follow-up with aggressive lubrication and antibiotic coverage; severely dry eyes may require a tarsorrhaphy; a conjunctival autograft may be performed if the injury is unilateral.

Key reference
1. Kunimoto DY, Kanitkar KD, Makar M: Chemical burns. In *The Wills eye manual*, ed 4, Philadelphia, 2004, Lippincott Williams & Wilkins, pp 14-16.

General references
Albert DM, Jakobiec FA, editors. *Principles and practice of ophthalmology*, vol 1, Philadelphia, 2000, Saunders.
American Academy of Ophthalmology: *Basic and clinical science*, section 8, San Francisco, 2006-2007, The Academy.
Wright K: *Textbook of ophthalmology*, Baltimore, 1997, Lippincott Williams & Wilkins.

DIAGNOSIS

Definition
Loss of vision and visual field from direct involvement of the optic chiasm, its blood supply, or the adjacent optic tract [1].

Synonyms
None.

Symptoms
Painless, asymmetric visual loss.

Hemifield slide phenomenon: in a complete bitemporal hemianopia, the intact nasal visual fields of each eye may overlap or separate; this can cause a sensory diplopia, or an object may seem to disappear from central vision.

Postfixation blindness: in a complete bitemporal hemianopia, when a patient converges to a point, the blind hemianopic visual fields align behind fixation; when the patient attempts to thread a needle, for example, the thread enters the eye of the needle but does not appear to exit on the other side.

Cerebrospinal fluid rhinorrhea (sphenoid sinus eroded by pituitary adenoma).

Headache.

Decreased libido, impotence.

Amenorrhea.

Galactorrhea, oligomenorrhea.

Infertility.

Asthenia.

Signs
Visual field loss that respects the vertical meridian.

Optic nerve dysfunction: may include visual acuity loss, relative afferent pupillary defect, dyschromatopsia, pallor of the neuroretinal rim of the optic disc, and dropout of the nerve fiber layer.

Acquired cupping (rare) **and neuroretinal rim pallor**.

Proptosis.

Investigations
Magnetic resonance imaging: sella optic chiasm, suprasellar cistern.

Endocrinologic evaluation: may include cortisol measurement for adrenal axis, thyroid tests, sex hormone measurement for gonadal axis, prolactin test, growth hormone assay, plasma and urine osmolality measurement for posterior pituitary, insulin tolerance test, and releasing hormone tests.

Complications
Pituitary adenoma can hemorrhage, become secondary, or undergo necrosis: this results in further visual loss as the optic nerve and chiasm are compressed. *Ophthalmoparesis* (usually third-nerve palsy) occurs as the enlarged tumor involves the cavernous sinus and subarachnoid space. There is a high mortality rate because of panhypopituitarism and subarachnoid hemorrhage. Immediate treatment is mandatory, with high-dose systemic corticosteroids and stabilization of electrolyte balance.

Pregnancy: *Sheehan's syndrome* refers to the postpartum infarction of a normal pituitary gland.

Differential diagnosis
Pseudo–visual field defect (e.g., from ptosis).
Bilateral cecocentral scotomas.
Enlarged blind spots.
Peripheral visual field contraction.
Retinitis pigmentosa.

Cause
Pituitary adenoma, 50%-55%.
Craniopharyngioma, 20%-25%.
Meningioma, 10%.
Gliomas, 7%.

Classification
- The *anterior chiasmal syndrome* refers to a central scotoma in one eye with superior temporal visual field loss respecting the vertical hemianopic meridian in the fellow eye.
- The *middle chiasmal syndrome* describes the bitemporal (often asymmetric) visual field defect.
- The *posterior chiasmal syndrome* is characterized by a central bitemporal hemianopia respecting the vertical hemianopic meridian, a bitemporal hemianopia respecting the vertical hemianopic line (more dense below than above), or an incongruous homonymous hemianopia resulting from the lesion affecting the junction of the optic tract at the optic chiasm.

Diagnosis continued on p. 66

TREATMENT

Diet and Lifestyle
- No special precautions are necessary.

Pharmacologic Treatment
- If the pituitary tumor is secreting prolactin, administration of bromocriptine is indicated.
- Replacement therapy: depending on hormonal involvement.

Treatment aims
To decompress the optic chiasm to regain vision or at least prevent further visual loss. To normalize pituitary function.

Prognosis
- Depends on the sellar lesion and the degree of involvement of the optic nerves and optic chiasm.

Follow-up and management
- Because of the recurrence of pituitary adenomas, craniopharyngiomas, and meningiomas, the patient must undergo at least yearly serial visual field testing and magnetic resonance imaging.

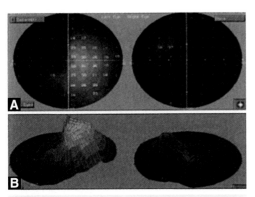

Figure 1 A, Visual field of 41-yr-old man who has progressively lost vision in his right eye. A temporal defect in his left eye respects the vertical hemianopic line. This is right anterior chiasmal syndrome. **B,** This three-dimensional visual representation demonstrates loss in the hill of vision in the same patient.

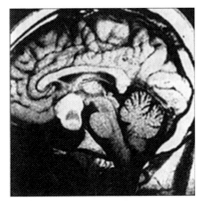

Figure 2 T1-weighted sagittal magnetic resonance image revealing pituitary adenoma with hemorrhage (pituitary apoplexy) compressing the chiasm from below.

Treatment continued on p. 67

DIAGNOSIS—cont'd

Pearls and Considerations
Varied and dependent on the etiology of the disease.

Referral information
Patients with chiasmal syndrome should be referred for imaging, blood work, and subspecialist consultation (e.g., endocrinologist, oncologist) depending on the etiology of the disease.

TREATMENT—cont'd

Nonpharmacologic Treatment

Transsphenoidal hypophysectomy.

Transfrontal craniotomy for large masses.

Radiation therapy: rarely used as a primary treatment.

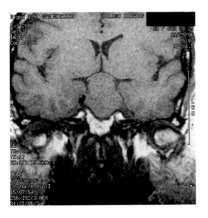

Figure 3   Pituitary adenoma with chiasmal compression. *(From Yanoff M, Duker J: Ophthalmology, ed 2, St Louis, 2003, Elsevier.)*

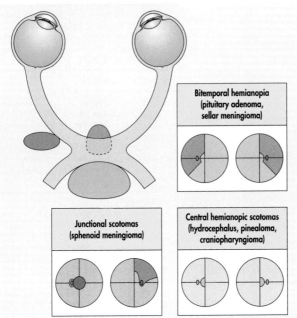

Bitemporal hemianopia (pituitary adenoma, sellar meningioma)

Junctional scotomas (sphenoid meningioma)

Central hemianopic scotomas (hydrocephalus, pinealoma, craniopharyngioma)

Figure 4   Localization and probable identification of masses by pattern of field loss. Junctional scotomas occur with compression of the anterior angle of the chiasm (sphenoid meningioma). Bitemporal hemianopia results from compression of the body of the chiasm from below (e.g., because of pituitary adenoma, sellar meningioma). Compression of the posterior chiasm and the decussating nasal fibers may cause central bitemporal hemianopic scotomas (e.g., because of hydrocephalus, pinealoma, craniopharyngioma). *(From Yanoff M, Duker J, editors: Ophthalmology, ed 2, St Louis, 2003, Elsevier.)*

Key reference

1. Ruben RM, Sadun AA, Pava A: Optic chiasm, parasellar region, and pituitary fossa. In Yanoff M, Duker JS, et al, editors: *Ophthalmology*, E-dition, St Louis, 2006, Elsevier.

General references

Foroozan R: Chiasmal syndromes, *Curr Opin Ophthalmol* 14(6):325-331, 2003.

Hedges TR: Optic chiasm field defects. In Walsh TJ, editor: *Visual fields: examination and interpretation*, San Francisco, 1990, American Academy of Ophthalmology, pp 151-177.

Trevino R: Chiasmal syndrome, *J Am Optometr Assoc* 66(9):559-575, 1995.

Chorioretinitis   (363.0)

DIAGNOSIS

Definition
Inflammation of the retina and choroid secondary to underlying infection or chronic granulomatous disease.

Synonyms
None; associated abbreviation: POHS (presumed ocular histoplasmosis syndrome).

Symptoms
Presumed Ocular Histoplasmosis

- Patients are usually asymptomatic; secondary **choroidal neovascularization** (CNV) may cause distortion, decreased vision, and scotomas.

Toxoplasmosis
Floaters, decreased vision, distortion of central vision.

Signs
Presumed Ocular Histoplasmosis

- Classic triad of clinical findings (*see* Fig. 1).
Peripapillary pigment alteration.
Multiple punched-out atrophic lesions in the peripheral fundus.
CNV in the macula.

Toxoplasmosis
Anterior-chamber inflammation: may be seen.
Vitreous cells.
Active retinitis: with an adjacent chorioretinal scar with overlying vitreous cells ("headlight in the fog") (*see* Fig. 2).
Subretinal hemorrhage, subretinal scar formation: from secondary CNV.
Macular or peripheral chorioretinal scar: implies a previous infection.

- Congenital cases may have associated microphthalmia, vitritis, glaucoma, and ocular palsies.
- Immunocompromised patients have a more severe retinochoroiditis that tends to be bilateral and multifocal.

Investigations
Presumed Ocular Histoplasmosis

Careful history: most patients with this disease have lived in the central and eastern river-valley regions of the United States.
Slit-lamp and dilated eye examination.
Fluorescein angiography: to determine the presence of active CNV.
Histoplasmin skin test: not helpful in making the diagnosis.

Toxoplasmosis

Careful history: previous exposure to cat feces, poorly cooked meats, raw eggs.
Careful slit-lamp and dilated fundus examination: necessary because the diagnosis is often clinical.
Immunoglobulin M and G titer: rising in acute infections; low or absent in chronic infections.

Differential diagnosis
Presumed ocular histoplasmosis
Idiopathic CNV.
Multifocal choroiditis.
Toxoplasmosis.
Sarcoidosis and multifocal choroiditis.

Cause
Presumed ocular histoplasmosis

- *Histoplasma capsulatum* is a dimorphic soil mold. Infection results from inhalation of spores and is usually asymptomatic.
- In immunocompromised individuals, disseminated disease (characterized by hepatosplenomegaly, lymphadenopathy, and pancytopenia) can occur.

Toxoplasmosis

- *Toxoplasma gondii* is an obligate intracellular parasite of humans and animals. The tachyzoite form invades tissue during an acute infection, which usually follows ingestion of contaminated meat or cat feces. Tachyzoites spread hematogenously; they can cross the placental barrier, causing acute infection in the fetus.

Epidemiology
Toxoplasmosis

- Congenital chorioretinitis infection has a propensity for the macular region and is bilateral in 85% of cases.
- 4% of seropositive individuals will show evidence of chorioretinal lesions on fundus examination [1].

Associated features
Toxoplasmosis

- Systemic features in acute infection include fever, headache, lymphadenopathy, fatigue, malaise, myalgias, urticaria, and erythematous macular rashes. Mild secondary leukopenia and pancytopenia are common. Patients with severe disease have pneumonitis, splenomegaly, encephalitis, and myocarditis.

Pathology
Presumed ocular histoplasmosis
Peripheral lesions: clinically they are 0.2-0.6 disc diameter in size, discrete, and often have pigmented borders; histologically, areas show varying degrees of inflammation with aggregates of lymphocytes in the choroid; eventually there is a loss of overlying retinal pigment epithelium and a degeneration of the rods and cones in this area [2].

Diagnosis continued on p. 70

TREATMENT

Diet and Lifestyle
Presumed Ocular Histoplasmosis

- No special precautions are necessary.

Toxoplasmosis

- Pregnant women need to avoid cat litter, undercooked meats, and foods made with raw eggs.

Pharmacologic Treatment
Presumed Ocular Histoplasmosis

- No pharmacologic treatment is recommended.

Toxoplasmosis

Standard dosage	Prednisone 40-80 mg/day depending on weight, with taper over 1-2 mo in addition to antibiotics.
	Sulfadiazine, 4-6 g divided in 4 daily doses for 4-6 wk.
Special points	If sulfadiazine is not available, clindamycin may be used (300 mg PO divided in 4 daily doses for 4-6 wk).

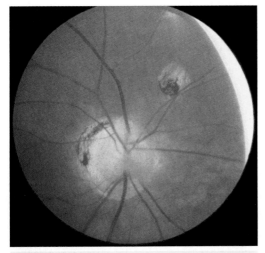

Figure 1   Presumed ocular histoplasmosis. Two components of the classic triad can be seen here: peripapillary atrophy and a peripheral punched-out lesion.

Treatment aims
Presumed ocular histoplasmosis
None.
Toxoplasmosis
To control reactivation.
To educate the patient on the possible secondary complications of glaucoma, cataract, macular edema, and CNV.

Prognosis
Presumed ocular histoplasmosis
Good, unless macular CNV occurs.
Toxoplasmosis

- Prognosis is good in adult patients when the lesion is peripheral.
- Macular reactivation can cause significant visual loss.
- Immunocompromised patients have a worse prognosis.
- Patients with congenital disease are often legally blind.

Follow-up and management
Presumed ocular histoplasmosis
Amsler grid to detect early signs of secondary CNV; otherwise, annual dilated eye examinations.
Toxoplasmosis

- Active lesions are followed closely until they subside.
- Chorioretinal scars can be followed on an annual basis.

Treatment continued on p. 71

DIAGNOSIS—cont'd

Complications
Presumed Ocular Histoplasmosis
Secondary CNV.

Toxoplasmosis

Permanent decreased vision: from macular scar formation from an active lesion or secondary CNV.

Cataracts, glaucoma, cystoid macular edema: caused by chronic active inflammation.

Pearls and Considerations

1. Lesions from histoplasmosis typically present as peripapillary atrophy, punched-out lesions of the periphery, and CNV of the macula (or resultant disciform scar after resolution of CNV).
2. Geographically, histoplasmosis is most common in the Ohio and Mississippi river valleys.
3. Systemic histoplasmosis and toxoplasmosis usually present as a mild to moderate respiratory infection.
4. Recurrence of toxoplasmosis infection is common because of the rupture of cysts, which form in any organ.
5. *Toxoplasma* infection can pass to infant (congenital toxoplasmosis) via transplacental transmission.

Referral Information

Refer to retinal specialist for oral medical therapy or laser photocoagulation.

TREATMENT—cont'd

Nonpharmacologic Treatment
Presumed Ocular Histoplasmosis

Laser photocoagulation to CNV, if extrafoveal location. For subfoveal CNV, consider photo-dynamic therapy or intravitreal avastin. [3].

Toxoplasmosis

- No nonpharmacologic treatment is recommended.

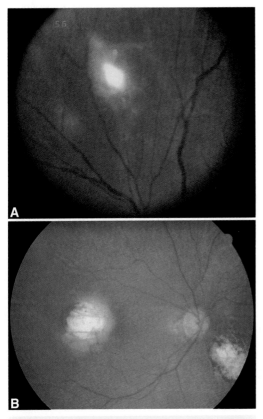

Figure 2 Toxoplasmosis. **A,** Active retinitis with an adjacent chorioretinal scar and overlying vitreous cells. **B,** Macular and peripheral chorioretinal scars in a patient with congenital toxoplasmosis.

Key references

1. Adams WH, Kindermann WR, Walls KW, et al: Toxoplasmic antibodies and retinochoroiditis in the Marshall Islands and their association with exposure to radioactive fallout, *Am J Trop Med Hyg* 36:315-320, 1987.
2. Makley TA, Craig EL, Werling K: Histopathology of ocular histoplasmosis, *Int Ophthalmol Clin* 23:1-18, 1983.
3. Saperstein DA, Rosenfeld PJ, Bressler NM, et al: Verteporfin therapy for CNV secondary to OHS, *Ophthalmology* 113:2371.e1-3, 2006.

General reference

Jabs DA, Nguyen QD: Ocular toxoplasmosis. In *Retina*, ed 4, E-dition, St Louis, 2006, Elsevier.

Chorioretinopathy, central serous (362.41)

DIAGNOSIS

Definition
A disease of the choroid and retina characterized by accumulation of clear fluid at the posterior pole of the fundus.

Synonyms
None; abbreviated CSC or CSR (central serous retinopathy)

Symptoms
Gradual decrease in vision.
Metamorphopsia.
Alteration in color vision.
Micropsia.

Signs
Shallow, round accumulation of subretinal fluid.
Subretinal precipitates.
Subretinal fibrin.
Changes in the retinal pigment epithelium (RPE): suggest a previous episode.
Extramacular RPE atrophic tracts.
Multiple bullous, serous, retinal, and RPE detachments.

Investigations
Fluorescein angiography: demonstrates pinpoint leakage that increases in size as the angiogram continues; late phases of the angiogram show pooling of dye into the subretinal space; a "smokestack" leakage pattern (*see* Fig. 2), although less common, is characteristic [1].

Complications
Permanently decreased vision: can occur with repeated bouts of CSC.
Secondary choroidal neovascularization.

Pearls and Considerations
1. Optical coherence tomography (OCT) can be useful in quantifying serous detachment and in tracking its resolution.
2. CSC has not been reported in patients under 20 yr of age.

Referral Information
Refer for photocoagulation if fluid does not resolve on its own.

Differential diagnosis
Pigment epithelial detachment.
Choroidal neovascularization.
Optic nerve pit with subretinal leakage.
Choroidal tumors.
Choroidal inflammation.
Choroidal ischemia.

Cause
- CSC is thought to result from focal leakage caused by alterations of the RPE that allow fluid from the choroidal layer to seep through to the subretinal space.
- There may be a correlation to stress.

Epidemiology
- More common in males age 25-50 yr.
- Spontaneously resolves over 6 mo.
- Can recur.
- Occurs bilaterally in 10% of cases.
- Has been seen in pregnant females.

Associated features
Migraine headaches.
Type A personality traits.
Hypochondria and hysteria [2].

Pathology
- Unknown, but believed to be multifactorial, in which one of the risk factors is stress; it is difficult to determine if CSC is a primary choroidal problem, a primary RPE problem, or combination of the two.

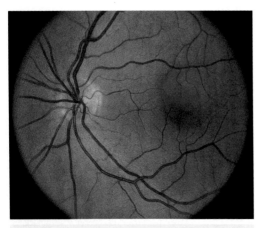

Figure 1   Serous elevation centered in the fovea.

TREATMENT

Diet and Lifestyle
- If related to stress, attempts to decrease stress may allow the disease to resolve more quickly.

Pharmacologic Treatment
- Oral steroids are contraindicated.

Nonpharmacologic Treatment
- If the fluid does not resolve over 4 mo or the patient's occupation requires clear binocular vision, laser photocoagulation to the leakage spot may be applied. Although laser photocoagulation does not improve the final visual outcome, it does allow the fluid to reabsorb more quickly.

Treatment aims
To resolve fluid.

Prognosis
- 80%-90% of patients resolve spontaneously.
Visual deterioration to less than 20/200 is uncommon.

Follow-up and management
- Patients should be followed periodically until the fluid resolves.
- Patients need to be educated on the risk of recurrence and involvement of the second eye.

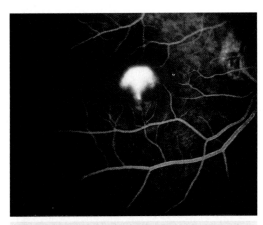

Figure 2 Classic "smokestack" fluorescein pattern in a patient with central serous chorioretinopathy.

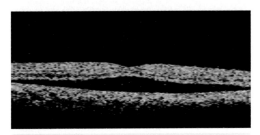

Figure 3 Optical coherence tomography demonstrates sub neuro sensory fluid with no intraretinal fluid. Foveal contour is preserved.

Key references
1. Folk J, Oh K: Chorioretinopathy, central serous, 2005, www.emedicine.com/oph/topic 689.htm.
2. Guyer DR, Gragoudas ES: Central serous chorioretinopathy. In Albert DM, Jakobiec FA: *Principles and practice of ophthalmology*, vol 2, Philadelphia, 1994, Saunders, pp 818-825.

General reference
Klais CM, Ober MD, Ciardella AP, Yanuzzi LA: Central serous chorioretinopathy. In *Retina*, ed 4, E-dition, St Louis, 2006, Elsevier.

Choroid dystrophies   (363.5)

DIAGNOSIS

Definition
Degeneration of the choriocapillaris caused by gene mutations affecting function of the retinal pigment epithelium (RPE), resulting in choroidal dystrophies (e.g., gyrate atrophy and choroideremia).

Symptoms
Gyrate Atrophy

Gradual decrease in vision to legal blindness: by age 40-55 yr.

Night blindness.

Choroideremia

Progressive visual loss, visual field constriction, and decreased night vision with advancing age: men >60 yr of age rarely retain central vision.

Signs
Gyrate Atrophy

Multiple sharply defined, scalloped areas of chorioretinal atrophy: separated from each other by thin margins of pigment; these lesions begin in the midperiphery, eventually coalescing to involve the entire fundus (*see* Fig. 1).

Choroideremia

Diffuse, progressive atrophy of the choriocapillaris and RPE: these changes start at the midperiphery and develop into scalloped edges that extend both anteriorly and posteriorly (*see* Fig. 2).

Retinal arteriolar attenuation.

Clumped pigment dispersed in the periphery.

Investigations
Gyrate Atrophy

Detailed family history: for decreased vision and blindness.

Slit-lamp and dilated fundus evaluation.

Visual field test: will show constriction.

Electroretinogram: will be abnormal or nonrecordable.

Abnormal dark adaptation.

Amino acid evaluation: decreased lysine levels; elevated plasma ornithine levels in all body fluids.

Choroideremia

Slit-lamp and dilated fundus examinations.

Dark adaptation thresholds: increase with age.

Visual field thresholds: demonstrate constriction over time.

Electroretinogram: will be greatly reduced.

Complications
Gyrate Atrophy

Legal blindness.

Choroideremia

Progressive, extensive visual loss.

Referral Information

Refer to eye care physician to rule out conditions that may mimic gyrate atrophy and choroideremia (e.g., retinitis pigmentosa).

Differential diagnosis
Gyrate atrophy
Choroideremia.
Paving-stone degeneration.
High myopia.
Thioridazine (Mellaril) retinopathy.
Choroideremia
Gyrate atrophy.
Retinitis pigmentosa.
Toxic retinopathy.
Albinism.

Cause
Gyrate atrophy
Autosomal recessive inheritance pattern.
Choroideremia
X-linked recessive trait found on the q21 band of the X chromosome.

Epidemiology
Choroideremia
- Asymptomatic carriers have normal visual acuity, dark adaptation, and visual fields. Fundus examination may show clumping of RPE and depigmentation of the pigment layer.

Associated features
Gyrate atrophy
- Seizures have been reported in some patients despite normal neurologic evaluation.
- Electron microscopy reveals morphologic changes in muscle fibers and hair shafts.

Pathology
Gyrate atrophy
- Swollen mitochondria in the retina lack ornithine ketoacid aminotransferase, the mitochondrial matrix that catalyzes the intraconversion of ornithine and α-ketoglutarate to pyrroline and glutamate; ornithine ketoacid aminotransferase is assigned to chromosome 10.
Choroideremia
- Irregular pigmentation with a well-defined zone of midperipheral depigmentation of the RPE; optic nerve and arterioles appear normal; atrophy of the outer segments of the photoreceptors; choriocapillaris atrophy; thickening of Bruch's membrane [1].

TREATMENT

Diet and Lifestyle
Gyrate Atrophy
- Reduce dietary protein consumption.
- Avoid arginine amino acid in food products.

Choroideremia
- No precautions are necessary.

Pharmacologic Treatment
Gyrate Atrophy

Standard dosage   Supplemental vitamin B_6 (pyridoxine), 20 mg/day PO to start; increase up to 500 mg/day.

Special points   A 30%-50% decrease in plasma ornithine levels will occur in 1 wk.

Choroideremia
- No pharmacologic treatment is recommended.

Nonpharmacologic Treatment
- No nonpharmacologic treatment is recommended.

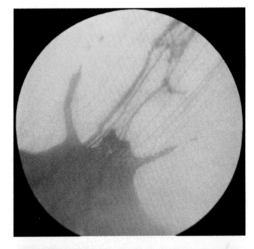

Figure 1 Gyrate atrophy. Note the scalloped, well-defined areas of chorioretinal atrophy in the midperipheral retina.

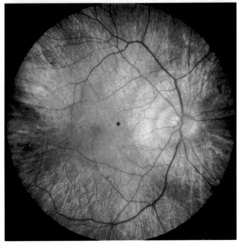

Figure 2 Choroideremia. This patient's eye has diffuse progressive atrophy of the choriocapillaris and retinal pigment epithelium, retinal arteriolar attenuation, prominent large choroidal vessels, and clumped pigment dispersed in the periphery.

Treatment aims
Choroideremia
- Unfortunately, there is no effective treatment. Low-vision aids may be of some benefit.

Gyrate atrophy
To lower plasma levels of ornithine through diet control (early detection is therefore of utmost importance), although the long-term benefit to visual preservation is unknown.

Other treatments
Darkly tinted sunglasses.
Genetic counseling.

Prognosis
Poor, because patients with either gyrate atrophy or choroideremia often lose vision to legal blindness.

Follow-up and management
Gyrate atrophy
- Ornithine levels need to be checked to determine the amount of vitamin B_6 needed to stabilize the ornithine levels.
- Serum ammonia levels are followed to monitor dietary arginine restriction.

Key reference
1. Flannery JG, Bird AC, Farber DB, et al: A histopathologic study of a choroideremia carrier, *Invest Ophthalmol Vis Sci* 31:229-236, 1990.

General reference
Berson EL: Retinitis pigmentosa and allied diseases. In Albert DM, Jakobiec FA, editors: *Principles and practice of ophthalmology*, vol 2, Philadelphia, 1994, Saunders, pp 1225-1226.

Choroidal detachment (after filtration surgery)   (363.70)

DIAGNOSIS

Definition
Displacement of the choroid from the sclera caused by accumulation of fluid in the virtual space between them.

Synonyms
None.

Symptoms
Decreased vision: visual acuity is typically decreased after filtration surgery for a few days to several weeks; however, choroidal detachment is associated with a loss of vision that becomes more profound than expected or a worsening of vision over time during the postoperative period; in the presence of a large choroidal detachment, patients may be aware of a black area in the field of vision corresponding to the location of the choroidal detachment.

Pain: pain associated with postoperative choroidal detachment is variable; many patients report no discomfort at all; some patients report mild to moderate pain with the onset of the choroidal detachment: if the detachment is hemorrhagic, pain may be quite severe.

Signs
Hypotony: choroidal detachments are generally associated with a very low intraocular pressure (IOP) postoperatively, usually caused by decreased ciliary body function due to the fluid collection in the suprachoroidal and supraciliary space; also, overfiltration may be associated with an abnormally large filtering bleb; a wound leak from the filtration site can be detected with the Seidel test; with a hemorrhagic choroidal detachment, the IOP may be elevated.

Shallowing of the anterior chamber: because of the fluid collection between the choroid and sclera and the associated anterior displacement of the ciliary body, and because of the hypotony, the anterior chamber will be abnormally shallow; there may be peripheral iris–cornea touch (grade 1), central iris–cornea touch (grade 2), or lens, implant, or vitreous–cornea touch (grade 3). Lens, implant, or vitreous–cornea touch will result in injury to the corneal endothelium, permanent corneal edema, and opacification if not corrected promptly.

Elevation of the choroid and retina: the choroid and overlying retina will be elevated; if the fundus can be seen, this will appear as a smooth, bullous, orange-brown elevation, usually arising from the inferior fundus; if the fundus cannot be seen, B-scan ultrasonography will usually reveal the detachment.

Investigations
Visual acuity testing: the visual acuity should be determined at each visit to monitor the effect of the choroidal detachment on vision.

Slit-lamp examination: the depth of the anterior chamber should be assessed and recorded at each visit using a recognized grading system; the size and appearance of the filtering bleb should be noted.

Seidel test: using a fluorescein strip to paint the bleb and conjunctival wound area, a Seidel test should be performed to look for aqueous leakage.

Intraocular pressure: the IOP should be measured at each postoperative visit.

Ultrasonography: B-scan ultrasonography is useful in the diagnosis of choroidal detachment (*see* figure) and the differentiation of choroidal from retinal detachment; B-scan ultrasonography can also be used to distinguish between hemorrhagic and serous choroidal detachments; ultrasonography will also help in monitoring the progress or resolution of the choroidal detachment as well as help plan the incision site for choroidal drainage surgery, if necessary.

Blood coagulation studies: in patients with hemorrhagic choroidal detachment, especially if there are recurrent episodes of hemorrhage, evaluation of clotting factors may reveal a cause for the hemorrhage.

Differential diagnosis
- The diagnosis of choroidal detachment following filtration surgery is usually fairly obvious. It is important to distinguish serous from hemorrhagic choroidal detachment. Differential diagnosis would include:
Retinal detachment.
Choroidal melanoma or metastatic tumor.

Etiology
- It is thought that the sudden decrease in IOP after filtration surgery causes the choroidal vessels to leak fluid into the suprachoroidal space. This sets up a vicious cycle because the resulting cilio-choroidal detachment prevents the ciliary body from producing aqueous. The resulting hypotony then tends to worsen the choroidal effusion, which in turn prolongs the hypotony.

Classification
- Choroidal detachments are classified as either *serous* (363.71) or *hemorrhagic* (363.72) depending on the nature of the fluid found in the suprachoroidal space.

Complications
Permanent loss of vision: choroidal detachment, especially if hemorrhagic, is often associated with injury to the photoreceptor cells of the retina and with varying degrees of permanent loss of vision.
Corneal edema and cataract: in severe cases of anterior-chamber shallowing, the corneal endothelium and lens epithelium may be damaged, leading to irreversible corneal edema and cataract formation.
Failure of filtration: if ciliary body shutdown caused by choroidal detachment is prolonged, the filtering bleb will flatten and become adherent to the sclera with scar formation, leading to failure of the filtration surgery.
Hypotonous maculopathy: prolonged hypotony may result in injury to the macula.

Diagnosis continued on p. 78

TREATMENT

Diet and Lifestyle
- No precautions are necessary.

Pharmacologic Treatment
Topical corticosteroids and atropine: these agents are useful in reducing inflammation and decreasing vascular permeability; the atropine also causes relaxation and posterior movement of the ciliary muscle, resulting in deepening of the anterior chamber.

Analgesics: systemic analgesics, including narcotics, may be necessary for severe pain.

Nonpharmacologic Treatment
Overfiltration: in cases of choroidal detachment associated with overfiltration, pressure patching, or the use of special contact lenses (e.g., the Simmons Compression Shell) may help reduce overfiltration, restore a normal IOP, and resolve the choroidal detachment; if this fails, surgery to resuture the sclerostomy may be necessary.

Treatment aims

To bring about a rapid resolution of the choroidal detachment while preserving the function of the retina, lens, cornea, and filtering bleb.

Prognosis

The prognosis is guarded. Serous choroidal detachments that are not associated with marked degrees of anterior-chamber shallowing will usually resolve without surgical treatment, but there is often some loss of central visual acuity. Hemorrhagic choroidal detachments are often associated with severe vision loss unless they are very small. Choroidal detachments that require surgery are often associated with loss of retinal function, corneal edema, cataract, and failure of filtration. Patients with choroidal detachment in the immediate postoperative period are at higher risk for developing late-onset choroidal detachment months or even years after glaucoma filtering surgery.

Follow-up and management

Patients should be followed frequently and carefully after filtration surgery. If the choroidal detachment resolves without complication, follow-up may be the same as for any postoperative glaucoma patient, but the patient must be monitored in case the choroidal detachment worsens or other complications develop that may require additional surgery.

Treatment continued on p. 79

DIAGNOSIS—cont'd

Pearls and Considerations

On B-scan ultrasonography, *choroidal* detachments appear as stable, fluid-filled, dome-shaped pockets and can be differentiated from *retinal* detachments, which are mobile and highly reflective.

Referral Information

If detachment persists beyond 7 days, consider referral for drainage of the suprachoroidal fluid.

TREATMENT—cont'd

Wound leak: in cases of choroidal detachment associated with a wound leak, a variety of treatments have been tried, including pressure patching, contact lenses, tissue glue, and injection of autologous blood into the bleb; if the wound leak persists, surgical repair is usually necessary.

Choroidal drainage and anterior chamber re-formation: in cases of persistent choroidal detachment or where the anterior-chamber shallowing has resulted in lens-cornea touch, surgical drainage of the suprachoroidal space and re-formation of the anterior chamber with a viscoelastic substance are usually required.

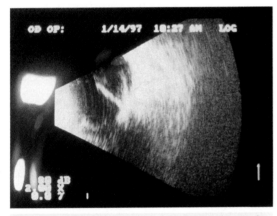

B-scan ultrasound demonstrating choroidal detachment after glaucoma filtering surgery.

General references

Bellows AR, Chylack LT, Hutchinson BT: Choroidal detachment: clinical manifestation, therapy and mechanism of formation, *Ophthalmology* 88:1107-1113, 1981.

Fourman S: Management of cornea-lens touch after filtering surgery for glaucoma, *Ophthalmology* 97:424-428, 1990.

Liebmann JM, Sokol J, Ritch R: Management of chronic hypotony after glaucoma filtration surgery, *J Glaucoma* 5:210-220, 1996.

Shields MB: Filtering surgery. In *Textbook of glaucoma*, ed 4, Baltimore, 1998, Williams & Wilkins, pp 518-527.

Traverso CE: Choroidal detachment, 2005, www.emedicine.com.

Choroidal rupture   (363.63)

DIAGNOSIS

Definition
Breaks in the choroid, Bruch's membrane, and retinal pigment epithelium (RPE) usually in the posterior pole; associated with blunt ocular trauma.

Synonyms
None.

Symptoms
Decreased vision after trauma.
Acute decreased vision: may be permanent if fovea is involved.
Central scotoma.

Signs
Yellow-white curvilinear streak(s): located around the optic nerve or in the papillomacular bundle.
Subretinal hemorrhage: may obscure the rupture initially.
Commotio retinae: white appearance to the retina.
Decreased intraocular pressure: if the rupture is large.
Subretinal fibrosis.
Subretinal neovascularization [1].

Investigations
Detailed history: for previous eye trauma.
Slit-lamp and dilated fundus evaluation.
Fluorescence angiography: will show early hypofluorescence because of damage to the choriocapillaries; late hyperfluorescent staining seen in the area of the break.

Complications
- Patients may experience permanent visual loss from the rupture itself if it involves the fovea or if the following complications occur:

Subretinal fibrosis.
Subretinal neovascularization.
Choroidal anastomosis [2].

Pearls and Considerations
1. Initially, the choroidal rupture may be obscured by overlying hemorrhage.
2. Deep choroidal vessels are usually spared.
3. Neovascularization is an expected part of the healing process and will usually resolve spontaneously.

Referral Information
Refer for laser photocoagulation if central vision is threatened.

Differential diagnosis
Angioid streaks: often emanate from the disc.
Lacquer cracks: associated with high myopia; appear as small, linear streaks in the macula.

Cause
Trauma.

Associated features
- The clinician should look for other signs of ocular trauma, such as:

Sclopetaria: pigment disruption in the peripheral retina from trauma.
Retinal detachment or retinal dialysis.
Cataract.
Iris sphincter tears.
Pigment on the surface of the lens.

Pathology
Splitting of Bruch's membrane and the choriocapillaris or entire choroid.
- The overlying RPE and neurosensory retina may be normal, atrophic, or ruptured (rarely).

TREATMENT

Diet and Lifestyle
Safety glasses during future sports activities.

Pharmacologic Treatment
- No pharmacologic treatment is recommended.

Nonpharmacologic Treatment
Laser photocoagulation to secondary choroidal neovascularization: may be necessary if it threatens the fovea.

Treatment aims
To stabilize vision.

Prognosis
Good, if fovea is not involved.
- Most secondary subretinal neovascular membranes resolve spontaneously and do not require treatment.

Follow-up and management
- Amsler grid testing daily to detect early distortion or visual loss from subretinal neovascularization.
- Fundus examination every 3-6 mo until findings are stable.

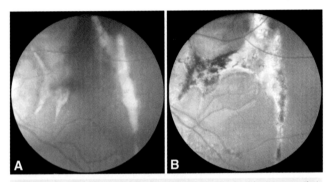

Figure 1 Choroidal rupture. **A,** The patient sustained a blunt trauma that resulted in choroidal ruptures in the posterior pole and in subneural retinal hemorrhages. Th optic nerve head is on the left in this eye. **B,** One year later, considerable scarring has taken place. These patients must be watched closely for the occurrence of subneural retinal neovascularization that may occur at the edge of the healed rupture.

Key references
1. Gass JDM: Specific choroidal diseases causing disciform macular detachment. In *Stereoscopic atlas of macular diseases*, ed 3, St Louis, 1987, Mosby, p 170.
2. Federman JL, Gouras P, Schubert RT, et al: Trauma. In Podos SM, Yanoff M, editors: *Textbook of ophthalmology*, London, 1994, Mosby, pp 15.2-15.6.

General references
Dugel PU, Win PH, Ober RR: Posterior segment manifestations of closed-globe contusion injury. In *Retina*, ed 4, E-dition, St Louis, 2006, Elsevier.
Wu L: Choroidal rupture, 2005, www.emedicine.com.

Commotio retinae (Berlin's edema)   (921.3)

DIAGNOSIS

Definition
A complication of blunt ocular trauma characterized by a milky opacification of the macular retina.

Synonyms
None.

Symptoms
Acute visual loss after trauma.

Signs
White discoloration to the outer retina: located in the posterior pole or peripheral retina (*see* figure).
Signs of trauma: hemorrhage, retinal detachment, sclopetaria.

Investigations
Careful history: to determine if the preceding trauma was blunt or from a penetrating injury; visual acuity.
Pupil examination: to look for an afferent pupillary defect indicating optic nerve or widespread retinal injury.
Slit-lamp and dilated retinal examination.
Fluorescence angiography: may show abnormal vascular permeability or blockage of choroidal fluorescence.

Complications
Loss of vision.

Pearls and Considerations
1. If only the outer segments of the photoreceptors are damaged, they will regenerate, and retinal and visual function will recover.
2. Optical coherence tomography (OCT) evaluation will demonstrate increased reflectivity at the level of the photoreceptors.

Referral Information
None; patients should be observed for resolution.

Differential diagnosis
Myelinated nerve fibers.
Central retinal artery occlusion.

Cause
Trauma to the eye.

Associated features
Other ocular findings seen with trauma (e.g., vitreous hemorrhage, retinal detachment, choroidal rupture).

Pathology
Disruption of the outer segments of the retina.
No evidence of actual retinal edema.

TREATMENT

Diet and Lifestyle
Safety glasses during sports-related activities.

Pharmacologic Treatment
• No pharmacologic treatment is recommended.

Nonpharmacologic Treatment
Observation.

Treatment aims
To observe patient.

Prognosis
• Depends on whether the macula is involved; there may be permanent damage to the retina and late pigmentary changes that lead to loss of vision.

Follow-up and management
• Depends on the extent of ocular damage from the trauma; once stable, a yearly dilated eye examination is indicated.

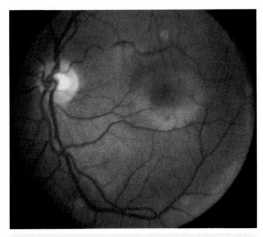

Patient who sustained blunt trauma to the left eye exhibits retinal whitening of the macula on fundus examination.

General references
Balles M: Traumatic retinopathy. In Albert DM, Jakobiec FA, editors: *Principles and practice of ophthalmology*, vol 2, Philadelphia, 1994, Saunders, pp 1027-1028.
Dugel PU, Win PH, Ober RR: Posterior segment manifestations of closed-globe contusion injury. In *Retina*, ed 4, E-dition, St Louis, 2006, Elsevier.
Sony P, Venkatesh P, Gadaginomath S, Garg SP: Optical coherence tomography findings in commotio retinae, *Clin Exp Ophthalmol* 34: 621-623, 2006.

Conjunctival degenerations: pinguecula (372.51) and pterygium (372.40)

DIAGNOSIS

Definition
Pinguecula: area of thickening of the bulbar conjunctiva adjacent to the limbus and within the palpebral fissure.
Pterygium: a growth of fibrovascular tissue onto the cornea from the conjunctiva.

Synonyms
None.

Symptoms
- Patients are usually asymptomatic.

Cosmetic concerns: common.
Photophobia, tearing, foreign body sensation: less common.
Decreased vision: if pterygium is close to visual axis or causing astigmatic changes (usually irregular astigmatism).

Signs
- Pingueculae are usually seen on the conjunctiva adjacent to nasal limbus: they have the appearance of yellow-white, amorphous, subepithelial deposits (*see* Fig. 1).
- Pterygium is a triangular-shaped fold of conjunctival and fibrovascular tissue that has advanced to the corneal surface (*see* Fig. 2).

Investigations
History.
Visual acuity testing: may be decreased from centralization of the pterygium, or irregular astigmatism.
Refraction: may have astigmatism from pterygium.
Intraocular pressure: usually normal.
Slit-lamp examination: may note an iron line (Stocker's line) in front of the pterygium, which usually indicates growth stabilization.
Dilated fundus examination: usually normal.

Complications
Dellen formation adjacent to pingueculae.
Corneal scarring: with pterygium.
Recurrence of pterygium: after excision.
Inflammation of the pinguecula: pingueculitis.

Pearls and Considerations
1. Pingueculae should be observed and noted at each exam as they may have the potential for progressing to pterygia.
2. Protective eyewear against ultraviolet (UV) radiation should be recommended to patients with either pinguecula or pterygia, possibly to impede further growth.

Referral Information
Refer for surgical excision as appropriate.

Differential diagnosis
Conjunctival intraepithelial neoplasia: unilateral jelly-like or white mass, often elevated, vascularized; not in a wing shape.
Dermoid.
Pannus.

Cause
Related to sun exposure, dust, and wind (chronic irritation).

Epidemiology
- Common in the 30-50 age group and in tropical climate.

Pathology
- The subepithelial tissue shows senile elastosis and dense subepithelial concretions not sensitive to elastase.

TREATMENT

Diet and Lifestyle
- Protect the eye from sun, dust, and wind (e.g., wear sunglasses or goggles).

Pharmacologic Treatment
Artificial tears or mild topical vasoconstrictor.
Mild topical steroid (if severe).

Nonpharmacologic Treatment
- Surgical removal may be considered if (1) the lesion interferes with contact lens wear, (2) patient experiences extreme irritation not relieved by the above treatments, (3) pterygium involves the visual axis or progresses, or (4) patient has cosmetic concerns.
- Surgery should not be performed casually because recurrent pterygia are often worse than primary ones. An estimated 40% recur; however, with conjunctival transplantation, the rate drops to 5%. Ipsilateral bulbar conjunction (usually from the superior region) is excised and grafted over the excised pterygium bed. Antiobiotic/steroid combination ointment is placed on the eye, and the eye is then patched until the next day. The patient is followed until epithelium heals over the cornea.
- Consider maintaining patients with large or recurrent pterygium on topical steroids for 3-6 mo to prevent recurrence. Any patient receiving topical steroids should be monitored regularly.

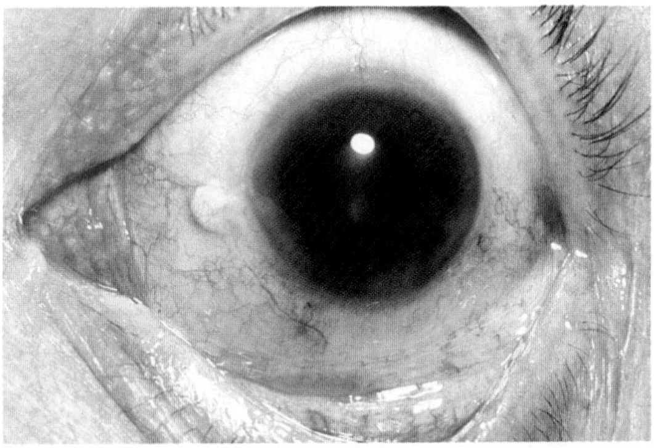

Treatment aims
To relieve symptoms and prevent worsening of visual acuity.

Other treatments
- Apply mitomycin-C (0.2 mg/cm^3) to bare sclera after excision (only in severe pterygium).
- Complications include scleral necrosis, cataract, persistent epithelial defects, and visual loss.

Prognosis
- Aggressive recurrence may occur after excision (minimized by conjunctival autograft).

Follow-up and management
- Asymptomatic patients may be checked every 1-2 yr.
- If treating with topical vasoconstrictor or topical steroid, check every 1-2 wk to monitor inflammation and intraocular pressure. Taper steroid dose over several days once the inflammation has abated.

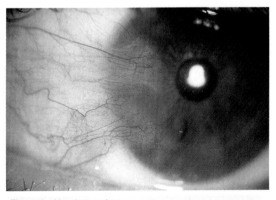

Figure 1   Nasal pinguecula.

Figure 2   Nasal pterygium.

General references
American Academy of Ophthalmology: *Basic and clinical science*, section 8, San Francisco, 2006-2007, The Academy.
Farjo QA, Sugar A: Conjunctival and corneal degenerations. In Yanoff M, Duker JS, editors: *Ophthalmology*, E-dition, St Louis, 2006, Elsevier.
Smolin G, Thoft RA: The cornea. In *Scientific foundation and clinical practice*, Boston, 2004, Little, Brown.
Wright K: *Textbook of ophthalmology*, Baltimore, 1997, Williams & Wilkins.

DIAGNOSIS

Definition
Inflammation of the conjunctiva of less than 4 wks' duration secondary to infection, allergen, toxin, or chemical insult.

Synonyms
"Pinkeye."

Symptoms
Discharge.
Eyelid sticking.
Red eye.
Foreign body sensation: of less than 4 wks' duration.

Signs
Severe purulent discharge, marked chemosis, conjunctival papillae, preauricular adenopathy: in gonococcal conjunctivitis.
Purulent discharge of moderate degree, conjunctival papillae: other bacterial conjunctivitis (*see* figure).
Mucus discharge, conjunctival follicles, preauricular adenopathy, subconjunctival hemorrhage, conjunctival pseudomembranes, subepithelial infiltrates (may be late sign): in viral conjunctivitis.
Thick ropy discharge, large conjunctival papillae under the upper lid or along the limbus, superior corneal-shield ulcer, limbal or palpebral raised white dots (Horner-Trantas dots): vernal/atopic conjunctivitis.
Chemosis, conjunctival papillae, scant mucus discharge, mild edema and erythema of eyelids: allergic conjunctivitis.

Investigations
History: Severe purulent discharge within 12 hr (gonococcal), recent upper respiratory tract infection or contact with someone who has red eye (adenoviral), seasonal recurrences (vernal), history of allergies (atopic or allergic).
Visual acuity test.
Slit-lamp examination.
Conjunctival swab for culture and sensitivities: e.g., blood agar, chocolate agar, Thayer-Martin plate, stat Gram stain if severe.

Complications
Corneal ulcer, scarring, perforation: gonococcal conjunctivitis.
Phlyctenules and marginal infiltrates.
Recurrence: herpes simplex infection.

Differential diagnosis
Episcleritis.
Scleritis.
Uveitis.
Acute angle-closure glaucoma.
Corneal ulcer.
Dural-cavernous fistulae.
Kawasaki syndrome.

Cause and classification
Infectious
Bacterial: *Staphylococcus aureus, Streptococcus pneumoniae, Haemophilus influenzae, Neisseria gonorrhoeae.*
Viral: adenovirus, herpes simplex.
Noninfectious
Allergic.
Vernal/atopic.

Diagnosis continued on p. 88

TREATMENT

Diet and Lifestyle
- In *adenoviral* conjunctivitis, wash hands frequently and avoid hand contacts.
- In *allergic* conjunctivitis, avoid allergen or eliminate the inciting agent.

Pharmacologic Treatment
For Adenoviral Conjunctivitis
- Administer artificial tears 4-8 times daily; apply cool compresses several times daily. Vasoconstrictor/antihistamines help itching.

Standard dosage   Fluorometholone or prednisolone acetate 0.125%, 4 times daily.

Special points   Used for pseudomembranes or corneal subepithelial infiltrate or if vision is reduced. Taper steroid slowly once resolved. Gently peel off membrane if present.

For Herpes Simplex Conjunctivitis
- Apply cool compresses several times daily.

Standard dosage   Trifluorothymidine (trifluridine) 1% (Viroptic) drops, 5 times daily.

For Bacterial Conjunctivitis (General)
Standard dosage   Ciprofloxacin drops or erythromycin ointment, 4 times daily for 7 days.

For *Haemophilus influenzae* Conjunctivitis
Standard dosage   Amoxicillin/clavulanate, 20-40 mg/kg/day PO in 3 divided doses.

Special points   Oral dose because of nonocular involvement (e.g., otitis media, pneumonia, meningitis).

For Gonococcal Conjunctivitis
- Treatment is initiated if the Gram stain shows gram-negative intracellular diplococci or if there is a high suspicion of gonococcal conjunctivitis clinically.

Standard dosage   Ceftriaxone, 1 g IM in single dose, *or* Ceftriaxone 1 g IV every 12-24 hr if severe with lid swelling and corneal involvement; patient should be hospitalized; duration based on clinical response.
Topical bacitracin or erythromycin ointment 4 times daily, *or* Ciprofloxacin drops every 2 hr.
Tetracycline or erythromycin, 250-500 mg PO 4 times daily for 2-3 wk.

Special points   Irrigate the eye with saline 4 times daily until the discharge is eliminated.

For Vernal/Atopic or Allergic Conjunctivitis
Mild infection
- Administer artificial tears.

Moderate infection
Standard dosage   Levocabastine (Livostin) or olopatadine HCl 0.1% (antihistamines), 4 times daily.
Ketorolac, 4 times daily.

Severe infection
Standard dosage   Fluorometholone, 4 times daily for 1-2 wk.

Special points   Add topical cromolyn sodium 4% or lodoxamide (Alomide) for vernal/atopic disease. If shield ulcer is present, add topical steroid and topical antibiotic (e.g., erythromycin ointment or Polytrim drops 4 times daily).

For Allergic Conjunctivitis
- Eliminate inciting factor if possible.
- Apply cool compresses 5 times daily.

Treatment continued on p. 89

Treatment aims
To relieve symptoms of adenoviral and atopic/vernal conjunctivitis.
To prevent corneal involvement in herpes simplex, gonococcal conjunctivitis.
To minimize symblepharon formation.

Prognosis
- Acute conjunctivitis has a duration of ≤4 wk and usually is self-limited except in gonococcal conjunctivitis.
- Recurrence of vernal/atopic conjunctivitis is common.

Follow-up and management
Adenovirus: every 1-3 wk.
Herpes simplex: every 2-3 days initially to monitor corneal involvement, then every 1-2 wk.
Bacterial: every 1-2 days initially, then every 2-5 days until resolved (gonococcal conjunctivitis needs to be followed daily until improvement noted, then every 2-3 days).
Vernal/atopic: every 1-3 days in the presence of a shield ulcer, otherwise every few weeks. Cromolyn sodium is maintained for the duration of the season.
Allergic: 1-3 wk to determine response to treatment. Continue to follow frequently if using topical steroids, until tapered.

DIAGNOSIS—cont'd

Pearls and Considerations

1. If herpetic infection is suspected, steroid treatment is contraindicated due to the potential for worsening the disease.
2. *Epidemic keratoconjunctivitis* (EKC) is highly contagious and easily spread to other patients through improperly disinfected slit lamps, tonometers, and other instruments. Careful disinfection of all instrumentation is critical in avoiding nosocomial infection of other patients.
3. Gonococcal conjunctivitis is an emergency, given possible rapid progression and risk of corneal perforation, that requires systemic treatment.

Referral Information

None.

TREATMENT—cont'd

Mild cases
- Administer artificial tears 4 times daily.

Moderate

Standard dosage   Olopatadine 0.1%,
Lodoxamide 0.1%,
Nedocromil 2%, *or*
Ketotifen 0.025%, twice daily.

Severe

Standard dosage   Multitopical steroid (loteprednol or fluorometholone) 4 times daily with taper.

Special points   Consider oral antihistamine if concomitant hay fever or systemic allergy symptoms for moderate or severe cases.

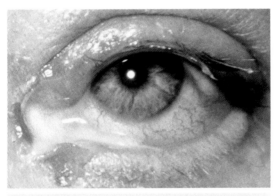

Conjunctival injection and purulent discharge in patient with bacterial conjunctivitis.

General references

Albert DM, Jakobiec FA, editors: *Principles and practice of ophthalmology*, vol 1, Philadelphia, 2000, Saunders.

American Academy of Ophthalmology: *Basic and clinical science*, section 8, San Francisco, 2006-2007, The Academy.

Stefkovicovaa M, Vicianova V, Sokolik J, Madar R: Causes and control measures in hospital outbreaks of epidemic keratoconjunctivitis, *Indoor Built Environ* 15:111-114, 2006.

Wright K: *Textbook of ophthalmology*, Baltimore, 1997, Williams & Wilkins.

Conjunctivitis, chronic   (372.1)

DIAGNOSIS

Definition
Inflammation of the conjunctiva of greater than 4 wks' duration secondary to toxin or infection.

Synonyms
"Pinkeye."

Symptoms
Discharge or eyelid sticking.

Red eye and ocular irritation: of longer than 4 wks' duration.

Signs
Chlamydial inclusion conjunctivitis: inferior tarsal conjunctival follicles, superior corneal pannus, palpable preauricular node (PAN), gray-white subepithelial infiltrates (SEI), and stringy mucus discharge.

Trachoma stage 1: superior tarsal follicles, mild superficial punctate keratitis, and pannus (often preceded by purulent discharge and tender PAN).

Trachoma stage 2: significant superior tarsal follicular reaction and papillary hypertrophy associated with pannus, SEI, and limbal follicles.

Trachoma stage 3: follicles and scarring of superior tarsal conjunctiva.

Trachoma stage 4: extensive conjunctival scarring.

Molluscum contagiosum: dome-shaped, umbilicated (usually multiple) nodules on the eyelid or eyelid margin; follicular conjunctival response from toxic viral products (*see* figure).

Toxic conjunctivitis: inferior papillary reaction, especially with aminoglycosides, antivirals, and preservatives; follicular response may be seen with atropine, miotics, epinephrine agents, topical glaucoma agents, and antiviral medications.

Investigations
History of exposure to sexually transmitted diseases (STDs): vaginitis, cervicitis, or urethritis may be present in chlamydial inclusion conjunctivitis.

History of exposure to areas with high incidence of trachoma: North Africa, Middle East, India, Southeast Asia.

History of eyedrop use: especially for glaucoma.

Visual acuity test.

Slit-lamp examination.

Dilated fundus examination.

Conjunctival scraping for Giemsa stain (basophilic and intracytoplasmic inclusion bodies in epithelial cell): chlamydial inclusion conjunctivitis and trachoma.

Complications
Corneal scarring and pannus: mild to severe.

Late complications of trachoma: severely dry eyes, trichiasis, entropion, keratitis, corneal scarring, superficial fibrovascular pannus, Herbert's pits (scarred limbal follicles), corneal bacterial superinfection, and ulceration.

Pearls and Considerations
Chronic follicular conjunctivitis may represent *Parinaud's oculoglandular syndrome*, an ocular manifestation of cat-scratch disease (CSD). A full dilated examination should be performed to rule out additional, more serious complications of CSD, including neuroretinitis (optic nerve swelling and macular star) and focal chorioretinitis.

Referral Information
Dependent on etiology and extent of ocular involvement.

Differential diagnosis
Herpes simplex conjunctivitis.

Cause
As described in Signs section; also allergic reactions (atropine, miotics, epinephrine, antivirals) and Reiter's syndrome.

Epidemiology
- Trachoma is endemic in North Africa, Middle East, India, Southeast Asia, and rarely the United States.

TREATMENT

Diet and Lifestyle

- Promote sanitary living conditions in trachoma-endemic areas.
- Patients with chlamydial inclusion conjunctivitis and their sexual partners should be evaluated by their medical physicians for other STDs.

Pharmacologic Treatment

For Chlamydial Inclusion Conjunctivitis

Standard dosage	Tetracycline, 250-500 mg PO 4 times daily; *or*
	Doxycycline, 100 mg PO 4 times daily; *or*
	Erythromycin, 250-500 mg PO 4 times daily; for 3 wk.
	Erythromycin ointment, 2-3 times daily for 2-3 wk.
	Azithromycin, 1 g for 1 dose.
Special points	These drugs should be given to patients and their sexual partners.

For Trachoma

- Treatment is same as for chlamydial inclusion conjunctivitis but for 3-4 wks' duration.

For Toxic Conjunctivitis

- Discontinue the offending agent, if possible.
- Artificial tears without preservatives should be administered 4-8 times daily.

Nonpharmacologic Treatment

For Molluscum Contagiosum

- Remove lesions by simple excision and curettage or by cryosurgery.

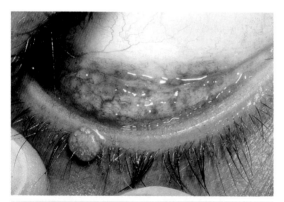

Eyelid nodule with follicular conjunctivitis in patient with molluscum contagiosum.

Treatment aims
- Treatment is usually curative.

Prognosis
- Trachoma must be treated in early stages to prevent significant corneal scarring.

Follow-up and management
- Every 1-3 wk, depending on the severity.

General references

Albert DM, Jakobiec FA, editors: *Principles and practice of ophthalmology,* vol 1, Philadelphia, 2000, Saunders.

American Academy of Ophthalmology: *Basic and clinical science,* section 8, San Francisco, 2006-2007, The Academy.

Cunningham ET, Keohler JE: Ocular bartonellosis, *Am J Ophthalmol* 130:340-349, 2000.

Wright K: *Textbook of ophthalmology,* Baltimore, 1997, Lippincott Williams & Wilkins.

Corneal abrasions (918.1) and foreign body (930.0)

DIAGNOSIS

Definition
A scratch of the corneal surface with or without an associated foreign body.

Synonyms
None.

Symptoms
Pain.
Photophobia.
Foreign body sensation.
Tearing.
Blurred vision.

Signs
Epithelial staining defect with fluorescein: conjunctival injection, swollen eyelid, mild anterior-chamber reaction (*see* figure).
Corneal foreign body, rust ring, or both.
Conjunctival injection.

Investigations
History: usually a history of scratching the eye, or foreign body arises from metal striking metal.
Visual acuity test.
Slit-lamp examination: with the use of fluorescein and eversion of the eyelids for foreign body; if there is a corneal whitening, rule out infection; there may be mild anterior-chamber reaction present, but if severe, rule out endophthalmitis.
Dilated fundus examination: rule out intraocular foreign body, especially with a history of striking metal against metal.

Complications
Infectious corneal infiltrate: with or without significant anterior-chamber reaction.
Decreased vision: secondary to central corneal scar.
Recurrent corneal erosions: occurs more often with a history of paper cut or fingernail abrasion.

Pearls and Considerations
The Seidel test can be used to rule out penetration and open-globe injury. Apply sodium fluorescein to the suspected site of penetration, and observe under a slit lamp for sign of streaming (diluted fluorescein running from the wound site). A positive Seidel sign indicates penetrating injury and open globe.

Referral Information
Refer for surgical evaluation if penetrating injury is suspected.

Differential diagnosis
Corneal laceration.
Corneal ulcer.
Corneal melt.

Etiology
Scratching the eye: fingernail, rubbing, paper cut, tree branch.
Iron shavings: most common foreign body.

Associated features
Sterile corneal infiltrate: need to rule out infection.

Pathology
Superficial epithelial defect or full epithelial defect.
Foreign body may or may not penetrate Bowman's membrane.

TREATMENT

Diet and Lifestyle
Safety goggles when striking metal on metal.

Pharmacologic Treatment
Corneal Abrasion
Cycloplegia: e.g., homatropine 5%.

Antibiotic ointment: e.g., erythromycin.

Pressure patch for 24 hr for clean corneal abrasions or recurrent erosions: should not be applied in cases of "dirty" trauma (such as fingernail or tree-branch scratch) or in a patient who wears contact lenses.

Corneal Foreign Body
Cycloplegia: e.g., homatropine 5%.

Antibiotic ointment: e.g., erythromycin, after removing the foreign body; pressure patch for 24 hr.

Nonpharmacologic Treatment
- Apply topical anesthetic (e.g., proparacaine) and remove the foreign body in one piece if possible with 25-gauge needle using the slit lamp. Rust ring can be removed with a drill. If the rust ring is too deep, leave it and allow time for the rust to migrate to the corneal surface.

Treatment aims
To prevent corneal infection.

Prognosis
- Corneal abrasions usually heal with no scarring.
- Removal of the foreign body usually leaves minimal scarring.

Follow-up and management
- Follow daily, and consider pressure patch with antibiotic ointment if epithelial defect is persistent. Avoid pressure patching in patients who wear contact lenses.
- If superficial punctate keratitis remains, treat with topical antibiotic for up to 4 days.
- If a corneal infiltrate is observed, appropriate smears and cultures should be obtained; treat as a corneal ulcer.

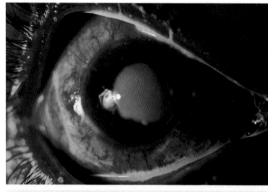

Central corneal abrasion staining with fluorescein.

General references
Albert DM, Jakobiec FA, editors: *Principles and practice of ophthalmology*, vol 1, Philadelphia, 2000, Saunders.
American Academy of Ophthalmology: *Basic and clinical science*, section 8, San Francisco, 2006-2007, The Academy.
Wright K: *Textbook of ophthalmology*, Baltimore, 1997, Lippincott Williams & Wilkins.

Corneal edema   (371.24)

DIAGNOSIS

Definition
Swelling of the corneal.

Synonyms
None.

Symptoms
Blurry vision.
Haloes.
Pain: if corneal epithelial defect is present.

Signs
Stromal edema.
Epithelial edema.
Bullous epithelial changes.
Endothelial corneal (Fuchs') dystrophy (cornea guttata) (*see* figure).
Abrasion.
Intraocular pressure (IOP): may be elevated.

Investigations
History: note any history of ocular surgery or trauma.
Visual acuity test: usually decreased relative to severity of edema.
Slit-lamp examination: pigmented guttata often visible in Fuchs' endothelial dystrophy and microcystic epithelial edema; bullous changes on the corneal surface are a sign of marked endothelial dysfunction. Carefully assess other eye for signs of Fuchs' dystrophy.
Intraocular pressure: may be low in patients with ocular ischemia and corneal edema as well as traumatic uveitis; may be elevated in phakic patients with angle closure caused by corneal edema and trauma.
Dilated fundus examination.

Complications
Corneal abrasion/ruptured bullae.
Infectious corneal ulcer.
Angle-closure glaucoma.

Pearls and Considerations
1. Corneal edema may also be associated with contact lens overwear. A thorough history of the patient's lens-wearing habits should be obtained.
2. Patients should be advised that Muro 128 stings/burns and that this is generally not a reason to discontinue use.

Referral Information
Varied and dependent on etiology.

Differential diagnosis
Interstitial keratitis.
Corneal scar.

Cause
- Endothelial dysfunction or elevated IOP related to the following:
  Pseudophakic/aphakic bullous keratopathy.
  Fuchs' endothelial dystrophy (common) and other endothelial dystrophies (rare).
  Trauma (e.g., Descemet's rupture/detachment).
  Slowly healing corneal abrasion.
  Corneal infiltrate.
  Herpetic disciform keratitis: associated with mild anterior uveitis.
  Corneal hydrops secondary to kerato-conus: usually with severe thickening of the cornea.
  Acute angle-closure glaucoma: associated with elevated IOP.
  Ocular ischemia: associated with hypotony, conjunctival injection, and anterior uveitis.

Pathology
Fuchs' endothelial dystrophy: Descemet's membrane with nodular excrescences (guttata) and decrease in endothelial cell numbers.
Trauma: discontinuation of Descemet's membrane with rolling of the edges.
Bullous keratopathy: fluid accumulating under epithelial tissue, elevating it to form a bullous appearance.

TREATMENT

Diet and Lifestyle
- No special precautions are necessary.

Pharmacologic Treatment
For Mild Cases (Nonglaucomatous)
- Sodium chloride (NaCl) 5% solution or ointment (e.g., Muro 128) 4 times daily; decrease IOP if elevated or in high teens with antiglaucoma medication.

For Acute Glaucoma
- Decrease IOP with antiglaucoma medication and topical as well as oral carbonic anhydrase inhibitors and hyperosmotic agents.

Nonpharmacologic Treatment
Bandage contact lens: for severe cases.
Corneal transplantation: ultimately may be needed for visual rehabilitation and comfort.
Laser peripheral iridectomy and trabeculectomy (if necessary): for corneal edema secondary to acute glaucoma.
For painful bullous keratopathy in eye with poor visual potential, consider anterior stromal puncture or amniotic membrane transplantation.

Treatment aims
To improve visual acuity.
To relieve pain.

Other treatments
Gundersen conjunctival flap (superior conjunctiva transposed over cornea): mainly performed to promote nonhealing abrasion and to relieve pain in eyes with poor visual potential.

Prognosis
- Good, after corneal transplantation.

Follow-up and management
Fuchs' endothelial dystrophy: every 1-3 mo.
Pseudophakic/aphakic bullous keratopathy: 1-3 mo.
Traumatic: weekly.
Nonhealing epithelial defect: every 3-5 days.
Acute angle-closure glaucoma: weekly after successful laser iridectomy or trabeculectomy.
Corneal hydrops: every 1-2 wk.

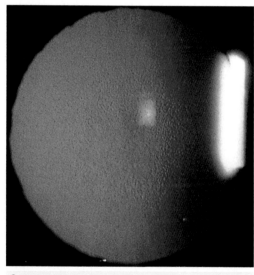

Cornea guttata seen in retroillumination.

General references
Albert DM, Jakobiec FA, editors: *Principles and practice of ophthalmology*, vol 1, Philadelphia, 2000, Saunders.
American Academy of Ophthalmology: *Basic and clinical science*, section 8, San Francisco, 2006-2007, The Academy.
Wright K: *Textbook of ophthalmology*, Baltimore, 1997, Lippincott Williams & Wilkins.

Cyclodeviations   (378.33)

DIAGNOSIS

Definition
A rotational deviation of the eye.

Synonyms
Cyclotropia, cyclophoria, torsional deviations.

Symptoms
Diplopia and visual confusion: in patients who cannot suppress.
Asthenopic symptoms.
- *Cyclodeviations do not cause head tilts.*

Signs
Objective Torsion
Fundus torsion: usually no externally apparent signs.

Subjective Torsion
Torsional results: on sensory testing.
Cyclo displacement of blind spot: on visual field testing.

Investigations
Objective Torsion

Fundus torsion: when viewed with fundus camera, fovea should be located one third of distance up from bottom of optic nerve; if fovea is located higher, it indicates intorsion of the fundus; if located lower, it indicates extorsion of the fundus; reverse for indirect ophthalmoscopic (usual) view (*see* figure).
Cover testing: no torsional "righting" of eye on cover testing; cyclotropia and cyclophoria behave identically.

Subjective Torsion

Maddox rod: throws line 90 degrees from direction of strong cylinders in rod; used singly before one eye, or differing colors used before both eyes (usually displaced with vertical prism).
Bagolini lenses: plano lenses with etching, throwing line 90 degrees from etching direction; usually used singly before each eye in turn; advantage of reproducing ordinary viewing conditions, and the wide viewing field permits input of peripheral fusion.
Lancaster red-green test: permits diagnosis but not quantitation of torsion.
Visual field test: torsional displacement of blind spot from usual position.

Complications
- Patients who have long-standing ocular cyclodeviations may not admit to target torsion on subjective testing, but they will have fundus torsion.

Differential diagnosis
- Patients who have dissociated vertical deviation will not have subjective or objective torsion in primary position.
- Patients who have oblique muscle dysfunction will have objective globe torsion in primary position and may have subjective torsional findings as well.

Cause
Primary and secondary oblique muscle dysfunctions.
Cyclovertical muscle palsies.
Fibrotic muscle syndromes (occasionally).
After strabismus surgery (especially oblique muscle surgery and rectus muscle translations for alphabet patterns).

Associated features
Oblique muscle dysfunctions.
Cyclovertical muscle palsies.

TREATMENT

Diet and Lifestyle
- No special precautions are necessary.

Pharmacologic Treatment
- No pharmacologic treatment is recommended.

Nonpharmacologic Treatment
- Many patients with cyclodeviations will have vertical deviations as well. Prism treatment of the latter often permits these patients to cyclofuse.
- Some patients will require strabismus surgery on oblique or rectus muscles for intorsion or extorsion.

Intorsion: recession or lengthening of superior oblique tendon, nasal translation of superior rectus muscle, temporal translation of inferior rectus muscle; and disinsertion of anterior half of superior oblique tendon.

Extorsion: Harada-Ito procedure, temporal translation of superior rectus muscle, nasal translation of inferior rectus muscle; weakening procedure on inferior oblique muscle; recession, disinsertion, myectomy, and advancement to inferior rectus insertion.

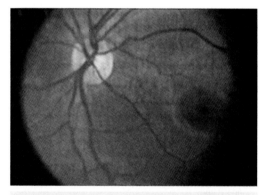

Extorsion of left eye as viewed with fundus camera.

Treatment aims
To achieve comfortable single binocular vision in all gaze positions.

Prognosis
- Medical and surgical treatment is generally effective.
- Patients must be warned about temporary postoperative torsional spatial distortion.

Follow-up and management
As above; individualized according to patient needs.

General references

Bixenmann W, von Noorden GK: Apparent foveal displacement in normal subjects and in cyclotropia, *Ophthalmology* 89:58-63, 1982.

Guyton DI, von Noorden GK: Sensory adaptations to cyclodeviations. In Reinecke RD, editor: *Strabismus*, New York, 1978, Grune & Stratton, pp 399-412.

Guyton DL: Clinical assessment of ocular torsion, *Am Orthop J* 33:7-12, 1983.

Locke JC: Heterotopia of the blind spot in ocular vertical muscle imbalance, *Trans Am Ophthalmol Soc* 65:306-316, 1967.

Dacryoadenitis   (375.0)

DIAGNOSIS

Definition
An inflammatory enlargement of the lacrimal gland.

Synonyms
None.

Symptoms
Pain.
Double vision: occasionally.

Signs
Swelling of the lid.
S-shaped appearance.
Nut-size mass (not connected to orbit or lid margin).
Conjunctival injection and chemosis.
Palpable preauricular nodes.
Ptosis.
Restriction of ocular motility: uncommon.
Proptosis: occasionally.

Investigations
Medical history.
Presence of other skin lesions.
Lymph node enlargement.
Computed tomography (CT) scan.
Biopsy: must be excisional if benign mixed tumor is suspected.
Blood count: to rule out elevated white blood cell counts or abnormal lymphoproliferative disorders.

Pearls and Considerations
Dacryoadenitis is usually representative of underlying systemic disease. A thorough history may shed light on its etiology.

Referral Information
1. Patients should be referred for biopsy, blood work, and imaging as appropriate.
2. Patients should be referred to the appropriate subspecialist for treatment of underlying systemic disease once identified.

Differential diagnosis
Chalazion.
Hordeolum.
Orbital cellulitis.
Prolapsed lacrimal gland.
Lymphoma.
Malignant or benign lacrimal tumors.
- Inflammation occurs in a 3:1 ratio to neoplastic swelling of the lacrimal gland.

Cause
Infectious disease (viral or bacterial).
Lymphoproliferative disease (e.g., mumps, infectious mononucleosis, influenza virus, herpes zoster).
Granulomatous disease (e.g., sarcoidosis).
Sjögren's syndrome, Graves' disease, Wegener's disease, lupus.

Classification
Acute: usually presents as unilateral swelling with pain and pressure.
Chronic: usually presents as a painless, nontender swelling present for >1 mo.

Pathology
- May result in lymphocytic infiltration of the gland with foci of granulomatous or nongranulomatous inflammation; underlying pathology depends on the systemic process (if present).

TREATMENT

Diet and Lifestyle
- Swelling can result from nutritional deficiencies, alcohol, diabetes, or drug use.

Pharmacologic Treatment
- Treat underlying disease process; may require systemic steroids.

Nonpharmacologic Treatment
Local treatment with heat, possible surgical incision, and drainage.
Evaluation and treatment of underlying disease processes.

Treatment aims
To resolve symptoms of inflammation and decrease swelling.

Other treatments
Treatment of possible underlying disease entities.

Prognosis
Dependent on underlying cause; if associated with systemic disease, prognosis may vary widely.

Follow-up and management
Dependent on underlying cause of glandular swelling; necessary for ancillary treatment of systemic illness.
- Refer patient to rheumatologist if collagen vascular disease is suspected.

General references
Fraunfelder F, Roy F, editors: *Current ocular therapy,* Philadelphia, 2000, Saunders.
Tasman W, Jaeger E, editors. In *Duane's clinical ophthalmology,* vol 2, Philadelphia, 1995, Lippincott-Raven.

Delayed visual-system maturation   (369.20)

DIAGNOSIS

Definition
A developmental delay in visual perception during the first year of life.

Synonyms
None.

Symptoms
Decreased visual acuity in a child <1 yr of age.

Signs
Decreased visual attentiveness: in setting of prematurity or developmental delay; often no fixational ability until 6 or 12 mo of age, occasionally later.

Normal or symmetrically sluggish pupils to light; no afferent pupillary defect.

No nystagmus.

Eyes are structurally normal.

Investigations
Electroretinogram: normal.

Visual-evoked response (VER) test: reported as normal, reduced, or absent; when compared with age-matched normal responses, most children with delayed visual maturation will have VERs normal for age; varying VER responses could represent different stages of resolution of the disorder.

Pearls and Considerations
1. This process will likely correct itself with time and further development. "Treatment" is often aimed at educating and reassuring the parents.
2. Should be considered a diagnosis of exclusion in young children with visual dysfunction. Underlying contributory pathology must be ruled out.

Referral Information
None.

Differential diagnosis
Cortical blindness: pupils usually are normally reactive to light, and patients do not develop nystagmus; occurs in same patient population (premature infants and developmentally delayed children); VER absent in most cases; may require nuclear magnetic resonance to separate from syndrome of delayed visual maturation; visual acuity does not improve with time.

Sedation: often children will be medicated for seizure disorder.

Inattention to targets because of developmental delay or deprivation.

Cause
Probably caused by delay in synaptic development; normal myelination is speculated.

Epidemiology
Most common in settings of prematurity and developmental delay; no racial or familial pattern.

Associated features
- Except for history of developmental delay and possible soft signs of cerebral palsy, no systemic associations are noted; more frequent in very premature infants.

TREATMENT

Diet and Lifestyle
- It is reasonable to visually stimulate these children, but such stimulation is of unproven benefit.

Pharmacologic Treatment
- No pharmacologic treatment has been proven effective. Withdrawal of seizure medication and sedatives as rapidly as possible seems reasonable.

Nonpharmacologic Treatment
- No nonpharmacologic treatment is recommended.

Treatment aims
No specific treatment is indicated.

Prognosis
- Spontaneous recovery without treatment is the typical outcome.

Follow-up and management
- Reassurance of parents and frequent (every 3 mo) follow-up.

General references

Cole GF, Hungerford J, Jones RB: Delayed visual maturation in infancy, *Arch Dis Child* 59: 107-110, 1984.

Hoyt CS, Jastrzebski G, Marg E: Delayed visual maturation in infancy, *Br J Ophthalmol* 67: 127-130, 1983.

Illingworth RS: Delayed visual maturation, *Arch Dis Child* 36:407-409, 1961.

Lambert SR, Kriss A, Taylor D: Delayed visual maturation: a longitudinal clinical and electro-physiological assessment, *Ophthalmology* 96:524-529, 1989.

Skarf B, Panton C: VEP testing in neurologically impaired and developmentally delayed infants and young children: ARVO Abstracts, *Invest Ophthalmol Vis Sci* 28(suppl):302, 1987.

Dermatochalasis   (374.87)

DIAGNOSIS

Definition
Drooping of the skin of the upper eyelid as a result of age-related skin laxity.

Synonyms
None.

Symptoms
Drooping of the eyelids: caused by aging, redundant eyelid skin (*see* figure).

Signs
Redundant skin: usually located on the outer two thirds of the lid; the skin may be so extensive that it can droop over the visual axis, obscuring vision.

Investigations
Visual acuity test.
Brow position.
Levator function.
Visual field test, with and without eyelids elevated/taped.
Slit-lamp examination: to rule out anterior segment abnormality.

Complications
Obscuration of the visual field.

Pearls and Considerations
Carbon dioxide (CO_2) laser resurfacing has been investigated for the treatment of dermatochalasis and may be considered a safe, effective, and less invasive treatment for patients uncomfortable with traditional treatment methods.

Referral Information
Refer for excisional blepharoplasty with patients who either experience limited superior visual field or who have related cosmetic concerns.

Differential diagnosis
Blepharochalasis: a true swelling of the eyelid resulting from recurrent inflammation.

Cause
Generalized change of aging.

Pathology
Involutional: stretching of skin.
- In *true* dermatochalasis, orbital septum is intact, as opposed to *blepharochalasis,* in which fat extrudes through orbital septum.

TREATMENT

Diet and Lifestyle
- No special precautions are necessary.

Pharmacologic Treatment
- No pharmacologic treatment is advised.

Nonpharmacologic Treatment
Surgical removal of the redundant skin and underlying fat.

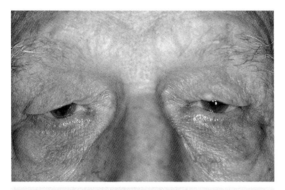

Redundant skin of the upper eyelids is present diffusely but most marked on the outer two thirds of the lids.

Treatment aims
To remove redundant skin to restore full visual (i.e., field) potential.

Prognosis
- After surgical removal, prognosis is good.

Follow-up and management
- Surgical removal of skin is curative unless further laxity occurs with increased age.

General references
Alster TS, Bellew SG: Improvement of dermatochalasis and periorbital rhytides with a high-energy pulsed CO_2 laser: a retrospective study, *Dermatol Surg* 30:483-487, 2004.
Fraunfelder F, Roy F, editors: *Current ocular therapy*, Philadelphia, 2000, Saunders.
Hornblass A: *Oculoplatic, orbital, and reconstructive surgery*, vol 2, Baltimore, 1990, Lippincott Williams & Wilkins.
Stewart W, editor: *Ophthalmic plastic and reconstructive surgery*, San Francisco, 1984, American Academy of Ophthalmology.

Diabetic retinopathy   (362.0)

DIAGNOSIS

Definition
Retinal vascular disease and visual loss associated with diabetes mellitus.

Synonym
PDR (proliferative diabetic retinopathy) and NPDR (nonproliferative diabetic retinopathy)

Symptoms
Gradual decreased vision.
Floaters.
Acute loss of vision.

Signs
Intraretinal hemorrhages: *see* Fig. 1.
Retinal edema.
Intraretinal microvascular abnormalities.
Cotton-wool spots: *see* Fig. 1.
Microaneurysms: *see* Fig. 1.
Neovascularization of the disc and elsewhere: *see* Fig. 2.
Venous beading.
Venous omega loops.
Vitreous hemorrhage.
Tractional retinal detachment.
Iris neovascularization.

Investigations
Careful slit-lamp examination: to rule out neovascularization of the iris.
Gonioscopy: if there is a suspicion for neovascular glaucoma.
Dilated fundus examination.
Fluorescein angiography: *see* Fig. 3.

Differential diagnosis
Ocular ischemic syndrome.
Hypertension.
Vasculitis.
Central, hemiretinal, or branch retinal vein occlusion.

Cause
Diabetes mellitus.

Epidemiology
- Diabetes accounts for 10% of new cases of legal blindness each year.
- Incidence of diabetic retinopathy depends on the age of patients, duration of the disease, and insulin-dependent versus non–insulin-dependent diabetes mellitus.
- 25%-50% of insulin-dependent patients of 10-15–yr duration will have signs of retinopathy [1].
- 23% of non–insulin-dependent patients of 11-13–yr duration will have signs of retinopathy [2].

Classification
Nonproliferative diabetic retinopathy: include microaneurysms, cotton-wool spots, retinal edema, intraretinal lipid, intraretinal microvascular abnormalities, venous beading, and venous omega loops.
Proliferative diabetic retinopathy: includes all the findings of nonproliferative disease plus neovascularization of the disc or elsewhere.

Pathology
Decrease in pericytes in the retinal vascular endothelium.
Progressive thickening of the retinal capillary basement membrane.
Vascular occlusion.
Microaneurysms form in the superficial retinal capillaries.
Dot and blot hemorrhages in the outer plexiform and inner nuclear layer of the retina.
Breakdown of the blood retinal barrier.
Intraretinal lipid exudates.

Diagnosis continued on p. 106

TREATMENT

Diet and Lifestyle
- Maintain a normal blood glucose level.
- Exercise.

Pharmacologic Treatment
For Neovascular Glaucoma

Standard dosage Nonselective β-blockers, 1 drop twice daily.

Selective β-blocker, 1 drop twice daily.

Topical carbonic anhydrase inhibitor, 1 drop 3 times daily.

Oral carbonic anhydrase inhibitor, 250 mg 4 times daily, or 500 mg twice daily.

- If there is evidence of iris neovascularization, administer atropine sulfate 1%. One drop twice daily is recommended to maintain long-term pupil dilation.

Nonpharmacologic Treatment

Focal laser therapy: for macular edema if it is within 500 μm of the fovea with or without intraretinal lipid, or if there is an area of macular edema that is equal or greater in size than one disc area within 1 disc diameter of the fovea [3].

Panretinal photocoagulation: for proliferative diabetic retinopathy if there is neovascularization of the disc or moderate to severe neovascularization elsewhere [4].

Pars plana vitrectomy: for nonclearing vitreous hemorrhage or tractional diabetic detachment that threatens the fovea.

Intravitreal triamcinolone injection: for macular edema involving the fovea that is affecting visual acuity and has not responded to macular laser [5].

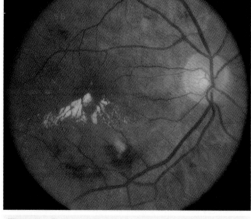

Figure 1 Background diabetic retinopathy. Note intraretinal lipid, microaneurysms, intraretinal hemorrhages, and cotton-wool spot.

Treatment aims
To stabilize vision or decrease the rate of visual loss.

To decrease macular edema.

To achieve regression of proliferative retinopathy.

To release traction if macula is threatened.

To clear vitreous hemorrhage if present ≥2 mo.

Prognosis
Depends on the severity of the disease.

Follow-up and management
- Yearly screening dilated fundus examinations should be performed on all diabetic patients.
- If diabetic retinopathy is detected, follow-up examinations may be as frequent as every 2-3 mo to observe the rate of progression.

Treatment continued on p. 107

DIAGNOSIS—cont'd

Complications
Cataracts.

Neovascular glaucoma secondary to ischemia with iris or angle neovascularization: *see* Pharmacologic Treatment.

Tractional retinal detachment.

Vitreous hemorrhage.

Preretinal hemorrhage.

Macular edema.

Optic nerve damage.

Pearls and Considerations
Even asymptomatic patients may need to be treated to prevent future visual loss from macular edema or neovascularization.

Referral Information
Patients need an annual diluted fundus examination, with or without symptoms.

TREATMENT—cont'd

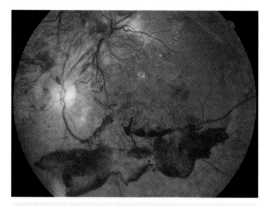

Figure 2   Proliferative diabetic retinopathy. Note neovascularization of the disc, preretinal fibrosis superiorly, and preretinal hemorrhage inferiorly.

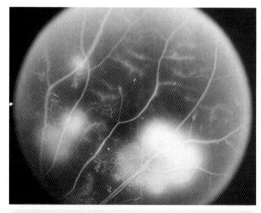

Figure 3   Fluorescein angiogram of the peripheral retina of a patient with proliferative diabetic retinopathy, showing hyperfluorescent leakage secondary to neovascularization elsewhere (white areas with poorly defined borders) and capillary loss (dark areas between the blood vessels).

Key references

1. Klein R, Klein BE, Moss SE, et al: The Wisconsin Epidemiologic Study of Diabetic Retinopathy. IX. Four-year incidence and progression of diabetic retinopathy when age of diagnosis is less than 30 years, *Arch Ophthalmol* 107:237-243, 1989.

2. Klein R, Klein BE, Moss SE, et al: The Wisconsin Epidemiologic Study of Diabetic Retinopathy. X. Four-year incidence and progression of diabetic retinopathy when age of diagnosis is 30 years or more, *Arch Ophthalmol* 107:244-249, 1989.

3. Aiello LM: Diagnosis, management, and treatment of nonproliferative diabetic retinopathy and macular edema, *Prin Pract Ophthal* 2:747-760, 1994.

4. Miller JW, D'Amico DJ: Proliferative diabetic retinopathy, *Prin Pract Ophthal* 2:760-782, 1994.

5. Martidis A, Duker JS, Greenberg PB, et al: Intravitreal triamcinolone for refractory diabetic macular edema, *Opthalmology* 109:920-927, 2002.

Duane syndrome   (378.71)

DIAGNOSIS

Definition
A congenital abnormality in which the palpebral fissure narrows and the globe retracts into the orbit when the eye is adducted.

Synonyms
Duane's retraction syndrome, retraction syndrome.

Symptoms
Cosmetic deformity on side gaze: *see* figure.
Loss of comfortable single binocular vision on side gaze.

Signs
General
- All patients with Duane syndrome have retraction of involved globe on adduction, attempted adduction ptosis on adduction, or attempted adduction.
- Many patients with Duane syndrome have overelevation or overdepression in adduction *(tether effect)*.

Specific
Duane I: absent abduction.
Duane II: absent adduction.
Duane III: limited abduction and adduction.

Investigations
Family history: specifically, age of onset of strabismus (if present) and any hearing deficiency.
Referral for skeletal examination: if appropriate.
Full motility examination: in all gaze positions.

Complications
Duane I: esotropia in 40% with head turn toward involved eye (always ≤30 prism diopters).
Duane II: exotropia in 20% with head turn away from involved eye.
Duane III: either esotropia or exotropia, usually small in magnitude.
Amblyopia may develop in patients who have strabismus and who abandon head turn.

Associated Syndromes
Klippel-Feil anomalad: cervical vertebral fusion, platybasia, spina bifida, scapular elevation.
Wildervanck syndrome: Klippel-Feil anomalad, congenital labyrinthine deafness.
Goldenhar syndrome: epibulbar dermoids, auricular appendages, microtia, mandibular and vertebral anomalies.
Vertical-retraction syndrome: monocular retraction of globe with narrowing of lid fissure on attempted up or down gaze; limitation of elevation or depression.
Synergistic divergence ("ocular splits"): simultaneous abduction of both eyes on gaze away from involved eye.
Speculated miswiring of horizontal recti: lateral rectus muscle innervated by both cranial nerve (CN) VI and branch of inferior division of CN III, with latter predominating.

Pearls and Considerations
Patients with Duane syndrome do not usually experience diplopia.

Referral Information
Surgical referral for extraocular muscle (EOM) surgery to limit retraction may be considered.

Differential diagnosis
Early-onset esotropia: >30 prism diopters.
Möbius syndrome: bilateral; no globe retraction or ptosis on adduction; associated CN VII and XII palsies.
CN VI palsies: no globe retraction or ptosis on adduction.

Cause
Duane I: depleted CN VI nucleus and absent CN VI; lateral rectus muscle innervated by branch of inferior division of CN III (proved by pathology).
Duane II: lateral rectus innervated by both CN VI and branch of inferior division of CN III (speculated).
Duane III: both medial and lateral recti muscles innervated by CN VI and branch of inferior division of CN III (speculated).

Epidemiology
- Duane syndrome represents 1% of all strabismus patients. Motility defect is congenital, but strabismus usually develops with age. Duane syndrome is unilateral in 80% of patients, bilateral in 20%.
- *Duane I* represents 85% of patients (60% of which are in the left eye, 60% of whom are female).
- *Duane II* represents 14% of patients.
- *Duane III* represents 1% of patients.
- Autosomal dominant form exists.
- Case reports of identical twins with Duane I (right eye in one twin, left eye in other twin).

Pathology
Duane I: depleted CN VI nucleus of absent nerve; lateral rectus partially or totally replaced with fibrous tissue.

TREATMENT

Diet and Lifestyle
- Many patients who have Duane syndrome and straight eyes in primary position will learn to turn the head to avoid cosmetic blemish in side gaze.

Pharmacologic Treatment
- No pharmacologic treatment is recommended.

Nonpharmacologic Treatment
- Surgery is indicated in patients with strabismus in primary position.

For Duane I: recede medial recti in both eyes.

For Duane II: recede lateral recti in both eyes.

For Duane III: as indicated.

- Surgery cannot reliably improve the duction limitation in this syndrome. Retraction can be improved with recession of both horizontal recti muscles in the involved eye. Tether effect can be improved by splitting the lateral rectus muscle to create a Y structure and reattaching each half to sclera in the oblique temporal quadrants.

Treatment aims

To achieve straight eyes in primary position with comfortable single binocular vision.

To ensure absence of overelevation or overdepression in adduction (tether effect).

To minimize globe retraction and ptosis on adduction or attempted adduction.

Prognosis

- Most patients will not develop strabismus in primary position; strabismus surgery effectively aligns the eyes in primary position of patients who do develop strabismus.

Follow-up and management

- Refractive errors and amblyopia should be managed as usual.

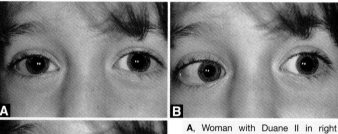
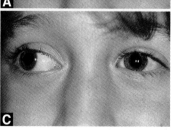

A, Woman with Duane II in right eye and Duane III in left eye. **B**, Note limitation of abduction in right eye. **C**, Abduction is limited in left eye.

General references

Hotchkiss MG, Miller NR, Clark AW, et al: Bilateral Duane's retraction syndrome: a clinico-pathologic report, *Arch Ophthalmol* 98:870-876, 1980.

Huber A: Electrophysiology of the retraction syndrome, *Br J Ophthalmol* 58:293-295, 1974.

Miller MT: Association of Duane retraction syndrome with craniofacial malformations, *J Craniofac Genet Dev Biol Suppl* 1:273-278, 1985.

Moster ML: Paresis of isolated and multiple cranial nerves and painful ophthalmoplegia. In Yanoff M, Duker JS, editors: *Ophthalmology*, E-dition, St Louis, 2006, Elsevier.

Pressman SH, Scott WE: Surgical treatment of Duane's syndrome, *Ophthalmology* 93:29-83, 1986.

Esotropia   (378.0)

DIAGNOSIS

Definition
Strabismus in which manifest deviation of the visual axis of one eye occurs toward that of the other eye, resulting in diplopia.

Synonyms
Convergent strabismus, internal strabismus, "cross-eye."

Symptoms
Asthenopia (headaches, irritability, visual discomfort): with onset of strabismus.
Probable loss of stereoscopic ability.
Possible cosmetic deformity.
- Children <7-9 yr of age who are binocular will develop sensory adaptations of suppression and anomalous retinal correspondence. They will also be asymptomatic.
- Children >7-9 yr of age who are binocular will develop diplopia and visual confusion.

Signs
Intermittent or constant inward deviation of the visual axes: especially when tired or ill.
Squinting or rubbing of one or both eyes: especially in bright sunlight.

Investigations
General medical and neurologic examinations: to exclude intracranial masses, myasthenia gravis, vascular disease, etc., as causes of esotropia.
History of other affected family members, trauma, recent immunizations (association with acute sixth-nerve palsy).
Age of onset, previous treatment, change in frequency and amplitude of deviation.
Sensory testing.
Measurement of alignment near, at distance, and in all gaze positions.
Evaluation of ductions and versions.

Complications
Amblyopia: if esotropia is not alternating and age of onset is <5 yr.
Probable loss of stereoptic ability while eyes are strabismic.
Cosmetic deformity.
Smaller extent of horizontal visual field than a normal patient.

Causes
Early-onset esotropia: either congenital lack of binocular vision with resultant esotropia or mismatch between sensory input and motor response systems with resultant esotropia.
Accommodative esotropia: either high hyperopia or increased ratio of accommodative convergence to accommodation (or both).
Duane syndrome: esotropia found in 40% of type I, with absence of sixth cranial nerve and miswiring of lateral rectus muscle by a branch of the lower division of the third cranial nerve; autosomal dominant form exists.
Cyclic esotropia: presumed inherent biologic clock.
Sixth-nerve palsy: increased intracranial pressure, mass, infection, or inflammation of cavernous sinus or Dorello canal; occlusion of vessel to nerve; pontine infarct or mass.
Sensory esotropia: poor acuity in one eye; often caused by congenital cataract, corneal opacity, strabismic or anisometropic amblyopia.
Möbius syndrome: unknown.
Strabismus fixus: presumably caused by congenital fibrosis of the medial recti.

Referral Information
Any child older than age 2 mo who has strabismus should be referred to an eye specialist.

Differential diagnosis
Early-onset esotropia: large angle; age of onset ~6 wk; no binocular vision unless eyes aligned <2 yr of age; risk of amblyopia ~40%.
Accommodative esotropia: initially greater deviation at near than at distance fixation; age of onset, mean ~18 mo.
Duane syndrome: congenital; no abduction in affected eye beyond midline; esotropia <30 prism diopters.
Cyclic esotropia: usually 24 hr of straight eyes followed by 24 hr of constant esotropia; usually congenital.
Sixth-nerve palsy: often associated with esotropia greater at distance than at near fixation; abduction in affected eye(s) may be limited.
Sensory esotropia: young children who have poor acuity in one eye.
Möbius syndrome: congenital large-angle esotropia with no abduction beyond midline in both eyes.
Strabismus fixus: congenital bilateral large-angle esotropia with no abduction.
Variable-angle esotropia: associated with developmental delay.

Epidemiology
Early-onset esotropia: 1% of live births; no gender or race predilection; 81% concordance in monozygous twins, 9% in dizygous twins; often found in families of patients with monofixation syndrome or accommodative esotropia.
Accommodative esotropia: 1% of live births; no gender or race predilection.
Duane syndrome: 1% of all strabismus cases; unilateral in 80%, bilateral in 20%; seen in left eye in 60%; women account for 60% of all patients; no race or gender predilection.
Cyclic esotropia: rare; about 200 cases reported in the literature; incidence is ~1:1000-30,000 childhood strabismus cases.
Möbius syndrome: rare; no known race or gender predilection; not inherited.

Pathology
Duane syndrome: in type I, absence of sixth cranial nerve from brainstem to muscle and innervation of lateral rectus muscle by branch of lower division of third cranial nerve.

TREATMENT

Diet and Lifestyle
- No special precautions are necessary.

Pharmacologic Treatment
- Infants and myopic patients can be treated for accommodative esotropia with phospholine iodide drops (0.125% in both eyes before each bedtime) to lower ratio of accommodative convergence to accommodation.
- Botulinum toxin injection into medial recti of affected patients usually requires general anesthesia in children; found to be less successful than surgery in most published series.

Nonpharmacologic Treatment
Glasses and contact lenses: foundation of initial treatment for accommodative esotropia; the full hyperopic correction with bifocals, if necessary, is prescribed for young children.

Base-out prisms: may be helpful in some patients with intermittent esotropia.

Strabismus surgery: necessary for eye alignment in most patients in whom glasses are not effective; procedures include symmetric medial rectus recessions, monocular recession of medial rectus and resection of lateral rectus, and symmetric lateral rectus resections.
- Many patients with esotropia are amblyopic and should be treated in the usual manner.

Associated Features
All forms: alphabet-pattern strabismus with greater esotropia in upgaze (A pattern) or downgaze (V pattern)

Early-onset esotropia: inferior oblique overaction (75%), superior oblique overaction (5%), dissociated vertical deviation (75%), latent nystagmus (50%), rotary nystagmus (20%), amblyopia (40%); deviation is the same at distance and at near fixations.

Accommodative esotropia: inferior oblique overaction (50%); deviation initially greater at near than at distance fixation.

Duane syndrome: esotropia (40% in type I); overelevation or overdepression in adduction; retraction of globe into orbit with adduction; pseudoptosis with adduction; may be associated with Klippel-Feil anomalad, Goldenhar syndrome, Wildervanck syndrome (Klippel-Feil anomalad, Duane syndrome, congenital labyrinthine deafness).

Möbius syndrome: upper-motor-neuron seventh-nerve palsies, lower-motor-neuron twelfth-nerve palsies, mental retardation, polydactyly, syndactyly, bradydactyly, clubbed feet, peculiar gait, peroneal muscle atrophy.

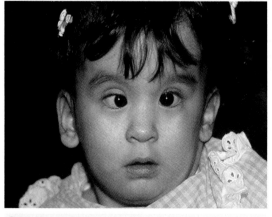

Congenital esotropia.

Treatment aims
To achieve excellent visual acuity in each eye.

To achieve straight eyes with comfortable single binocular vision and stereopsis.

To remove cosmetic deformity.

To expand horizontal binocular visual field.

Prognosis
Early-onset esotropia: early strabismus surgery results in development of binocular vision in ~90% of patients, but central binocularity and normal stereopsis rarely develop.

Accommodative esotropia: 50% of patients can be completely weaned from wearing glasses, but ~25% will require strabismus surgery to regain eye alignment.

Duane syndrome: strabismus surgery will result in straight eyes in primary position in almost all patients, but abduction beyond primary position cannot be attained.

Cyclic esotropia: strabismus surgery will be successful in almost all patients and can be performed on a day when the eyes are esotropic.

Möbius syndrome: strabismus surgery will result in straight eyes in primary position in almost all patients, but abduction beyond primary position will rarely be obtained.

Sixth-nerve palsy: prognosis depends on the cause.

Follow-up and management
- Care is individualized depending on cause and type of esotropia.

General references
Baker JD, Parks MM: Early-onset accommodative esotropia, *Am J Ophthalmol* 90:11-18, 1980.

Henderson JC: The congenital facial diplegia syndrome: clinical feature, pathology, and etiology: a review of 61 cases, *Brain* 62:381-384, 1939.

Hitchkiss MG, Miller NR, Clark AW, et al: Bilateral Duane's retraction syndrome: a clinical-pathologic report, *Arch Ophthalmol* 98:870-890, 1980.

Ing MR: Early surgical alignment for congenital esotropia, *Trans Am Ophthalmol Soc* 79:625-633, 1981.

DIAGNOSIS

Definition
Abnormal protrusion of the globe from the bony orbit.

Synonym
Bulging eye.

Symptoms
Swelling/pressure.
Red, painful eye: if exophthalmos is excessive, exposure keratitis may cause redness and pain in the eye.
Tearing.
Blurred vision.
Strabismus and diplopia (double vision).

Signs
Exophthalmos (ocular proptosis): a lesion within the muscle cone causes more exophthalmos than a similar-sized lesion outside the muscle cone; paresis of the extraocular muscles as a result of inflammation (ophthalmoplegia) can cause 2.0 mm of ocular proptosis.
Chemosis of conjunctiva: may be so severe that the chemotic conjunctiva protrudes through the semiclosed eyelids.
Lid swelling.
Redness: neoplasms (e.g., rhabdomyosarcomas) may present initially with redness and swelling of the lids, causing a misdiagnosis of orbital cellulitis.
Strabismus and diplopia (double vision).

Investigations
History: especially presence of breast or lung cancer, lymphoma, or leukemia.
- *Duration.* Benign neoplasms (e.g., orbital cavernous hemangioma [the most common primary orbital neoplasm that causes exophthalmos and benign mixed tumor; *see* Figs. 1 and 2]) tend to have a long history of slow growth, whereas malignant neoplasms (e.g., adenoid cystic carcinoma of lacrimal gland or rhabdomyosarcoma [the most frequent primary mesenchymal malignant neoplasm of the orbit]) tend to have a rapid, short course.
- *Age at onset.* Congenital orbital tumors (e.g., dermoids) usually are diagnosed at a very early age. Cavernous hemangioma, although congenital, is not usually diagnosed until the fourth or fifth decade. The vast majority of orbital rhabdomyosarcomas occur before age 20 yr. Other malignant tumors, such as fibrosarcoma and adenoid cystic carcinoma, tend to occur in middle-aged to elderly individuals.
- Orbital metastasis from lung cancer usually occurs early in the course of the disease. Conversely, orbital metastasis from breast cancer tends to occur late in the disease.
Ocular examination: visual acuity, ocular motility, complete external examination, exophthalmometry (measurement of exophthalmos by an exophthalmometer), intraocular pressure, undilated and dilated slit-lamp examination and dilated fundus examination.
General examination: physical examination and any indicated laboratory test.
Special examination: orbital imaging by computed tomography, magnetic resonance imaging, and orbital ultrasound is the benchmark of orbital tumor diagnosis; this type of imaging often is diagnostic of the process and allows for anatomic delineation of the tumor from a surgical point of view.

Differential diagnosis
Benign neoplasms
Cavernous hemangioma (most common), lymphangioma, orbital varix, dermoid, hemangiopericytoma, reactive fibrous proliferations, fibrous dysplasia, neurofibroma, neurilemmoma, meningioma, optic nerve glioma, benign mixed tumor of lacrimal gland, Langerhans granulomatoses, sinus histiocytosis.
Malignant neoplasms
Kaposi's sarcoma, fibrous histiocytoma, rhabdomyosarcoma, adenoid cystic carcinoma and malignant mixed tumors of lacrimal gland, lymphoma, leukemia.

Cause
Unknown in most cases.

Epidemiology
- All orbital neoplasms, benign and malignant, are extremely rare.
- Cavernous hemangioma is the most common benign tumor, followed by orbital dermoid.
- Rhabdomyosarcoma is the most common primary mesenchymal orbital malignant tumor, followed by lymphoma and leukemia.
- Lung, breast, and neuroblastoma are the most common metastatic tumors in men, women, and children, respectively.

Classification
- Orbital tumors can be classified as primary or secondary or according to tissue of origin.
- Hamartomas (e.g., cavernous hemangiomas) are congenital tumors of tissue normally present in the orbit.
- Choristomas (e.g., dermoids) are congenital tumors of tissue not normally present in the orbit.

Associated features
Depend on the cause (e.g., metastatic orbital tumors have systemic findings; Kaposi's sarcoma usually is associated with AIDS).

Pathology
Depends on the type of lesion present in the orbit; basically, soft tissue tumor pathology is involved.

Diagnosis continued on p. 114

TREATMENT

Diet and Lifestyle
- No special precautions are necessary.

Pharmacologic Treatment
- In general, pharmacologic treatment is ineffective, except in special cases of chemotherapy (e.g., for rhabdomyosarcoma).

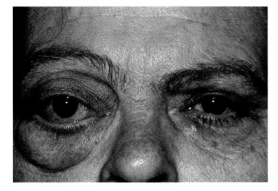

Figure 1 Exophthalmos of the right eye caused by a cavernous hemangioma of the orbit.

Treatment aims
To preserve vision.
To eradicate the tumor.

Other treatments
- If the tumor is part of a systemic process (e.g., metastatic tumor, neurofibromatosis, Langerhans granulomatoses), further study is indicated.

Prognosis
- Prognosis depends on the type of tumor and whether it is benign or malignant.

Follow-up and management
- Close initial follow-up is essential to monitor effectiveness of therapy.
- Long-term follow-up is necessary to recognize any early recurrence.

Treatment continued on p. 115

DIAGNOSIS—cont'd

Complications

Visual loss.

Exposure keratitis.

Cosmetic appearance (permanent exophthalmos).

Strabismus and diplopia.

Morbidity and mortality: if caused by malignant neoplasm.

Pearls and Considerations

1. Orbital metastasis from lung usually occurs early in the disease, whereas from breast usually occurs late.
2. Generally, a difference of >2 mm protrusion between the two eyes is considered abnormal.
3. An average exophthalmometry reading is 21 mm, although this figure is somewhat variable by race and gender.

Referral Information

Refer to appropriate subspecialist (e.g., oncologist, endocrinologist) for management of underlying systemic pathology.

TREATMENT—cont'd

Nonpharmacologic Treatment

- Orbital biopsy usually is necessary for diagnosis, especially of malignant tumors.
- Local excision is adequate for most benign tumors, whereas exenteration may be necessary for malignant tumors.
- Radiation therapy may be appropriate for certain malignant neoplasms (e.g., malignant lymphomas).

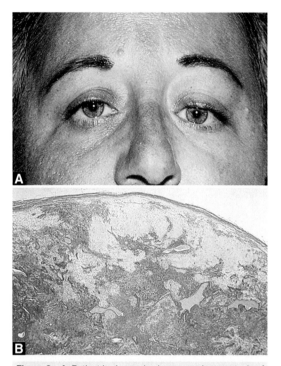

Figure 2   A, Patient had very slowly progressive proptosis of the left eye for a long time. **B,** Histologic section shows the characteristic diphasic pattern, consisting of a pale background that has a myxomatous stroma and a relatively amorphous appearance contiguous with cellular areas that contain mainly epithelial cells, characteristic of a benign mixed tumor (pleomorphic adenoma).

General references

Demirici H, Shields CL, Shields JA, et al: Orbital tumors in the older population, *Ophthalmology* 109(2):243-248, 2002.

Kodsi SR, Shetlar DJ, Campbell RJ, et al: A review of 340 orbital tumors in children during a 60-year period, *Am J Ophthalmol* 117:177-182, 1994.

Mercandetti M, Cohen AJ: Exophthalmos, 2004, www.emedicine.com.

Sharara N, Holden JT, Woho TH, et al: Ocular adnexal lymphoid proliferations: clinical, histologic, flow cytometric, and molecular analysis of forty-three cases, *Ophthalmology* 110(6): 1245-1254, 2003.

Shields CL, Shields JA: Rhabdomyosarcoma: review for the ophthalmologist, *Surv Ophthalmol* 48(1):39-57, 2003.

Exotropia (378.1)

DIAGNOSIS

Definition
Strabismus in which manifest deviation of the visual axis of one eye occurs away from that of the other eye, resulting in diplopia.

Synonyms
Divergent strabismus, external strabismus, "walleye."

Symptoms
Asthenopia (headaches, irritability, visual discomfort): with onset of strabismus.
Probable loss of stereoscopic ability: when strabismic.
Possible cosmetic deformity.
- Children <7-9 yr of age who are binocular will develop sensory adaptations of suppression and anomalous retinal correspondence. They will also be asymptomatic.
- Children <7-9 yr of age who are binocular will develop diplopia and visual confusion.

Signs
Intermittent or constant outward deviation of the visual axes: especially when tired or ill.
Squinting or rubbing of one or both eyes: especially in bright sunlight.

Investigations
General medical and neurologic examinations: as appropriate to exclude intracranial masses, myasthenia gravis, vascular disease, etc., as cause of exotropia.
History of other affected family members, trauma.
Age of onset, previous treatment, change in frequency and amplitude of deviation.
Sensory testing.
Measurement of alignment near, at distance, and in all gaze positions.
Evaluation of ductions and versions.

Complications
Amblyopia: if exotropia is not alternating and age of onset is <5 yr.
Probable loss of stereoptic ability while eyes are strabismic.
Cosmetic deformity.

Associated Features
Early-onset exotropia: risk of amblyopia 40%; overaction of inferior oblique muscles (50%), but dissociated vertical deviation is rare; often spontaneously resolves by 1 yr of age.
Intermittent exotropia: overaction of inferior oblique muscles (35%), overaction of superior oblique muscles (15%), amblyopia (25%); alphabet-pattern strabismus with greater exotropia in upgaze (V pattern) or downgaze (A pattern).
Third-nerve palsy: pupillary dilation and paralysis of accommodation, simultaneous fourth-, fifth-, and sixth-nerve palsies; involved eye exotropic, hypotropic with ptosis; limitation of elevation, depression, adduction.
Consecutive exotropia: consider slipped or lost medial rectus muscle if postoperative patient and if adduction is limited.
Exotropia associated with osteologic or facial abnormalities: overelevation in adduction caused by horizontal rectus muscle displacement from horizontal meridians; absent superior rectus or superior oblique muscles or tendons.
Duane syndrome: type II associated with limitation of adduction, full abduction, retraction of globe on attempted adduction, overelevation or depression of globe on attempted adduction.

Differential diagnosis
Early-onset exotropia: large angle; age of onset is ~6 wk; no binocular vision unless eyes aligned <2 yr of age.
Intermittent exotropia: typical age of onset is ~18 mo; exotropia greater at distance than at near fixation in most patients.
Third-nerve palsy.
Consecutive exotropia: after treatment (usually surgical) for esotropia.
Exotropia associated with osteologic, cranial, and facial disorders: Crouzon, Apert, Pfeiffer, and Carpenter syndromes.
Duane syndrome: type II associated with exotropia in 20%.

Cause
Early-onset exotropia: either congenital lack of binocular vision with resultant exotropia or mismatch between sensory input and motor response systems with resultant exotropia.
Intermittent exotropia: deficient fusional convergence amplitudes.
Third-nerve palsy: midbrain masses or infarcts, infection or inflammation of cavernous sinus, occlusion of vessels to third cranial nerve.
Consecutive exotropia: after surgery for exotropia.
Duane syndrome: type II postulated to occur because of combined innervation of lateral rectus muscle by sixth cranial nerve and branch of lower division of third nerve.

Epidemiology
Early-onset exotropia: 10% as frequent as early-onset esotropia; no gender or race predilection.
Intermittent exotropia: 1% of children; no race or gender predilection.
Duane syndrome: type II uncommon; no race, gender, or eye predilection.

TREATMENT

Diet and Lifestyle
- No special precautions are necessary.

Pharmacologic Treatment
- No pharmacologic treatment is recommended.

Nonpharmacologic Treatment

Glasses or contact lenses: may be effective in myopic exotropic patients by stimulating accommodative convergence.

Base-in prisms: may be helpful in some patients with intermittent exotropia.

Fusional training exercises: may be helpful in some patients with intermittent exotropia, especially those who have convergence insufficiency (greater exotropia at near than distance fixation).

Alternate-eye occlusion: has been helpful in some patients with intermittent exotropia.

Strabismus surgery: will be necessary for those patients in whom the previous treatments are unsuccessful; procedures include symmetric lateral rectus muscle recessions, monocular lateral rectus recession combined with medial rectus resection, and symmetric medial rectus resections; occasionally, patients will require a single lateral rectus recession.

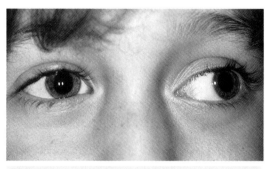

Constant exotropia at distance fixation.

Treatment aims

To achieve excellent visual acuity in each eye.

To achieve straight eyes with comfortable single binocular vision and stereopsis.

To remove cosmetic deformity.

Prognosis

Early-onset exotropia: about one third of cases will spontaneously resolve before 1 yr of age; strabismus surgery is ~70% successful after one operation, 90% after two.

Intermittent exotropia: approximately one third of patients will respond to medical treatment; two thirds will require strabismus surgery; surgery is ~85% successful.

Third-nerve palsy: depends on cause and severity of involvement; total palsy is difficult to treat.

Consecutive exotropia: usually responds to medical or surgical treatment.

Duane syndrome: surgery for type II will result in straight eyes in primary position in almost all patients, but adduction beyond primary position will rarely be obtained.

Follow-up and management

- Care is individualized depending on cause and type of exotropia.

General References

Gregeeson E: The polymorphous exo patient: analysis of 231 consecutive cases, *Acta Ophthalmol* 47:579-583, 1969.

Hardesty HH, Boynton JR, Kennan JP: Treatment of intermittent exotropia, *Arch Ophthalmol* 96:268-280, 1978.

Hoyt WF, Nachtigaller H: Anomalies of the ocular motor nerves: neuroanatomic correlates of paradoxical innervation in Duane's syndrome and related congenital oculomotor disorders, *Am J Ophthalmol* 60:443-451, 1965.

Moore S, Cohen RL: Congenital exotropia, *Am Orthop J* 35:68-74, 1985.

Raab EL, Parks MM: Recession of the lateral recti: early and late postoperative alignments, *Arch Ophthalmol* 82:203-211, 1969.

Eyelid ectropion   (374.1)

DIAGNOSIS

Definition
An outward turn (eversion) of the lid margin and lashes.

Synonyms
None.

Symptoms
Corneal irritation.
Foreign body sensation.
Blurred vision.
Tearing.

Signs
Conjunctival chemosis
Conjunctivitis (chronic).
Corneal exposure.
Corneal drying.

Investigations
Visual acuity test.
Evaluation of lid/lash position.
Slit-lamp examination: to evaluate cornea for ulceration.
Fluorescein staining of cornea: for exposure.

Complications
Corneal scarring: from chronic irritation.
Corneal ulcerations.
Thickening of the lid margin.
Keratinization of conjunctival surface (*see* figure).

Pearls and Considerations
1. Patients with ectropion may be constantly wiping their eyes, which will exacerbate lid laxity and ectropion.
2. Interim bandage contact lens treatment is often helpful in maintaining patient comfort and minimizing corneal desiccation.

Referral Information
Consider oculoplastics referral for surgical repair.

Differential diagnosis
Flaccid types: involutional, paralytic.
Cicatricial: traumatic, spastic.
Mechanical: tumor, swelling.

Cause
Involutional: most common type; relaxation of the orbicularis muscle.
Cicatricial: history of burns, scars from lacerations, complications of blepharoplasty; results in shortening of the anterior lid lamella.
Mechanical: caused by weight of lid tumors.
Paralytic: such as in cases of Bell's palsy or seventh-nerve palsy.

Classification
Congenital (rare).
Cicatricial.
Involutional.

Pathology
See Cause section.

TREATMENT

Diet and Lifestyle
• No special precautions are necessary.

Pharmacologic Treatment
Artificial tears, lubrication.

Nonpharmacologic Treatment
Surgical repair depending on type and cause; possible surgery includes diathermy, lazy-T resection, V-Y–plasty or Z-plasty, horizontal shortening, and canthal tendon surgery.

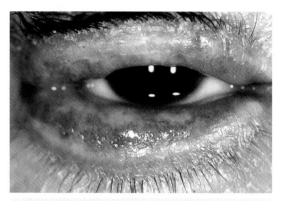

Ectropion of lower lid with keratinization of palpebral conjunctiva in child with ichthyosis congenita.

Treatment aims
To restore the lid tensions and positions to allow proper apposition of the lid and redirection of tear flow.

Prognosis
• The variety of procedures shows that no single repair will work at all times. Care must be taken to tailor an appropriate functional and anatomic result for the individual patient.

Follow-up and management
As needed.

General references
Fraunfelder F, Roy F, editors: *Current ocular therapy*, Philadelphia, 2000, Saunders.
Hornblass A: *Oculoplastic, orbital, and reconstructive surgery*, vol 2, Baltimore, 1990, Lippincott Williams & Wilkins.
Ing E: Ectropion, 2005, www.emedicine.com.
Tasman W, Jaeger E, editors: *Duane's clinical ophthalmology*, vol 5, Philadelphia, 1995, Lippincott-Raven.

DIAGNOSIS

Definition
An inward turn (inversion) of the lid margin and lashes.

Synonyms
None.

Symptoms
Corneal irritation.
Foreign body sensation.
Blurred vision.
Tearing.

Signs
Conjunctival chemosis: caused by irritation from internal turning of lid margin against the eye (*see* Fig. 1).
Conjunctivitis (chronic).
Corneal ulcerations.
Abnormal eyelash position (*see* Fig. 2).

Investigations
Visual acuity test.
Evaluation of lid/lash position.
Slit-lamp examination: to evaluate cornea for ulceration.
Fluorescein staining: of cornea for abrasion.

Complications
Corneal scarring: from chronic irritation.
Corneal ulcerations.

Pearls and Considerations
1. Small amounts of botulinum toxin may be useful in managing spastic entropion.
2. It is important to identify and aggressively treat any blepharitis to reduce risk of corneal infection.

Referral Information
Consider oculoplastics consult for surgical repair.

Differential diagnosis
Epiblepharon (extra fold of skin).
Trichiasis (abnormal or misdirected lashes).
Distichiasis (extra row of lashes).

Cause
Congenital: rare.
Cicatricial: history of ocular inflammation (Stevens-Johnson syndrome, trachoma, chemical or heat burns), resulting in the shortening of the posterior lid surface.
Spastic: found with recent intraocular surgery or inflammation.
Involutional (senile): most common; results from dysfunction of the lower-lid retractor, preseptal orbicularis overriding the pretarsal muscle, or weakness of the inferior preseptal muscle.

Classification
Congenital.
Cicatricial.
Spastic.
Involutional.

Pathology
See Cause section.

TREATMENT

Diet and Lifestyle
- No special precautions are necessary.

Pharmacologic Treatment
Artificial tears, lubrication.

Nonpharmacologic Treatment
Taping of the lid to evert the margin.
Surgical repair.

Treatment aims
To restore the lid anatomy to allow proper positioning of the lids and lashes.

Prognosis
- The abundance of surgical repair procedures shows that no single treatment is always sufficient to reestablish the lid contours. Care must be taken, therefore, to evaluate the cause and to tailor the procedure to the patient's functional and anatomic needs.

Follow-up and management
As needed.

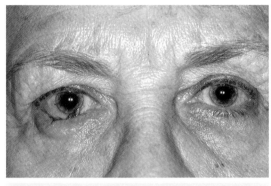

Figure 1   The margin of the right lower lid is turned inward.

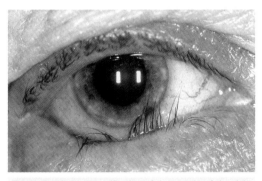

Figure 2   Higher magnification of the margin of the right lower lid. Note the eyelashes rubbing against the cornea.

General references
Fraunfelder F, Roy F, editors: *Current ocular therapy*, Philadelphia, 2000, Saunders.
Hornblass A: *Oculoplastic, orbital, and reconstructive surgery*, vol 2, Baltimore, 1990, Lippincott Williams & Wilkins.
Tasman W, Jaeger E, editors: *Duane's clinical ophthalmology*, vol 5, Philadelphia, 1995, Lippincott-Raven.

Eyelid hemorrhage   (374.81)

DIAGNOSIS

Definition
Subepidermal bleeding of the skin around the eye.

Synonyms
Ecchymosis, "black eye."

Symptoms
Swelling.
Periorbital pressure.
Pain.
Lid discoloration.
Itching.

Signs
Lid edema, lid ecchymosis (*see* figure).
Ptosis.
Double or blurred vision.

Investigations
Inspection of lids: to rule out traumatic injury.
Palpation of lids: to rule out occult malignancy.
History of drug use.
Visual acuity test.
Ocular motility.
Slit lamp examination.
Dilated fundus examination.

Complications
Secondary ptosis: as a result of inflammation.
Associated orbital fractures.
Associated orbital hemorrhage: with compressive neuropathy.

Pearls and Considerations
1. Evaluation of traumatic ecchymosis should include full dilated examination to rule out further ocular trauma and ocular motility testing to evaluate for orbital blow-out fracture or muscle entrapment.
2. Anticoagulation therapy is a common pharmacologic cause of ecchymosis and occurs in up to 25% of patients receiving this therapy.

Referral Information
None, unless further trauma requires care.

Differential diagnosis
Usually easily distinguished by history. With unknown cause, occult tumor should be ruled out.

Cause
- Most common cause is trauma.
- Rule out drug-induced side effect.
Multiple drugs have been associated with spontaneous lid bleeding.
- Hutchinson's syndrome (adrenal cortex neuroblastoma with orbital metastasis) is rare.

Immunology
- No immunologic factors have been associated with lid bleeding.

TREATMENT

Diet and Lifestyle
- No special precautions are necessary.

Pharmacologic Treatment
Modification (if possible) of any medications that may precipitate eyelid bleeding.

Nonpharmacologic Treatment
Nonspecific treatment with use of cool compresses to decrease swelling and for increased comfort over 24-48 hr; warm compresses can be considered after 48 hr.

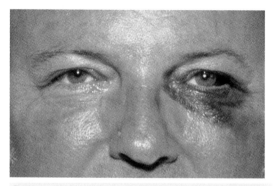

Ecchymosis of the left eye. Trauma to the left eye causes hemorrhage mainly into left lower lid. Note also that the same trauma caused a conjunctival hemorrhage temporarily in the left eye.

Treatment aims
To relieve lid swelling and discomfort.

Other treatments
Cessation of any drugs (e.g., aspirin), if possible based on other medical issues, that may induce capillary fragility, leading to hemorrhage with even minimal trauma.

Prognosis
- If isolated findings are related to drug use or trauma, resolution should result in no permanent disfigurement or ocular dysfunction.

Follow-up and management
- As needed to ensure that complete resolution occurs without residual ptosis from disruption of the levator muscle complex.

General references
Kaiser RS, Williams GA: Ocular manifestations of hematologic diseases. In Tasman W et al, editors: *Duane's clinical ophthalmology* (CD-ROM), Baltimore, 2004, Lippincott Williams & Wilkins.
Patel B: Lids. In *Ocular differential diagnosis*, Baltimore, 1997, Lippincott Williams & Wilkins.
Tasman W, Jaeger E, et al: *Duane's clinical ophthalmology*, vol 5, Philadelphia, 1995, Lippincott-Raven.

Eyelid noninfectious dermatoses   (373.3)

DIAGNOSIS

Definition
Inflammation of the eyelid skin by other than an infectious agent.

Synonyms
None.

Symptoms
Irritation.
Itching.
Tearing.

Signs
Chemosis (*see* figure).
Watery discharge.
Punctate keratopathy.
Lid crusting.
Lid swelling.
Scaling.
Lichenification.

Investigations
History of exposure to potential irritants.
Slit-lamp examination: to rule out conjunctival papillary responses or corneal changes.
For atopic types: history of food allergy or respiratory allergy; elevated immunoglobulin E (IgE) levels.

Pearls and Considerations
Treatment of periorbital dermatoses with steroids carries a risk for serious side effects (e.g., glaucoma, cataract) with prolonged use. Care should be taken to choose a steroid with minimal penetration.

Referral Information
None.

Cause
Contact dermatitis: results from exposure to a wide variety of environmental substances, including dyes, resins, drugs, and metals; certain eye medications (neomycin, atropine) act as sensitizing agents.
Irritant type: results from substances with irritant properties that cause excessive moisture; there is no allergy response in this type.
Allergic type: occurs in sensitized individuals and involves T-cell–mediated responses.

Epidemiology
- Atopic is most likely in younger individuals.

Classification
- Allergic versus contact.

Immunology
- Allergic types require prior sensitization and T-cell–mediated responses.
- Atopic reactions have high IgE levels.

TREATMENT

Diet and Lifestyle
- Avoid inciting agents, if any.

Pharmacologic Treatment
Steroid lotions and creams.
Cromolyn drops (for atopic types).
Antihistamines.

Nonpharmacologic Treatment
- Caution against rubbing of eyes after exposure to potentially irritating substances, such as chemicals, soaps, detergents, dyes, and plants.
- Apply cold compresses for symptomatic relief.

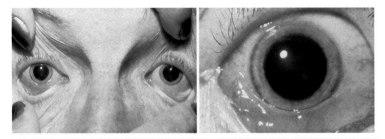

Chemosis and mild eyelid erythema in patient with allergy to dilating drops.

Treatment aims
To alleviate irritation and remove inciting agent.

Prognosis
- Removal of the noxious stimulus should result in resolution of the irritant condition.

Follow-up and management
- Avoid known allergens or irritants; topical treatments prevent scarring.

General references
Fraunfelder F, Roy F, editors: *Current ocular therapy*, Philadelphia, 2000, Saunders.
Hornblass A: *Oculoplastic, orbital, and reconstructive surgery*, vol 2, Baltimore, 1990, Lippincott Williams & Wilkins.
Tan MH, Lebwohl M, Esser AC, Wei H: Penetration of 0.005% fluticasone propionate ointment in eyelid skin, *J Am Acad Dermatol* 45(3):392-396, 2001.

Foreign body, intraocular   (871.6)

DIAGNOSIS

Definition
An object embedded within the internal space of the eye.

Synonyms
None.

Symptoms
Pain.
Floaters.
Decreased vision.
Red eye.
Lid swelling.

Signs
Entrance wound on the cornea, sclera (*see* Fig. 1).
Subconjunctival hemorrhage.
Iris transillumination defect.
Cataract.
Peaked pupil.
Vitreous hemorrhage.
Evidence of an intraocular foreign body: when viewing the anterior segment or posterior segment of the eye.

Investigations
History.
Careful slit-lamp examination: looking for an entrance site.
Seidel test: to check for a wound leak.
B-scan ultrasound: if the view of the fundus is obscured by cataract or corneal pathology or vitreous hemorrhage.
Computed tomography: if metallic foreign object is suspected (*see* Fig. 2).
Magnetic resonance imaging: if looking for glass, wood, or other vegetable matter.

Complications
Endophthalmitis: about 10.7% [1].
Cataract formation.
Retinal detachment.
Uveal prolapse.
Vitreous loss.
Choroidal rupture, hemorrhage, or detachment.
Optic nerve damage.
Secondary glaucoma.
Loss of vision.
Loss of eye.
Phthisis.
Toxic reaction to metal: copper alloy metals at high concentration: calchosis, Kayser-Fleischer ring, sunflower cataract; copper pure: massive reaction, endophthalmitis; iron ionizes: siderosis bulb; zinc and lead: chronic nongranulomatous reaction; gold, silver, aluminum, and glass: almost inert, little or no reaction.

Differential diagnosis
Ruptured globe secondary to blunt trauma.

Cause
- Mechanisms of injury include:
Hammering metal on metal.
Projectile weapon.
Explosion.
Auto accident with shattered glass.
Machine tool.
Gardening accident.
Tree branch.
Metal dart.

Epidemiology
- Most intraocular foreign bodies are secondary to hammering metal on metal.
- Most patients retain a final visual acuity of 20/40 or better.

Classification
- Classification is based on location:
Corneal.
Anterior chamber.
Iris.
Vitreal.
Retinal (*see* Fig. 3).

Diagnosis continued on p. 128

TREATMENT

Diet and Lifestyle
Safety glasses.

Pharmacologic Treatment
Topical antibiotics: e.g., ciprofloxacin or ofloxacin.

Topical cycloplegics: e.g., atropine sulfate 1%.

Intravitreal antibiotics: if endophthalmitis is suspected; usually amikacin and vancomycin are used; if the foreign body is vegetable matter, be concerned about fungus.

Topical steroids: to decrease inflammation.

Consider IV fluoroquinolone.

Nonpharmacologic Treatment
Emergency surgery: to remove foreign body from the eye; if the foreign body is metallic, a rare-earth magnet is often used at surgery to localize the foreign body and aid in its removal.

Treatment aims
To remove foreign body promptly.

Prognosis
- Prognosis is good if the foreign body is removed promptly and is small. The larger the foreign body, the more potential damage to intraocular contents, which will affect final visual outcome.
- Prognosis is more guarded if secondary endophthalmitis ensues.

Follow-up and management
Frequent follow-up visits in the postoperative period to look for signs of endophthalmitis, retinal detachment, or other possible complications.

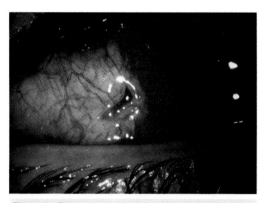

Figure 1   Entrance wound on the sclera of a patient secondary to intraocular glass fragment from a motor vehicle accident.

Treatment continued on p. 129

DIAGNOSIS—cont'd

Pearls and Considerations
1. Although often difficult, visual acuity should be recorded at initial presentation of ocular trauma patients. It is a valuable indicator of long-term visual prognosis.
2. Patients must be thoroughly educated regarding the importance of protecting the fellow eye.

Referral Information
Refer for appropriate imaging and surgical intervention as each patient requires.

TREATMENT—cont'd

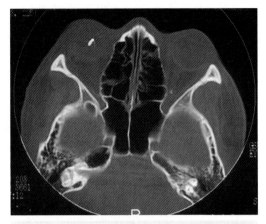

Figure 2   Computed tomography scan of a patient with an intraocular metallic foreign body caused by an injury related to a gunshot wound.

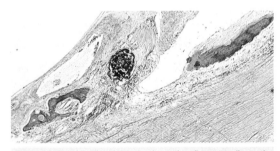

Figure 3   Iron foreign body in the retina (hematoxylin-eosin stain).

Key reference

1. Flynn H: Current management of endophthalmitis, *Int Ophthalmol Clin* 44(4):115-137, 2004.

General references

Hartstein ME, Fink SR: Traumatic eyelid injuries, *Int Ophthalmol Clin* 42(2):123-134, 2002.

Lit ES, Young LH: Anterior and posterior segment intraocular foreign bodies, *Int Ophthalmol Clin* 42(3):107-120, 2002.

Rubsamen PE: Posterior segment ocular trauma. In Yanoff M, Duker JS, editors: *Ophthalmology*, E-dition, St Louis, 2006, Elsevier.

Fourth-nerve palsy (trochlear) (378.53)

DIAGNOSIS

Definition
Paralysis or paresis of the fourth cranial nerve (CN IV, trochlear).

Synonyms
None.

Symptoms
Vertical diplopia.
Head tilt.
Reading material held down and out.
Patient reads into the next line of print.

Signs
Hyperphoria or tropia: increases across from the higher eye or on ipsilateral head tilt.

Investigations
Measurement of the hyperphoria/hypertropia: in cardinal positions of gaze.
Measurement of subjective cyclotorsion: with Maddox rods and Bagolini striated lenses.
Assessment of objective cyclotorsion: with ophthalmoscopy or fundus photographs.
Old photographs: to identify head tilt.
Neuroimaging.
Vasculopathic workup.

Pearls and Considerations
1. To distinguish from ipsilateral inferior oblique fibrosis: vertical deviation of a patient with fourth-nerve palsy will worsen in downgaze, and vertical imbalance of a patient with inferior rectus fibrosis will worsen in upgaze.
2. Except in cases of trauma, trochlear nerve (CN IV) palsy is much less common than oculomotor (CN III) or abducens (CN VI) palsy.

Referral Information
Surgical referral for extraocular muscle (EOM) realignment only in select patients.

Differential diagnosis
Loss of vertical fusional reserves
Skew deviation
Myasthenia gravis
Graves' orbitopathy
Contralateral third-nerve palsy

Cause
Adults
Trauma.
Idiopathic.
Ischemic.
Neoplastic.
Aneurysm.
Children
Trauma.
Congenital.

Classification
Knapp's classification
Class I: hypertropia is greatest in the action of the overacting inferior oblique muscle.
Class II: hypertropia is greatest in the action of the paretic superior oblique muscle.
Class III: hypertropia is the same in the entire opposite field.
Class IV: hypertropia is the same in the entire opposite field and in downgaze (L-shaped pattern).
Class V: hypertropia is the same across downgaze.

Associated features
See table.

Anatomic localization of a "complicated" fourth-nerve palsy: the checklist examination

What to look for	Anatomic localization	Cause
Contralateral Horner's sign	Locus ceruleus (nuclear)	Trauma, neoplasm
Contralateral internuclear ophthalmoplegia	Medial longitudinal fasciculus (nuclear)	Infarct
Ipsilateral relative afferent pupillary defect	Brachium of superior colliculus (fascicular)	Tumor
Dorsal midbrain syndrome (vertical gaze palsy, eyelid retraction, tectal pupils, convergence-retraction nystagmus)	Anterior medullary velum (fascicular)	Trauma
Bilateral fourth-nerve palsies	Anterior medullary velum	Trauma, tumor, infarct
Truncal ataxia and ipsilateral dysmetria	Superior cerebellar peduncle	Trauma
Ipsilateral third and sixth nerves, CN VI, and oculosympathetic nerves	Cavernous sinus	Tumor

TREATMENT

Diet and Lifestyle
- No special precautions are necessary.

Pharmacologic Treatment
- No pharmacologic treatment is recommended.

Nonpharmacologic Treatment
Surgical Treatment by Knapp's Classification
Class I: inferior oblique muscle weakening.

Class II: superior oblique muscle tuck.

Class III: superior oblique tuck and inferior oblique weakening.

Class IV: superior oblique tuck, inferior oblique myectomy, and resection of ipsilateral inferior rectus muscle.

Class V: superior oblique tuck and tenectomy of contralateral superior oblique muscle.

Nonsurgical Treatment
Base-down prism before the hypertropic eye.

Eye patch.

Treatment aims
To restore and maintain single, simultaneous, binocular vision in primary position at distance and near.
To eliminate head tilting.

Prognosis
- Vasculopathic fourth-nerve palsies resolve in 3 mo.
- Traumatic fourth-nerve palsies may require 12 mo.
- No surgical intervention should be undertaken in a traumatic fourth-nerve palsy for 1 yr unless secondary contracture is occurring.

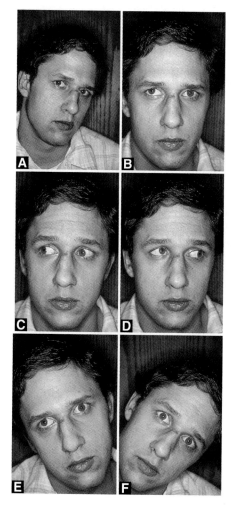

Figure 1 A, This man has a long-standing right fourth-nerve paresis with a left head tilt. **B,** Head straightened. **C** and **D,** Right hypertropia diminishes in right gaze and increases in left gaze. **E,** Significant right hypertropia on right head tilt. **F,** Minimal hypertropia on left head tilt.

General references
Bielschowsky A: Etiology, prognosis, and treatment of ocular paralyses, *Am J Ophthamol* 22: 723-734, 1943.

Chen CH, Hwang WJ, Tsai TT, Lai ML: Midbrain hemorrhage presenting with trochlear nerve palsy, *Chung Hua Hsueh Tsa Chih/Chinese Med J* 63(2):138-143, 2000.

Glaser JS, Siatkowski RM: Infranuclear disorders of eye movement. In Tasman W et al, editors: *Duane's clinical ophthalmology* (CD-ROM), Baltimore, 2004, Lippincott Williams & Wilkins.

Yanoff M, Duker J, editors: *Ophthalmology*, St Louis, 2003, Elsevier.

Fuchs' heterochromic iridocyclitis   (364.21)

DIAGNOSIS

Definition
An uncommon form of anterior uveitis. Generally, there is unilateral low-grade inflammation of the iris and ciliary body leading to iris depigmentation with fine keratic precipitates and secondary cataract.

Synonyms
Fuchs' heterochromic uveitis, Fuchs' syndrome.

Symptoms
Decreased vision: most patients are asymptomatic in the early stages; cataract is typically seen in Fuchs' heterochromic iridocyclitis and will result in decreased vision; in patients with glaucoma, decreased vision may be noticed if the glaucoma is far advanced at presentation; unlike in many other forms of uveitis, hyperemia, pain, and photophobia are not reported.

Heterochromia: the patient or a family member may notice the difference in iris color between the two eyes.

Age at onset: the disease is usually diagnosed in young and middle-aged adults; most cases are advanced at diagnosis, so onset must be considerably earlier; rarely diagnosed in children or adolescents.

Signs
Heterochromia: the involved iris is typically lighter (*see* figure), although patients who already have very lightly pigmented irises may have the darker iris on the involved side.

Keratic precipitates: numerous characteristic "stellate-shaped" keratic precipitates are seen diffusely on the corneal endothelium.

Anterior-chamber flare and cells: a mild to moderate, chronic anterior-chamber reaction is seen; characteristically, this reaction is unresponsive to topical steroids; unlike in many other forms of anterior uveitis, posterior synechiae do not form.

Fine vessels in the anterior-chamber angle: fine blood vessels are seen in the angle on gonioscopy; they may bleed, producing a hyphema after intraocular surgery; rarely they may bleed spontaneously.

Investigations
Uveitis workup: the diagnosis of Fuchs' heterochromic iridocyclitis is usually obvious, and extensive laboratory and radiologic testing is not necessary.

Complications
Cataract: a cataract usually develops in the involved eye with long-standing disease; the cataract usually begins as a cortical or subcapsular opacity that generally progresses to a mature or hypermature state.

Glaucoma: common, but not an inevitable complication; 25%-50% of patients with Fuchs' heterochromic iridocyclitis develop glaucoma.

Differential diagnosis
- The differential diagnosis includes other forms of uveitis that are typically unilateral, including:

Glaucomatocyclitic crisis.
Herpes simplex.
Herpes zoster.

- Other causes of heterochromia include:

Horner's syndrome.
Iris tumors.
Hereditary heterochromia.
Trauma.
Neovascularization.
Siderosis.

Cause
- The cause is unknown. Some evidence indicates sympathetic denervation in involved eyes, suggesting an abiotrophy (late manifestation of a congenital defect).
- Possible role of herpes simplex virus (HSV) infection and ocular toxoplasmosis.

Epidemiology
- The disease is relatively rare and usually sporadic.
- Most patients are diagnosed between 35 and 40 yr of age.

Associated features
- Reported association with certain neural tube abnormalities (e.g., status dysraphicus, syringomyelia).

Immunology
- High incidence of seropositivity for antibodies against certain corneal epithelial proteins, but the significance of this is unclear.

Pathology
- Atrophy of the iris stroma with loss of melanocytes. A nongranulomatous inflammatory reaction in the trabecular meshwork, iris, and ciliary body is characterized by lymphocytic and plasma cell infiltration.

TREATMENT

Diet and Lifestyle
- No special precautions are necessary.

Pharmacologic Treatment
Corticosteroids
- One of the characteristic features of Fuchs' heterochromic iridocyclitis is nonresponsiveness to treatment with corticosteroids. Because steroids carry a significant risk of side effects and are of no benefit, their use in patients with this disease is contraindicated.

Aqueous Suppressants and Prostaglandin Analogs
- In patients with glaucoma, medical treatment is often very effective. As with most other forms of uveitis, miotics should be avoided. Aqueous suppressants should be the first line of treatment. The role of prostaglandin analogs in glaucoma associated with inflammation is unclear because of the possible increase in inflammation, which is theoretically possible with prostaglandin treatment. Until more is known, prostaglandin analogs should probably be avoided.

Nonpharmacologic Treatment
Cataract surgery: in patients with a visually significant cataract, surgery with lens implantation is indicated and usually produces good results; the risk of postoperative inflammation or increased intraocular pressure is higher than in the usual cataract patient; intraoperative or postoperative intraocular hemorrhage is a significant risk.

Laser trabeculoplasty: usually not effective in the glaucoma associated with Fuchs' heterochromic iridocyclitis and is contraindicated because of the risk of increased inflammation.

Filtering surgery: aqueous shunt devices usually have good results; because of the chronic inflammatory response, antifibrotic agents such as 5-fluorouracil or mitomycin-C should be used.

Treatment aims
- The inflammatory response in Fuchs' heterochromic iridocyclitis cannot be suppressed with currently available treatments. Thus, unlike for most other forms of uveitis, suppression of inflammation is not a treatment goal. In patients with cataract, the aim of treatment is to restore useful vision. In patients with glaucoma, preservation of vision and control of intraocular pressure are the main treatment aims.

Prognosis
- The prognosis in most patients is good. Cataract surgery is usually successful, and the glaucoma can often be controlled with treatment to prevent severe vision loss.

Follow-up and management
- Patients not showing evidence of cataract or glaucoma may be followed annually without treatment to watch for the development of complications.

Patients with cataract or chronic glaucoma should be managed as any other patient with these conditions.

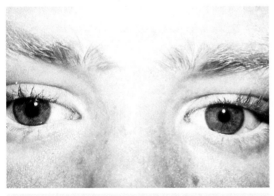

Fuchs' heterochromic iridocyclitis. The lighter-colored iris indicates the involved eye.

General references
Barequet IS, Li Q, Wang Y, et al: Herpes simplex virus DNA identification from aqueous fluid in Fuchs' heterochromic iridocyclitis, *Am J Ophthalmol* 129(5):672-673, 2000.

Jones NP: Fuchs' heterochromic uveitis: an update, *Surv Ophthalmol* 37:253-272, 1993.

La Hey E, de Vries J, Langerhorst CT, et al: Treatment and prognosis of secondary glaucoma in Fuchs' heterochromic iridocyclitis, *Am J Ophthalmol* 116:327-340, 1993.

Glaucoma associated with anterior-chamber anomalies   (365.41)

DIAGNOSIS

Definition
Glaucoma resulting from congenital malformations within the anterior chamber.

Synonyms
None; often associated with Axenfeld's and Rieger's anomalies.

Symptoms
- As in most chronic glaucomas, patients are usually asymptomatic.
- **Decreased vision:** depending on the age of onset and severity of the glaucoma, some patients will note decreased vision.
- **Ocular and skeletal deformities:** some patients or parents of patients may note the ocular or skeletal deformities in severe cases.

Signs
Cornea: prominent and anteriorly displaced Schwalbe's line (posterior embryotoxon).

Anterior-chamber angle: prominent, large iridocorneal adhesions attached to Schwalbe's line; between these adhesions, the angle appears to be open.

Iris: may appear normal in Axenfeld's anomaly (743.44); in Rieger's anomaly (743.44) there may be areas of stromal thinning and atrophy, hole formation (polycoria), or distortion and displacement of the pupil (corectopia).

Glaucoma: 50%-60% of patients with Axenfeld's or Rieger's anomaly will develop glaucoma with elevation of intraocular pressure and typical optic disc cupping and visual field loss; age of onset varies from infancy to adulthood, with most cases developing during childhood or adolescence.

Investigations
Complete eye examination including gonioscopy: patients with glaucoma who are old enough should have perimetry and optic disc imaging.

Pediatric evaluation: children should be examined by a pediatrician to rule out any systemic anomalies.

Associated Features
- Some patients with Rieger's anomaly will have dental abnormalities or hypoplasia of the facial bones; this is called *Rieger's syndrome*. Other systemic anomalies involving the pituitary, central nervous system, heart, ears, umbilicus, and genitourinary system have been reported.

Pearls and Considerations
1. Other anterior-chamber anomalies that may result in glaucoma include aniridia and Peters' anomaly.
2. Often, Axenfeld's and Rieger's anomalies are grouped together under the term *Axenfeld-Rieger syndrome*.
3. When Axenfeld's anomaly is associated with glaucoma, it is called *Axenfeld's syndrome*.

Referral Information
1. Refer to pediatrician to rule out further systemic anomalies.
2. Refer for glaucoma surgery as appropriate.

Differential diagnosis
Iridocorneal epithelial syndrome.
Posterior polymorphous corneal dystrophy.
Peters' anomaly.
Aniridia, congenital iris hypoplasia, oculo-dentodigital dysplasia, ectopia lentis et pupillae, congenital ectropion uvea and previous uveitis with peripheral anterior synechiae.

Cause
- It is thought that there is a developmental arrest of structures in the anterior segment derived from neural crest cells. As a result, there is retention of the primordial endothelium and the basement membrane, which leads to iris and angle changes and obstructs the outflow of aqueous. Many pedigrees demonstrate an autosomal dominant mode of inheritance. Spontaneous cases are often associated with chromosomal anomalies.

Pathology
- Schwalbe's line is unusually prominent. Peripheral iris strands are adherent to the corneoscleral junction. A cellular layer with a basement membrane is seen over the iris. The iris stroma is hypoplastic in some areas. Trabecular meshwork is attenuated and hypocellular. Schlemm's canal is not developed completely.

TREATMENT

Diet and Lifestyle
- No precautions are necessary.

Pharmacologic Treatment
- Any of the medications available for treating chronic glaucoma may be used (*see* Appendix A).
- As in many childhood glaucomas, medical treatment is often ineffective.

Nonpharmacologic Treatment
Filtering Surgery
Many patients with severe glaucoma will require filtering surgery. Because such surgery often fails in children or young adults, 5-fluorouracil or mitomycin-C is often used. If filtration surgery fails, an aqueous tube-shunt device may be tried. In severe, recalcitrant cases, cyclodestruction may become necessary. Laser trabeculoplasty is ineffective in these cases.

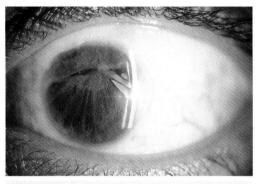

Rieger's anomaly.

Treatment aims
To control the intraocular pressure.
To preserve visual function.

Prognosis
- Depends on the severity of the glaucoma. In the absence of glaucoma or severe congenital anomalies, the Axenfeld-Rieger anomaly causes only cosmetic problems. If the glaucoma can be controlled, the prognosis is quite good. In severe cases, treatment is often not effective, and severe loss of visual function ensues.

Follow-up and management
- Patients are managed as any chronic glaucoma patient, with regular optic disc evaluations and perimetry.

General references
Beck AD, Lynch MG: Pediatric glaucoma. In *Focal points clinical modules for ophthalmologists*, vol 15, no 5, section 2, San Francisco, 1997, American Academy of Ophthalmology.
Shields MB, Buckley E, Klintworth GK, Thresher R: Axenfeld-Rieger syndrome: a spectrum of developmental disorders, *Surv Ophthalmol* 29:387-409, 1985.
Waring GO III, Rodrigues MM, Laibson PR: Anterior chamber cleavage syndrome: a stepladder classification, *Surv Ophthalmol* 20:3-27, 1975.

DIAGNOSIS

Definition

Elevated intraocular pressure (IOP) or optic neuropathy as a symptom of an underlying congenital anomaly (systemic disease).

Synonyms

None; associated anomalies include neurofibromatosis and Sturge-Weber syndrome.

Symptoms

Glaucoma Associated with Neurofibromatosis

- Children with plexiform neuromas involving the lids often present with a unilateral congenital or childhood glaucoma. Occasionally there may be bilateral involvement. Other congenital anomalies (e.g., iris neuromas [Lisch nodules], congenital ectropion uveae, anterior-chamber anomalies) may be present.

Glaucoma Associated with Sturge-Weber Syndrome

Cosmetic blemish: the most noticeable manifestation is the large hemangioma involving the face (*see* figure).

Signs

Glaucoma Associated with Neurofibromatosis

See Symptoms.

Glaucoma Associated with Sturge-Weber Syndrome

Port-wine hemangioma of the face: typically present at birth, unilateral, and in the distribution of the trigeminal nerve.

Dilated episcleral and conjunctival veins: easily seen with the slit lamp and often visible grossly.

Choroidal hemangioma: will be visible ophthalmoscopically.

Heterochromia: involvement of the iris with the uveal hemangioma may produce darker iris on the involved side.

Congenital glaucoma: in ~50% of patients in whom the facial hemangioma involves the ophthalmic and maxillary branch of the trigeminal nerve, glaucoma will be present; typical features include corneal and ocular enlargement, elevated IOP, and optic disc cupping.

Investigations

Glaucoma Associated with Neurofibromatosis

- Children with neurofibromatosis should have a complete medical and neurologic evaluation. Central nervous system (CNS) tumors and a variety of other systemic anomalies may be found.

Glaucoma Associated with Sturge-Weber Syndrome

Examination under anesthesia: *see* Glaucoma, congenital.

Neurologic evaluation: vascular CNS anomalies are common; evaluation by a pediatrician or pediatric neurologist is indicated.

Complications

Glaucoma Associated with Neurofibromatosis

- Involvement of the iris, angle, limbus, or choroid may make filtering surgery difficult.

Glaucoma Associated with Sturge-Weber Syndrome

Loss of vision: a risk in any child with a congenital glaucoma; fortunately, Sturge-Weber syndrome is usually unilateral, and the contralateral eye is rarely involved.

Exudative retinal detachment: may develop over the choroidal hemangioma.

Expulsive choroidal hemorrhage: patients with large choroidal hemangiomas have a significant risk of expulsive hemorrhage after intraocular surgery.

Pearls and Considerations

Topic too broad for specific recommendations.

Referral Information

Refer to appropriate subspecialist based on etiology and underlying systemic disease.

Differential diagnosis

With neurofibromatosis
Other hamartomas with ocular involvement. Orbital and lid tumors. Primary congenital glaucoma.
With Sturge-Weber syndrome
None.

Cause

With neurofibromatosis
- Most cases of neurofibromatosis are inherited as autosomal dominant. The glaucoma is thought to result from incomplete development of the angle, with persistence of embryonic tissue, as well as maldevelopment of Schlemm's canal.

With Sturge-Weber syndrome
- The cause is unknown, but heredity does not seem to be a factor in most cases. The mechanism of the glaucoma is controversial. In infants the mechanism appears to be caused by a developmental anomaly of the angle, as in congenital glaucoma. In older patients, elevated episcleral venous pressure may play a role.

Epidemiology

With neurofibromatosis
- Neurofibromatosis is estimated to occur in 1:2500-3300 births.

With Sturge-Weber syndrome
- Most cases are spontaneous without any apparent familial, racial, or gender preference. The condition is uncommon but not rare.

Classification

With neurofibromatosis
- Two forms have been described:

Neurofibromatosis *type 1* is more common and is characterized by proliferation of neuromas and astrocytes, with mainly cutaneous and peripheral nerve involvement. The gene has been localized to chromosome 17.

Neurofibromatosis *type 2* is characterized by the proliferation of many cell types and involves mainly the CNS. The gene has been localized to chromosome 22.

TREATMENT

Diet and Lifestyle
- No special precautions are necessary.

Pharmacologic Treatment
Glaucoma Associated with Neurofibromatosis
- Pharmacologic treatment for any chronic glaucoma should be tried. In children with congenital glaucoma, pharmacologic treatment is often not effective.

Glaucoma Associated with Sturge-Weber Syndrome
- The severity of the glaucoma in Sturge-Weber syndrome varies greatly. If ocular enlargement is not present, medical treatment may be successful in controlling IOP. Drugs that suppress aqueous production are generally most useful.

Nonpharmacologic Treatment
Glaucoma Associated with Neurofibromatosis
- In patients with severe lid and ocular involvement, surgery is often unsuccessful. Filtering surgery, tube-shunt devices, or cyclodestructive procedures may be considered in severe cases, depending on the extent of lid and ocular involvement with neurofibromas.

Glaucoma Associated with Sturge-Weber Syndrome
Argon laser trabeculoplasty: some success has been reported in adult patients with late onset of glaucoma; in young children, however, trabeculoplasty is usually not effective.

Trabeculotomy, goniotomy: these procedures may be tried in infants with congenital glaucoma, but success rates are lower in Sturge-Weber syndrome than in primary congenital glaucoma.

Filtering surgery: some success has been reported with trabeculectomy; in younger patients, mitomycin-C or 5-fluorouracil may be used; cyclophotocoagulation or aqueous tube-shunt devices may be tried in recalcitrant cases, but there is little reported experience with the modalities; all surgery in these cases carries a risk of choroidal hemorrhage.

Other Treatments
Glaucoma Associated with Sturge-Weber Syndrome
- A variety of laser treatments for the skin are available to improve the patient's appearance by blanching the port-wine hemangioma on the face.

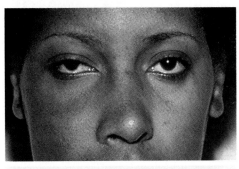

Sturge-Weber syndrome showing facial hemangioma.

Treatment aims
With neurofibromatosis
To control IOP.
To preserve visual function.
- In patients with plexiform neuromas, cosmesis is often a severe problem, and surgery to improve the patient's appearance may be indicated.

With Sturge-Weber syndrome
To control IOP.
To preserve vision.

Prognosis
With neurofibromatosis
- In patients with plexiform neuroma of the lid and glaucoma, the prognosis is quite poor, and most patients have marked loss of visual function.

With Sturge-Weber syndrome
- The prognosis depends on the age of onset and severity of the glaucoma. Generally, the later in life the glaucoma develops, the better the prognosis. Patients with extensive choroidal, iris, and angle hemangiomas tend to have a worse outcome.

Follow-up and management
With neurofibromatosis
- Careful, lifelong follow-up as for any chronic childhood glaucoma is required.

With Sturge-Weber syndrome
- As with any juvenile glaucoma, careful and frequent follow-up throughout life is required. Patients should be carefully monitored for the development of CNS manifestations. Patients with known cerebral or spinal meningeal hemangiomas are at significant risk from general or spinal anesthesia for any surgical procedure.

General references
Iwach AG, Hoskins HD, Hetherington J, Shaffer RN: Analysis of surgical and medical management of glaucoma in Sturge-Weber syndrome, *Ophthalmology* 97:904-909, 1990.

Weiss JS, Ritch R: Glaucoma in the phakomatoses. In Ritch R, Shields MB, Krupin T, editors: *The glaucomas,* ed 2, St Louis, 1996, Mosby, pp 899-907.

Glaucoma associated with elevated episcleral venous pressure   (365.82)

DIAGNOSIS

Definition
Elevated intraocular pressure (IOP) and optic neuropathy caused by increased pressure in the episcleral veins, inhibiting uveoscleral aqueous outflow.

Synonyms
None.

Symptoms
- In milder cases with slow onset, the patient may be asymptomatic.

Pain: depending on the cause of the elevated episcleral venous pressure and the rapidity of onset, patient may have pain that varies from mild to severe.

Decreased vision: in acute conditions (e.g., carotid-cavernous fistulae), significant loss of vision may occur at the onset of the episcleral venous pressure elevation; in chronic conditions the glaucomatous damage to the optic nerve may progress to symptomatic visual loss.

Tinnitus: with arteriovenous (AV) shunting the patient may be aware of a pulsatile tinnitus corresponding to the heartbeat.

Signs
Hyperemia: elevated episcleral venous pressure, whether from venous obstruction or AV shunting, is associated with dilation of the episcleral venous plexus.

Elevated IOP.

Blood in Schlemm's canal: the increased venous pressure results in increased blood in Schlemm's canal visible by gonioscopy.

Optic disc cupping and visual field loss: may be seen in the presence of chronic elevations of IOP.

Proptosis, limitations of eye movements: some causes of episcleral venous pressure elevation are associated with orbital neoplastic, inflammatory, or vascular diseases that may produce proptosis or extraocular muscle restriction.

Audible bruit: some AV shunts may be associated with an audible vascular bruit over the orbit or temple.

Investigations
Measurement of episcleral venous pressure: several devices are available for measurement of episcleral venous pressure on the surface of the eye; this may be useful for diagnosis in doubtful cases.

Orbital imaging: radiography, computed tomography scan, magnetic resonance imaging, and ultrasound are often useful in diagnosing orbital processes associated with elevated episcleral venous pressure.

Arteriography: carotid and cerebral angiography may also be useful for diagnosing carotid-cavernous fistulae and other conditions.

Differential diagnosis
Conditions associated with ocular hyperemia and glaucoma (e.g., uveitis, keratitis, scleritis).

Cause
Aqueous leaves the eye through the aqueous collector channels that drain aqueous from Schlemm's canal to the episcleral venous plexus on the surface of the eye. In order for aqueous to flow from the anterior chamber into the venous system, IOP must be greater than episcleral venous pressure. The relationship between IOP and episcleral venous pressure is expressed by Goldmann's equation, $P_i = F/C + P_{ev}$ (where P_i is intraocular pressure, F is aqueous flow rate, C is the facility of outflow, and P_{ev} is the episcleral venous pressure). This equation shows that elevation of episcleral venous pressure will elevate the IOP independently of aqueous production or outflow, and that IOP cannot fall below episcleral venous pressure in the intact eye.

Associated features
- The associated features will depend on the underlying cause.

Diagnosis continued on p. 140

TREATMENT

Pharmacologic Treatment

- Because the effects of episcleral venous pressure are largely independent of aqueous dynamics, medical treatment is often unsuccessful. In milder, more chronic cases, aqueous suppressants have shown some success.

Treatment aims

To treat the underlying disease (e.g., carotid-cavernous fistulae; orbital, neck, or thoracic tumors): a priority.

To control IOP and preserve visual function.

Prognosis

- The prognosis depends on the nature of the underlying cause, the severity and time course of the onset, and the duration of the glaucoma. Patients with a chronic elevation of episcleral venous pressure that cannot be relieved generally have a poor long-term prognosis.
- Relatively abrupt onset of elevated episcleral venous pressure (as in carotid-cavernous fistula or thyroid ophthalmopathy) may produce acute irreversible injury to the optic nerve.

Follow-up and management

- Patients with a chronic glaucoma should be followed with frequent and regular optic disc and visual field evaluation.

Treatment continued on p. 141

DIAGNOSIS—cont'd

Complications

Optic neuropathy: elevated episcleral venous pressure may damage the optic nerve by two mechanisms: (1) in the presence of elevated IOP, cupping may develop as in any glaucoma, and (2) many conditions are associated with compressive effects in the orbit that may produce a picture resembling ischemic or compressive optic neuropathy.

Classification

Causes of Episcleral Venous Pressure Elevation

Venous obstruction.
Orbital tumors.
Thyroid ophthalmopathy.
Superior vena caval syndrome.
Congestive heart failure.
Cavernous sinus or orbital vein thrombosis.
Episcleral or orbital vein vasculitis.
Jugular vein obstruction.
Arteriovenous shunts.
Carotid-cavernous fistula (traumatic, aneurysmal).
Orbital varix.
Sturge-Weber syndrome.
Orbital meningeal shunt (*see* figure).
Carotid-jugular shunt.
Intraocular vascular shunts.
Idiopathic.
Sporadic.
Familial (usually transmitted as autosomal dominant).

Pearls and Considerations

Topic is too broad for specific recommendations; each underling cause is unique.

Referral Information

Refer for imaging and laboratory tests to determine underlying cause, and then refer to appropriate subspecialist for treatment as appropriate.

TREATMENT—cont'd

Nonpharmacologic Treatment

Treatment of the underlying disease: as noted in the Classification section, many cases of episcleral venous pressure elevation are secondary to another disease process; in many patients the glaucoma will resolve after treatment of the underlying disease.

Filtering surgery: often necessary to relieve elevated IOP; there is a substantial risk of expulsive suprachoroidal hemorrhage after filtering surgery in eyes with elevated episcleral venous pressure.

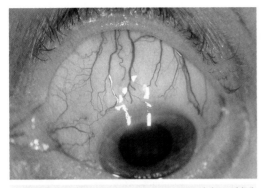

Elevated episcleral venous pressure caused by orbital meningeal shunt. Note marked dilation of episcleral veins.

General references

Fiore PM, Latina MA, Shingleton BJ, et al: The dural shunt syndrome. I. Management of the glaucoma, *Ophthalmology* 97:56-62, 1990.

Moses RA, Grodzki WJ Jr: Mechanism of glaucoma secondary to increased episcleral venous pressure, *Arch Ophthalmol* 103:1701-1703, 1985.

Weinreb RN, Karwatowski WSS: Glaucoma associated with elevated episcleral venous pressure. In Ritch R, Shields MB, Krupin T, editors: *The glaucomas,* ed 2, St Louis, 1996, Mosby, pp 1143-1155.

Glaucoma associated with ocular inflammation   (365.62)

DIAGNOSIS

Definition
Elevated intraocular pressure (IOP) and optic neuropathy secondary to uveitis.

Synonym
Uveitic glaucoma.

Symptoms
- All symptoms are highly variable depending on the acuteness of the process, the severity of the inflammation, and the level and duration of IOP elevations.

Pain: most inflammatory diseases of the eye are accompanied by some degree of discomfort.

Photophobia: variable symptom that is often present in acute inflammations, but may be absent in many cases of chronic uveitis.

Loss of vision: may be profound; in some cases, loss of vision may be minimal, and patients may not complain.

Redness: most ocular inflammatory disease is accompanied by some degree of hyperemia.

Signs
Elevated IOP: glaucomas secondary to uveitis are characterized by moderate to marked elevations of IOP.

Decreased vision and visual field loss: many patients will have decreased visual acuity; uveitis may produce loss of vision by several mechanisms; corneal, lenticular, or vitreous opacities may occur; if IOP is acutely elevated, corneal edema may result; involvement of the retina or choroid may also affect vision; in patients with chronic elevations of IOP, cupping of the optic nerve with associated visual field loss will be found.

Corneal changes: corneal edema may be present; in some cases (e.g., caused by herpes simplex or zoster), epithelial or stromal keratitis may be present; keratic precipitates are often seen in cases of anterior uveitis; chronic uveitis is often associated with a band keratopathy.

Anterior-chamber flare and cells: some degree of anterior-chamber flare and cells is seen in most cases of uveitis associated with glaucoma (*see* figure).

Iris changes: posterior synechiae may be present; areas of iris atrophy, sometimes resulting in heterochromia, may be seen.

Anterior-chamber angle: the angle may be either open or closed; in some patients the angle may appear normal; in others, inflammatory debris or excessive pigment may be seen in the angle; the angle may be partially or completely closed with peripheral anterior synechiae; in cases of iris bombé caused by extensive posterior synechiae, the angle may be closed by a secondary pupillary-block mechanism.

Investigations
Systemic evaluation: in some patients the cause of the uveitis may be obvious on ocular examination; other patients may not have an apparent cause for their uveitis; if the uveitis is severe, recurrent, or chronic, the patient should have a systemic evaluation to detect any underlying infectious, autoimmune, or inflammatory disease that might be associated with a uveitis.

Differential diagnosis
Other acute inflammatory glaucomas (e.g., acute angle-closure glaucoma, neovascular glaucoma, phacolytic and phacomorphic glaucoma).

Cause
"Uveitis" is a nonspecific term used for any inflammation involving the choroid, ciliary body, or iris. In some cases the cause of a uveitis is known (e.g., infection of herpes simplex virus). In other cases there is an associated underlying disease (e.g., ankylosing spondylitis, Crohn's disease). Uveitis can produce glaucoma by several mechanisms. Open-angle glaucoma may be caused by inflammation, edema, and dysfunction of the trabecular meshwork or by clogging of the meshwork with protein, cells, or other inflammatory material. Nonpupillary-block angle closure may be seen in the presence of extensive peripheral anterior synechiae. Pupillary-block glaucoma may be seen in the iris bombé syndrome, with extensive posterior synechiae completely obstructing the flow of aqueous from the posterior chamber through the pupil into the anterior chamber.

Classification
Idiopathic uveitis
Acute hypertensive iritis, chronic iridocyclitis.
Ocular conditions
Fuchs' heterochromic iridocyclitis, Posner-Schlossman syndrome (glaucomatocyclitic crisis), intermediate uveitis (pars planitis), sympathetic ophthalmia, traumatic iritis.
Systemic disease associated with uveitis
Rheumatologic disease (ankylosing spondylitis, Reiter's syndrome, juvenile rheumatoid arhthritis), sarcoidosis, Vogt-Koyanagi-Harada syndrome, Behçet's disease, Crohn's disease.
Infectious diseases
Viral (herpes simplex, herpes zoster, rubella, mumps, influenza, AIDS [HIV]).
Bacterial (syphilis, Lyme disease, leprosy, tuberculosis).
Protozoal and parasitic (toxoplasmosis, onchocerciasis [river blindness]).

Immunology
- Most uveitis is thought to represent an autoimmune antigen-antibody response to uveal tissue.

Diagnosis continued on p. 144

TREATMENT

Diet and Lifestyle
- No special precautions are necessary.

Pharmacologic Treatment
For Glaucoma
- Miotics should be avoided in inflammatory glaucomas because they tend to increase vascular permeability, synechiae formation, and discomfort.
- Some object to the use of prostaglandin analogs in theory because prostaglandins are an important mediator of inflammation and may aggravate an existing uveitis. There are few studies, however, on the use of prostaglandin analogs in uveitis glaucoma.
- Aqueous suppressants (e.g., β-blockers, α-agonists, carbonic anhydrase inhibitors) are the mainstay of glaucoma treatment in uveitis. Hyperosmotics may be useful in acute situations.

For Uveitis
- Treatment of the underlying uveitis is extremely important. If a specific cause can be identified, specific treatment may be indicated. For example, herpes simplex may be treated with antivirals. Nonspecific antiinflammatory treatment is usually required. Topical and systemic steroids, nonsteroidal antiinflammatory agents, and immunosuppressives are the principal agents used.
- Pupillary dilation with the use of cycloplegics and sympathomimetics is beneficial. Pupillary dilation aids in the prevention and breakup of posterior synechiae and possible pupillary block.

Treatment aims
To suppress the inflammatory response.
To control IOP.
To preserve visual function.

Prognosis
- The prognosis varies depending on the nature, severity, and duration of the uveitis and the glaucoma. In some conditions (e.g., Posner-Schlossman syndrome) the prognosis for long-term retention of vision is quite good. In other conditions (e.g., juvenile rheumatoid arthritis) the prognosis is quite poor.

Follow-up and management
- As with any chronic or recurrent disease, patients with uveitic glaucoma require careful, lifelong follow-up.

Treatment continued on p. 145

DIAGNOSIS—cont'd

Complications
Cataracts: many cases of uveitis are associated with the development of lenticular opacities; the chronic use of steroids may also be responsible for cataracts in some patients.

Retinal changes: chronic uveitis is often associated with cystoid macular edema.

Pathology
- Uveitis may be either granulomatous or nongranulomatous. Any type of inflammatory cell infiltrate may be seen, depending on the type and duration of the uveitis.

Pearls and Considerations
1. When treating the underlying inflammation, patients must be carefully monitored for additional steroid-response elevation in IOP.
2. Glaucoma will occur in up to 25% of patients with chronic ocular inflammation.
3. Glaucoma associated with uveitis may be either open angle or angle closure, with open angle the more common finding.

Referral Information
Uveitis specialist, rheumatologist, glaucoma specialist; or refer to primary care physician to rule out underlying systemic causes and infectious diseases.

TREATMENT—cont'd

Nonpharmacologic Treatment

Laser iridectomy: treatment of choice for pupillary block in the iris bombé syndrome; iridectomy may be technically difficult to perform in some of these eyes; the iridectomy may become occluded from synechiae formation on the edge of the iridectomy to the lens if the inflammation is not adequately suppressed.

Argon laser trabeculoplasty: trabeculoplasty is generally ineffective in uveitic glaucoma and is contraindicated because of its tendency to increase inflammation.

Filtering surgery: has a high rate of failure in uveitic glaucomas; antifibrotics such as mitomycin-C or 5-fluorouracil are generally indicated; in severe, recalcitrant cases, aqueous tube-shunt implantation or cyclophotocoagulation may be useful.

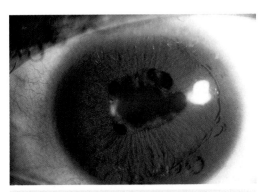

Uveitic glaucoma with extensive posterior synechiae, which may lead to iris bombé.

General references

Dunn JP: Uveitis in children. In *Focal points: clinical modules for ophthalmologists,* vol 13, no 4, San Francisco, 1995, American Academy of Ophthalmology.

Goldstein DA, Tessler HH: Complications of uveitis and their management. In Tasman W et al, editors: *Duane's clinical ophthalmology* (CD-ROM), Baltimore, 2004, Lippincott Williams & Wilkins.

Herndon L: Glaucoma, uveitic, 2006, www.emedicine.com.

Kass MA. Wilensky JT, Ruderman JM: Chronic uveitis and glaucoma, *J Glaucoma* 3:84-91, 1994.

Moorthy RS, Mermoud A, Baerveldt G, et al: Glaucoma associated with uveitis, *Surv Ophthalmol* 41:361-394, 1997.

Nussenblatt RB, Whitcup SM, Palestine AG: *Uveitis fundamentals and clinical practice,* ed 2, St Louis, 1996, Mosby.

Samples JR: Management of glaucoma secondary to uveitis. In *Focal points: clinical modules for ophthalmologists,* vol 13, no 4. San Francisco, 1995, American Academy of Ophthalmology.

Shields MB: Glaucoma associated with ocular inflammation. In *Textbook of glaucoma,* ed 4, Baltimore, 1998, Lippincott Williams & Wilkins, pp 308-322.

Weinreb RN: Management of uveitis and glaucoma, *J Glaucoma* 3:174-176, 1994.

Glaucoma associated with ocular trauma (365.65)

DIAGNOSIS

Definition

- Ocular trauma is a broad topic. Trauma to the eye may be caused by contusion (blunt), penetrating, or chemical injury. During the acute phase of any injury, intraocular pressure (IOP) may be elevated. Severely injured eyes may also develop chronic elevation of IOP. The management of elevated IOP in these situations is only one aspect of the overall management of the severely traumatized eye.
- For the purposes of this book, the following discussion is limited to the *late-onset glaucoma* that follows a contusion injury and is associated with anterior-chamber angle recession.

Synonyms
None.

Symptoms

- Glaucoma associated with the late effects of a contusion injury presents as a chronic open-angle glaucoma, and patients are often asymptomatic (*see* Glaucoma, primary open-angle and normal-tension).
- **History of trauma:** patients will usually recall an episode of blunt trauma to the eye; the trauma may have occurred many years before the detection of the glaucoma; in these cases, or when the trauma occurred in childhood, the patient may not remember.
- **Loss of vision:** in severe cases or in cases diagnosed late in the course of the disease, the patient may become aware of a loss of visual field or central vision in the involved eye.

Signs

- **Elevated intraocular pressure:** IOP is typically moderately elevated, but very high pressures may also be found; most blunt injuries are unilateral, so the late glaucoma typically involves one eye; in some patients (e.g., boxers, abused spouses), bilateral trauma is more common; the IOP elevation may occur any time after the trauma, even more than 20 years later.
- **Asymmetry of anterior-chamber depth:** the anterior chamber on the involved side may appear appreciably deeper than that of the uninvolved eye.
- **Optic disc cupping and visual field loss:** as with any chronic glaucoma, cupping and visual field loss are found; because the disease is usually unilateral and asymptomatic, glaucomatous damage is often far advanced at diagnosis.
- **Gonioscopic findings:** the gonioscopic appearance of the angle recession is characteristic; the ciliary body band is abnormally wide and is irregular in width (*see* figure); the iris root appears displaced posteriorly; there are often fine, gray or white linear scars in the trabecular meshwork and face of the ciliary body; there is often heavy pigment.

Associated Features

- Hyphema is often seen during the acute phase after blunt injury. Almost all patients with traumatic hyphema will have a detectable angle recession, but most of these do not develop glaucoma. Other signs of blunt trauma may be seen, including cataract, subluxed lens, iris sphincter tears, iridodialysis, cyclodialysis, and retinal tears or detachment. Blunt trauma resulting in orbital fractures is often associated with ocular trauma.

Pathology

- The inner part of the pars plicata and the iris root are displaced posteriorly. Scar tissue is seen in the trabecular meshwork and on the anterior face of the ciliary body. There may be endothelial proliferation of the angle with production of abnormal Descemet's membrane.

Pearls and Considerations

1. May occur early (acute glaucoma) or late (chronic glaucoma).
2. Acute glaucoma may occur with or without a hyphema present.
3. Chronic glaucoma may result from a variety of processes, including angle recession, peripheral anterior synechiae (PAS), and posterior synechiae.

Referral Information

1. Refer to glaucoma specialist for surgery as appropriate.
2. Refer to appropriate subspecialist for any other associated trauma.

Differential diagnosis

- The differential diagnosis includes other forms of chronic glaucoma without signs of active inflammation:
Primary open-angle glaucoma.
Pigmentary glaucoma.
Pseudoexfoliative glaucoma.
- Chronic angle-closure glaucoma should also be considered.

Cause

- When the eye is struck, aqueous is forcefully displaced toward the peripheral portion of the anterior chamber. If the force is sufficient, the trabecular meshwork and face of the ciliary body may be torn. Degenerative changes occur that eventually interfere with aqueous outflow.

Epidemiology

- Ocular trauma is primarily a disease of young men; most cases of angle-recession glaucoma therefore occur in men. Populations at high risk include athletes in contact and racquet sports, abused spouses, and people living in areas where crime and violence are common. Not all cases of angle recession associated with contusion injury result in glaucoma. It is estimated that delayed-onset glaucoma occurs in only 5%-20% of cases. Some evidence indicates that the fellow, uninjured eye is at greater risk for the development of primary open-angle glaucoma, suggesting that the eyes that develop angle-recession glaucoma are prone to IOP elevation.

Classification

- Glaucoma associated with ocular trauma is classified by the nature of the trauma: contusion injuries, penetrating trauma, chemical injury, radiant energy.

TREATMENT

Diet and Lifestyle

- High-risk populations should take steps to prevent ocular trauma. Athletes, particularly children and amateurs, should wear proper eye protection. Industrial workers, construction workers, and "do-it-yourselfers" who use power tools should also wear eye protection.

Pharmacologic Treatment

- Angle-recession glaucoma is treated pharmacologically similar to primary open-angle glaucoma (*see* Glaucoma, primary open-angle and normal-tension).
- In angle-recession glaucoma, outflow through the trabecular meshwork is limited. This uveal-scleral outflow plays a larger role in IOP control. Miotics decrease uveal-scleral outflow and thus are less useful.

Nonpharmacologic Treatment

Laser trabeculoplasty: the results are poor for angle-recession glaucoma, so it is not recommended. There have been reports of postprocedural IOP spikes.

Filtering surgery: many patients with severe disease and extensive angle recession are unresponsive to medical or laser treatment, making filtering surgery necessary.

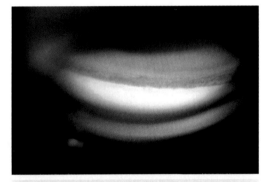

Gonioscopic photograph of traumatic angle recession showing abnormally and irregularly widened ciliary body.

Treatment aims
To control IOP and preserve visual function.

Prognosis
- In cases detected early or in cases with incomplete angle recessions, control of the glaucoma is often possible with treatment. In more advanced cases or in cases with 360 degrees of angle recession, the prognosis for preservation of vision is often poor.

Follow-up and management
- Patients should be followed with regular, frequent optic disc and visual field evaluations as in any chronic glaucoma.

General references

Berke SJ: Post-traumatic glaucoma. In Yanoff M, Duker JS, editors: *Ophthalmology*, E-dition, St Louis, 2006, Elsevier.

Goldberg I: Argon laser trabeculoplasty and the open-angle glaucomas, *Aust N Z J Ophthalmol* 13(3):243-248, 1985.

Herschler J: Trabecular damage due to blunt anterior segment injury and its relationship to traumatic glaucoma, *Ophthalmology* 83:239-248, 1977.

Kaufman JH, Tolpin DW: Glaucoma after traumatic angle recession: a ten-year prospective study, *Am J Ophthalmol* 78:648-654, 1974.

Mermoud A, Heuer DK: Glaucoma associated with trauma. In Ritch R, Shields MB, Krupin T, editors: *The glaucomas*, ed 2, St Louis, 1996, Mosby, pp 1259-1275.

Robin AL, Pollack IP: Argon laser trabeculoplasty in secondary forms of open-angle glaucoma, *Arch Ophthalmol* 101(3):382-384, 1983.

Salmon JF, Mermoud A, Levy A, et al: The detection of post-traumatic angle recession by gonioscopy in a population-based glaucoma survey, *Ophthalmology* 101:1844-1850, 1994.

Tesluk GC, Spaeth GL: The occurrence of primary open-angle glaucoma in the fellow eye of patients with unilateral angle-cleavage glaucoma, *Ophthalmology* 92:904-911, 1985.

Glaucoma associated with other anterior-segment anomalies   (365.43)

DIAGNOSIS

Definition
Elevated intraocular pressure (IOP) and optic neuropathy secondary to deformation of the anterior segment.

Synonyms
None.

Symptoms
Loss of vision: patients present in infancy with congenital corneal opacity and usually cataract; loss of vision is usually profound; patients with congenital glaucoma may have epiphora, photophobia, and blepharospasm.

Signs
Central corneal opacity: patients are born with a dense central corneal opacity in both eyes associated with stromal thinning and absence of Descemet's membrane and corneal endothelium centrally *(Peters' anomaly)*.

Congenital cataract: the lens is often opacified, but may be clear in mild cases.

Glaucoma: in severe cases, glaucoma is often present at birth with associated buphthalmos; in milder cases, glaucoma may not develop until later in childhood; *see* figure.

Investigations
Examination under anesthesia: as in congenital glaucoma, examination under anesthesia is usually necessary.

B-scan ultrasonography: because the fundus usually cannot be seen, B-scan ultrasonography is required to evaluate the posterior segment of the eye.

Electroretinography: may be indicated if there are concerns about the function of the retina.

Pearls and Considerations
1. Other anterior-chamber anomalies that may result in glaucoma include aniridia and Peters' anomaly.
2. Often, Axenfeld's and Rieger's anomalies are grouped together under the term *Axenfeld-Rieger syndrome.*
3. When Axenfeld's anomaly is associated with glaucoma, it is called *Axenfeld's syndrome.*

Referral Information
1. Refer to pediatrician to rule out further systemic anomalies.
2. Refer for glaucoma surgery as appropriate.

Differential diagnosis
Congenital glaucoma
Birth trauma.
Mucopolysaccharidoses.
Congenital hereditary corneal dystrophy.
Posterior keratoconus.
Intrauterine infections.
Congenital corneal leukoma.

Cause
- The cause is unknown. Most cases are spontaneous, although some familial cases with either autosomal recessive or autosomal dominant patterns of inheritance have been reported.

Classification
Type I: not associated with keratolenticular contact or cataract; most often unilateral.
Type II: associated with keratolenticular contact or cataract; most often bilateral.

Associated features
- *Krause-Kivlin syndrome:* systemic association of Peters' anomaly with short stature, facial dysmorphism, developmental delay, and delayed skeletal maturation; autosomal recessive inheritance.
- *Peters-plus syndrome:* Peters' anomaly with syndactyly, genitourinary anomalies, brachycephaly, central nervous system anomalies, cardiac disease, or deafness; uncertain inheritance pattern.
- *Fetal alcohol syndrome:* association with Peters' anomaly.
- *PAX-6 mutations:* found in some Peters' anomaly patients.

Pathology
- Descemet's membrane and corneal endothelium are absent centrally. The overlying stroma is thinned and opaque. There may be iris adhesions to the borders of the corneal defect. The lens epithelium and capsule are deficient at the anterior pole, and the lens may be adherent to the cornea. The lens often has a characteristic "top hat" shape.

TREATMENT

Diet and Lifestyle
- No special precautions are necessary.

Pharmacologic Treatment
- Most children with Peters' anomaly are rather severely affected and require surgical treatment. Older children with a chronic glaucoma may be treated pharmacologically, as for any patient with chronic glaucoma.

Nonpharmacologic Treatment
- Depending on the severity of the corneal opacity, lenticular involvement, and glaucoma, children may require keratoplasty, cataract surgery, and filtering surgery. In some children with glaucoma without keratolenticular contact, trabeculotomy may be effective. Otherwise, filtering surgery, a tube-shunt device, or cyclodestructive procedures may be necessary.

Treatment aims
To restore vision by removing any corneal or lenticular opacities.
In treating the glaucoma, to control IOP and preserve visual function.

Prognosis
- The prognosis depends on the severity of the anomaly. In mild to moderate cases, prognosis may be quite good. In more severely affected children, marked visual disability is common.

Follow-up and management
- Children should be followed regularly, as in patients with congenital glaucoma (see Glaucoma, congenital).
- Special education and programs for blind children should be recommended.

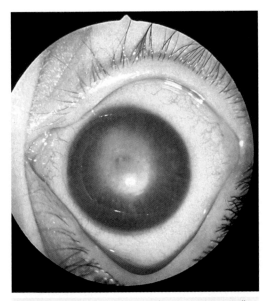

Glaucoma associated with anterior-segment anomalies (Peters' anomaly).

General references

Hanson IM, Fletcher JM, Jordan T, et al: Mutations at the PAX 6 locus are found in heterogeneous anterior segment malformations including Peters' anomaly, *Nat Genet* 6:168-173, 1994.

Heon E, Barsoum-Homsy M, Cevrette L, et al: Peters' anomaly, the spectrum of associated ocular malformations, *Ophthalmic Pediatr Genet* 13:137-143, 1992.

Mayer UM: Peters' anomaly and combination with other malformations, *Ophthalmic Pediatr Genet* 13:131-135, 1992.

Miller MT, Epstein RJ, Sugar J, et al: Anterior segment anomalies associated with the fetal alcohol syndrome, *J Pediatr Ophthalmol Strabismus* 21:8-18, 1984.

Mirzayans F, Pearce WG, MacDonald IM, Walter MA: Mutation of the PAX 6 gene in patients with autosomal dominant keratitis, *Am J Hum Genet* 57:539-548, 1995.

Traboulsi EL, Maumenee IH: Peters' anomaly and associated congenital malformations, *Arch Ophthalmol* 110:1739-1742, 1992.

Waring GO III, Rodrigues MM, Laibson PR: Anterior chamber cleavage syndrome: a stepladder classification, *Surv Ophthalmol* 20:3-27, 1975.

Glaucoma associated with scleritis (365.62) and episcleritis (379.0)

DIAGNOSIS

Definition

Elevated intraocular pressure (IOP) and optic neuropathy secondary to inflammation of the sclera or episclera.

Synonyms

None.

Symptoms

Pain: prominent symptom of scleral and episcleral inflammations; may vary from mild to moderate discomfort in episcleritis to severe in scleritis; the pain associated with scleritis is among the most severe of all ocular conditions.

Loss of vision: unusual in episcleritis; scleritis, particularly the necrotizing and posterior varieties, may be associated with profound vision loss; in patients who develop a secondary glaucoma, cupping and visual field loss may also produce loss of vision.

Signs

Hyperemia: marked dilation of the episcleral and conjunctival vessels is a prominent feature; episcleritis is characterized by a localized patch of hyperemia either nasally or temporally; scleritis is characterized by a diffuse, generalized hyperemia.

Tenderness: marked tenderness of the globe on palpation is a common sign.

Scleromalacia: recurrent or long-standing scleritis may produce thinning and atrophy of the sclera, allowing the underlying uvea to become visible as blue or slate-gray patches on the surface of the eye.

Elevated IOP: most patients with scleritis do not develop glaucoma; those who do, however, often have marked elevation of IOP.

Investigations

Rheumatologic evaluation: patients with scleritis often have an underlying connective tissue or autoimmune disease; a complete medical and rheumatologic evaluation is indicated.

Complications

Uveitis: most patients with scleritis do not have clinical evidence of an anterior-chamber reaction; in some patients an iridocyclitis may develop.

Keratitis: stromal or sclerosis keratitis has been reported; in some cases, corneal vascularization may develop.

Cataract.

Classification

Episcleritis: simple (379.01), nodular (379.02).

Scleritis: anterior diffuse (379.03), anterior nodular (379.03), anterior necrotizing with inflammation (379.03), anterior necrotizing without inflammation (scleromalacia perforans, 379.04), posterior (379.07).

Associated Features

Underlying or systemic diseases associated with scleritis include rheumatoid arthritis, relapsing polychondritis, systemic lupus erythematosus, polyarteritis nodosa, polymyalgia rheumatica, giant cell arteritis, ankylosing spondylitis, Wegener's granulomatosis, ulcerative colitis, Crohn's disease, Behçet's disease, herpes zoster, herpes simplex, tuberculosis, syphilis, Raynaud's disease, gout, sarcoidosis, acne rosacea, and psoriasis.

Pearls and Considerations

Patients treated with topical or systemic steroids must be monitored for further elevation in IOP as a side effect of this therapy.

Referral Information

1. Refer to rheumatologist in all cases of scleritis to determine underlying systemic cause.
2. Refer to glaucoma specialist for ongoing management of IOP (surgical or pharmacologic as deemed appropriate).

Differential diagnosis

Other glaucomas associated with inflammation and hyperemia (e.g., uveitic glaucoma, elevated episcleral venous pressure).

Cause

- Episcleral and scleral inflammation may produce glaucoma by several different mechanisms.

Open-angle glaucoma

Associated with inflammation (limbal scleritis with possible involvement of trabecular meshwork, Schlemm's canal, or aqueous collector channels; uveitis, glaucoma associated with episclera vessel vasculitis).

Elevated episcleral venous pressure.

Steroid-induced glaucoma.

Preexisting open-angle glaucoma.

Angle-closure glaucoma

Acute pupillary block may occur in susceptible eyes because of pain.

Nonpupillary block caused by edema and forward rotation of the ciliary body (sometimes with choroidal effusion).

Immunology

- Scleritis is thought to represent an autoimmune reaction in which antibodies to other antigens (e.g., viruses, endogenous connective tissue) cross-react with scleral antigens. Many patients will have serum antibodies (e.g., rheumatoid factor, antinuclear antibody) that suggest immunologic abnormalities.

Pathology

- Marked scleral edema and inflammation are present. The inflammation may be either granulomatous or nongranulomatous, depending on the underlying cause. In granulomatous types, marked areas of scleral thickening may develop. In other types, the sclera may become quite thin. In severe cases or in the necrotizing variety, areas of scleral necrosis may be seen.

TREATMENT

Diet and Lifestyle
- No special precautions are necessary.

Pharmacologic Treatment

Antiinflammatory Drugs
- Episcleritis usually responds to topical steroids. Scleritis is often treated with systemic non-steroidal antiinflammatory drugs (e.g., indomethacin, ibuprofen). In some cases, systemic steroids may be necessary. Topical steroids may be useful, but there is a risk of scleral melting and perforation.

Immunosuppressives
- In severe cases of scleritis, immunosuppressive agents (e.g., methotrexate, cyclosporine) may be necessary to suppress the inflammatory response.

For the Underlying Systemic Disease
- If an underlying systemic disease can be identified, appropriate treatment may be very beneficial in resolving the scleral inflammation.

For Glaucoma
- Aqueous suppressants are the drugs of choice. As in any inflammatory glaucoma, miotics and prostaglandin analogs should be avoided.

Nonpharmacologic Treatment
Laser iridectomy: in the occasional patient who develops pupillary-block glaucoma in association with scleritis or episcleritis, laser iridectomy should be performed.

Filtering surgery: because of the scleral inflammation, trabeculectomy often fails. The use of mitomycin may be associated with additional scleral thinning and necrosis. In patients with scleritis-associated glaucoma who require filtration, the use of an aqueous tube-shunt device may be the safest option.

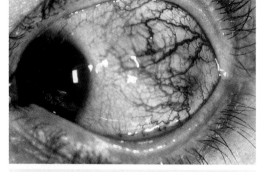

Scleritis with secondary glaucomas showing marked deep and superficial hyperemia.

Treatment aims
To suppress the inflammatory response, which often resolves the glaucoma.

Other treatments
Ciliary body ablation: in severe, recalcitrant cases, laser cyclophotocoagulation may prove useful in lowering IOP.

Prognosis
- The prognosis depends on the ease with which the inflammation can be controlled; if the scleritis can be adequately treated, the glaucoma can usually be well managed.

Follow-up and management
- Patients who develop a chronic glaucoma should be followed with regular optic disc and visual field evaluations. Patients who have an underlying systemic disease or who require systemic treatment with antiinflammatories or immunosuppressives should be followed in conjunction with a primary care physician.

General references
De la Maza MS, Foster CS, Jabbur NS: Scleritis associated with rheumatoid arthritis and with other systemic immune-mediated diseases, *Ophthalmology* 101:1281-1288, 1994.

De la Maza MS, Jabbur NS, Foster CS: An analysis of therapeutic decision for scleritis, *Ophthalmology* 100:1372-1376, 1993.

De la Maza MS, Jabbur NS, Foster CS: Severity of scleritis and episcleritis, *Ophthalmology* 101:389-396, 1994.

Dubord PJ, Chalmers A: Scleritis and episcleritis: diagnosis and management. In *Focal points: clinical modules for ophthalmologists,* vol 13, no 9, San Francisco, 1995, American Academy of Ophthalmology.

Legmann A, Foster CS: Noninfectious necrotizing scleritis, *Int Ophthalmol Clin* 36:73-80, 1996.

Wilhelmus KR, Grierson I, Watson PG: Histopathologic and clinical associations of scleritis and glaucoma, *Am J Ophthalmol* 91:97-705, 1981.

Glaucoma, congenital (365.14)

DIAGNOSIS

Definition
Elevated intraocular pressure (IOP) and optic neuropathy present from birth secondary to improper development of the aqueous outflow system.

Synonyms
None.

Symptoms
Epiphora, blepharospasm, photophobia: infants with congenital glaucoma behave as if their eyes are painful and irritated; tearing is a frequent early symptom; blepharospasm, especially in brightly lit environments, is also common.

Enlargement of the eye: parents may observe that one or both of their infant's eyes are unusually large and prominent or that the cornea is not clear (*see* figure).

Decreased vision: infants and children may behave as if they cannot see.

Signs
Enlargement of the cornea: characteristic of congenital glaucoma; the normal newborn cornea should be <10.5 mm in diameter and <12 mm at 1 year; any corneal diameter larger than this is abnormal and may indicate glaucoma.

Enlargement of the globe: in addition to the cornea, an infant's entire eye enlarges in response to elevated IOP; in neglected or unresponsive cases, the eye may become grossly enlarged (a condition called *buphthalmos*); the abnormal enlargement of the eye is also often associated with high degrees of myopia.

Elevated intraocular pressure: IOP measurement in an infant or young child usually requires sedation or anesthesia but will normally be found to be <24 mm Hg; pressures >24 mm Hg are unusual in normal infants and children.

Corneal edema: clouding of the cornea from stromal and epithelial edema is common in congenital glaucoma; slit-lamp examination may reveal characteristic vertical or concentric breaks in Descemet's membrane called *Haab's striae.*

Abnormal iris insertion: on gonioscopy the iris may appear to be inserted high on the trabecular meshwork; the iris insertion may have a scalloped appearance; the trabecular meshwork appears unusually thick and seems to be covered by a membrane; in many cases of congenital glaucoma, however, the appearance of the angle cannot be distinguished from that of a normal newborn.

Cupping of the optic disc: prominent feature of all glaucomas; in congenital glaucoma the cupping is usually concentric and often reversible if IOP is promptly brought under control.

Investigations
Complete pediatric evaluation: primary congenital glaucoma is an isolated finding in an otherwise-healthy child and is not usually associated with other anomalies; however, many congenital anomalies and syndromes are associated with a congenital glaucoma; therefore, patients should arrange a thorough physical examination by a pediatrician experienced in the evaluation of children with congenital or hereditary abnormalities.

Examination under anesthesia: for infants suspected of having congenital glaucoma: IOP measurement before deep anesthesia, corneal diameter measurement, gonioscopy, axial length measurement, retinoscopy, and fundus examination.

Differential diagnosis
Congenital and acquired abnormalities associated with infantile glaucoma (see Classification section).

Other causes of corneal clouding or enlargement (e.g., megalocornea, polysaccharidoses, neonatal infections, hereditary endothelial dystrophy, obstetric trauma).

Other causes of epiphora or photophobia (e.g., nasolacrimal obstruction, conjunctivitis, trauma).

Congenital optic nerve anomalies.

Cause
- The disease is believed to have a genetic basis. Although most cases are sporadic, familial cases are common, usually showing an autosomal recessive inheritance pattern.

Epidemiology
- Congenital glaucoma is uncommon, estimated to occur in about 1:10,000 live births. It is a significant cause of blindness in children, estimated to account for ~10% of patients in institutions for the blind. Approximately two thirds of affected patients are male.

Classification
Isolated congenital glaucoma.

Glaucomas associated with other congenital abnormalities:

Aniridia, Sturge-Weber syndrome, neurofibromatosis, Marfan syndrome, Pierre Robin syndrome, homocystinuria, goniodysgenesis, Lowe syndrome, microcornea, microspherophakia, rubella, chromosomal abnormalities (including trisomy 21), broad thumb syndrome, persistent hypoplastic vitreous.

Acquired glaucoma in infants:

Retinopathy of prematurity, tumors (retinoblastoma, juvenile xanthogranuloma), intrauterine and neonatal infections and inflammations (especially rubella), trauma.

Pathology
- The iris, ciliary body, and anterior-chamber angle have the appearance of arrested development, resembling that of a fetus of 6-8 mo of gestation rather than that of a normal newborn. The iris and ciliary body are anteriorly placed and overlap the posterior portion of the trabecular meshwork.
- Most cases of primary congenital glaucoma occur sporadically. Most inherited cases show a recessive pattern. Two major loci of recessively inherited primary congenital glaucoma (GLC-3A and GLC-3B) have been identified.

Diagnosis continued on p. 154

TREATMENT

Diet and Lifestyle
• No special precautions are necessary.

Pharmacologic Treatment
• Medical treatment is generally ineffective, and surgery is the primary treatment of choice.

Nonpharmacologic Treatment
Goniotomy: performed by passing a knife through clear cornea, across the anterior chamber, and into the angle; this is done with a gonioscope lens.

Treatment aims
To preserve vision and control IOP.

Other treatments
• In severe cases diagnosed later in childhood or in patients in whom goniotomy or trabeculotomy has failed, filtering surgery may be attempted using (1) antifibrotics such as 5-fluorouracil or mitomycin-C, (2) aqueous shunt devices, or (3) ciliodestructive procedures. Treatment for amblyopia is extremely important in preserving vision after definitive surgery has been performed.

Prognosis
• The prognosis is generally good in patients in whom the diagnosis has been prompt and goniotomy or trabeculotomy has achieved good results. In cases diagnosed late or in patients resistant to initial treatment, prognosis is poor, and severe vision loss often results.

Follow-up and management
• Patients must be carefully followed at regular intervals for life because corneal decompensation, cataract, and elevated IOP may occur in later years.

Treatment continued on p. 155

DIAGNOSIS—cont'd

Complications

Corneal opacification: in severe or neglected cases, chronic corneal edema may develop with vascularization and permanent opacification of the cornea.

Buphthalmos: gross enlargement of the eye may result; thinning of the sclera may result in anterior staphyloma formation.

Amblyopia: because the disease is often asymmetric, significant anisometropia with amblyopia may result.

Pearls and Considerations

1. The disease is bilateral in approximately three fourths of cases.
2. The classic triad of symptoms in infants with congenital glaucoma is *blepharospasm, photophobia,* and *epiphora.*

Referral Information

Refer to pediatric glaucoma specialist immediately for the earliest possible intervention.

TREATMENT—cont'd

Trabeculotomy: performed by making an external incision at the limbus and identifying Schlemm's canal; a small probe is placed into the lumen of Schlemm's canal and rotated into the anterior chamber, thus rupturing the overlying trabecular meshwork; done when no clear view exists through the cornea.

- Either surgical procedure may be used to cut through the abnormal trabecular meshwork and allow aqueous access to Schlemm's canal. Both procedures have high success rates, and excellent results are obtained when diagnosis and treatment are not unduly delayed.

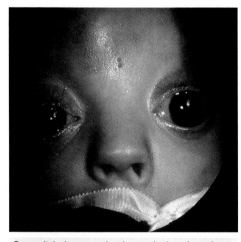

Congenital glaucoma showing marked ocular enlargement, especially of the left eye.

General references

Anderson DR: Trabeculotomy compared to goniotomy for glaucoma in children, *Ophthalmology* 90:805-806, 1983.

Barsoum-Homsy M, Chevrette L: Incidence and prognosis of childhood glaucoma, *Ophthalmology* 93:1323-1327, 1986.

Beck AD, Lynch MG: Pediatric glaucoma. In *Focal points: clinical modules for ophthalmologists,* vol 15, no 5, San Francisco, 1997, American Academy of Ophthalmology.

Cibis GW, Urban RC, Dahl AA: Glaucoma, primary congenital, 2006, www.emedicine.com.

Glaucoma, phacolytic   (365.51)

DIAGNOSIS

Definition
Elevated intraocular pressure (IOP) resulting from ocular inflammation caused by a hypermature cataract.

Synonyms
None.

Symptoms
Pain, hyperemia, loss of vision: phacolytic glaucoma typically presents as an acute inflammatory glaucoma with severe pain, redness, and marked loss of vision; the patient usually has a history of a longer, gradual loss of vision for several months or years preceding the acute episode.

Signs
Greatly elevated IOP.

Corneal edema: as in any acute glaucoma, corneal epithelial edema (and sometimes stromal edema) is present.

Ocular inflammation: there is a marked inflammatory response with conjunctival and episcleral hyperemia, a heavy anterior-chamber flare and cellular response, and a marked degree of pain and tenderness (*see* figure).

Loss of vision: vision loss is usually profound, rarely better than being able to distinguish hand motions; phacolytic glaucoma is one of the few conditions in which a patient may present with no light-perception vision and yet recover vision after treatment.

Mature cataract: the cataract is almost always mature or hypermature; pupil appears white; lens may appear shrunken, and there may be wrinkles in the anterior lens capsule; chunk-like pieces of white material may appear on the lens capsule or in the aqueous.

Deep anterior chamber and open angle: on gonioscopy, characteristic of phacolytic glaucoma.

Investigations
B-scan ultrasonography: because the fundus cannot be seen through the opaque lens, B-scan ultrasonography is indicated to rule out gross abnormalities of the vitreous or retina (e.g., retinal detachment, malignant melanoma).

Pearls and Considerations
The lens capsule may be ruptured or just abnormally leaky.

Referral Information
Refer for cataract extraction.

Differential diagnosis
Other acute lens-induced glaucomas (e.g., phacomorphic or subluxed lens, acute angle-closure glaucoma).
Other acute inflammatory glaucomas (e.g., uveitis, iris bombé, neovascular glaucoma).

Cause
- As the lens proteins degenerate in a maturing cataract, they become soluble and leak into the aqueous through the intact lens capsule. In the aqueous, these proteins provoke an inflammatory response characterized by macrophages that phagocytize the lens proteins and collect in the trabecular meshwork. The macrophages laden with lens protein obstruct the outflow of aqueous.
- An alternative theory is that the soluble high-molecular-weight lens protein itself can obstruct the meshwork without being phagocytized by macrophages.

Epidemiology
- The condition is the result of neglected cataracts. Two or three decades ago, phacolytic glaucoma was much more common, and it is still seen frequently in medically underserved parts of the world. In modern North America, where cataracts are rarely allowed to develop beyond the early stage without surgery, phacolytic glaucoma has become quite unusual.

Immunology
- The lens is an immunologically privileged site. The lens proteins are isolated by the lens capsule and are not recognized by the body's immune system. When lens proteins are released into the ocular fluids, they generally provoke an immunologic response that leads to inflammation. After cataract surgery, in which lens material is not completely removed from the eye, a condition similar to phacolytic glaucoma called *lens-particle glaucoma* may be seen. *Phacoanaphylaxis*—a severe, granulomatous, foreign body–type inflammatory reaction—may occur after trauma to the lens.

Pathology
- Fragmentation and globule formation are seen in the lens cortex, consistent with a mature cataract. Macrophages filled with eosinophilic lens material are seen in the aqueous and trabecular meshwork.

TREATMENT

Diet and Lifestyle
- No special precautions are necessary.

Pharmacologic Treatment
- Oral or intravenous hyperosmotics should be given to lower IOP acutely before surgery.
- Treatment with agents that suppress aqueous formation are also useful acutely to lower IOP.
- Topical steroids and atropine should be given to suppress the inflammatory response.
- Because phacolytic glaucoma is often an extremely painful condition, analgesics (including narcotics, if necessary) are indicated for relief of pain.

Nonpharmacologic Treatment
Cataract extraction: immediate removal of the lens on an emergency basis is usually the definitive treatment; if the condition has not been neglected for a long time, the resolution of the pain, inflammation, and elevated IOP is usually dramatic.

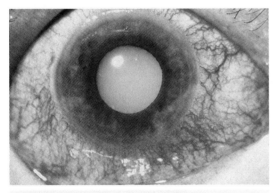

Phacolytic glaucoma caused by a completely mature cataract with marked ocular inflammation.

Treatment aims
To eliminate the lens, which is the source of the protein provoking the inflammatory response.

Prognosis
- The prognosis depends of the duration of the disease. In patients treated within 24 hr, the prognosis for resolution of inflammation and restoration of vision is good. With longer duration, the risk of permanent damage to the trabecular meshwork or optic nerve increases.

Follow-up and management
- Once the lens has been removed, the major problem is visual rehabilitation. If an intraocular lens was implanted at the original surgery, visual rehabilitation is usually accomplished with a simple refraction. If not, aphakic correction with spectacles or a contact lens may be required. Secondary lens implantation is also an option. If the IOP is controlled after lens extraction, subsequent problems with glaucoma are unusual.

General references
Lane SS, Kopietz LA, Lindquist TD, Leavenworth N: Treatment of phacolytic glaucoma with extracapsular cataract extraction, *Ophthalmology* 95:749-753, 1988.
Layden WE: Cataract and glaucoma. In Tasman W et al, editors: *Duane's clinical ophthalmology* (CD-ROM), Baltimore, 2004, Lippincott Williams & Wilkins.
Richter CU: Lens-induced open-angle glaucoma. In Ritch R, Shields MB, Krupin T, editors: *The glaucomas*, ed 2, St Louis, 1996, Mosby, pp 1023-1031.

DIAGNOSIS

Definition
Elevated intraocular pressure (IOP) secondary to accumulation of pigment granules on the inner surface of the anterior chamber.

Synonyms
None.

Symptoms
- Most patients are asymptomatic and unaware of any ocular problem.

Decreased vision: if the disease is far advanced at diagnosis, the patients may be aware of the loss of vision.

Blurred vision with exercise: some patients will complain of blurred vision after vigorous exercise because of pigment shedding in the anterior chamber.

Signs
Elevated IOP: usually significantly elevated and often extremely asymmetric.

Optic disc cupping: indistinguishable from other forms of open-angle glaucoma.

Visual field loss: resulting from defects in the nerve fiber bundle, as in other forms of open-angle glaucoma.

Excessive pigment dispersion in the anterior segment: pigment on the endothelial surface of the cornea assumes a triangular or spindle shape (Krukenberg's spindle); pigment dotting on the anterior surface of the iris is seen; gonioscopy shows heavy pigment on the trabecular meshwork as well as pigment on Schwalbe's line and the endothelial surface of the peripheral cornea; the uniform, homogeneous trabecular pigment helps differentiate pigment dispersion from pseudoexfoliation, which has patchy trabecular pigment; pharmacologic dilation of the pupil often produces shedding of a large amount of pigment into the aqueous; pigment may also be seen on the lens zonules and on the equator of the lens (Scheie's line) by performing gonioscopy with a widely dilated pupil.

Iris transillumination and backward bowing: slitlike defects occurring in the midperiphery of the iris pigment epithelium can be seen to transilluminate the anterior chamber and often appear unusually deep; the peripheral iris appears bowed posteriorly.

Myopia: most patients have moderate to high degrees of myopia.

Investigations
B-scan ultrasound biomicroscopy: may reveal areas of iris-zonular or iris–ciliary process contact.

Complications
See Glaucoma, primary open-angle and normal-tension.

Differential diagnosis
- Other conditions in which loss of iris pigment, heavy pigmentation of the trabecular meshwork, and glaucoma may be seen:
  Uveitis.
  Exfoliative glaucoma.
  Posttraumatic glaucoma.
  Ocular melanosis.
  Postsurgical glaucomas.
  Iris or ciliary body cysts and melanomas.

Cause
The disease is thought to result from abnormal posterior displacement of the peripheral iris. The iris rubs on the lens zonules or ciliary processes. The pigment in the iris pigment epithelium is released into the anterior segment. The trabecular meshwork is phagocytized by the trabecular endothelial cells. The pigment-laden endothelial cells do not function normally, and the IOP becomes elevated.

Epidemiology
- Pigmentary glaucoma is thought to represent 1%-2% of all glaucomas in Europe and North America. The disease is most often diagnosed in young adults. Important risk factors include myopia and male gender. White patients are also at risk, and the disease is uncommon in nonwhite populations.
- 25%-50% of patients with pigment dispersion syndrome develop pigmentary glaucoma.
- Autosomal dominance inheritance.

Pathology
- Reverse–pupillary-block mechanism.
- Iris pigment epithelial cells and pigment are absent in areas corresponding to the transillumination defects. Trabecular meshwork endothelial cells are heavily laden with phagocytized pigment and show signs of degeneration and disintegration. There is collapse of the trabecular beams, loss of intertrabecular spaces, and collection of cellular debris in the outflow pathway.

Diagnosis continued on p. 160

TREATMENT

Diet and Lifestyle
- No special precautions are necessary.

Pharmacologic Treatment
- Treatment is similar to that for open-angle glaucoma (*see* Glaucoma, primary open-angle and normal-tension). Because these patients are younger than most glaucoma patients, miotics may produce more side effects of brow ache, ciliary spasm, and blurred vision. Use of pilocarpine gel or Ocuserts (Alza Pharmaceuticals, Palo Alto, Calif) is often helpful.

Treatment aims
To control IOP and prevent loss of visual function.

Prognosis
- Prognosis with adequate treatment is usually good. Pigment dispersion tends to decrease with age; thus the need for treatment may diminish as the patient grows older.

Follow-up and management
- Patients should be followed at regular intervals with optic disc evaluation and perimetry as for open-angle glaucoma (*see* Glaucoma, primary open-angle and normal-tension). The frequency of the follow-up will depend on the severity of the disease.

Treatment continued on p. 161

DIAGNOSIS—cont'd

Classification

Pigment Dispersion Syndrome

- Characterized by signs of pigment dispersion without elevated IOP evidence of optic nerve damage.

Active phase: evidence of active pigment shedding, or increasing iris transillumination over time.

Inactive phase: no evidence of active pigment shedding, or decreasing iris transillumination over time.

Pigmentary Glaucoma

- Pigmentary glaucoma is characterized by signs of pigment dispersion syndrome with evidence of elevated IOP and signs or risk of optic nerve damage.

Pearls and Considerations

1. Pigmentary glaucoma is thought to be an autosomal dominant inherited condition.
2. Active pigment dispersion usually ceases in these patients at 45-50 yr of age.
3. Pigmentary glaucoma is considered to be an "ocular-only" disease, meaning that it has no associated underlying systemic conditions.

Referral Information

Refer for glaucoma surgery as appropriate.

TREATMENT—cont'd

Nonpharmacologic Treatment

Argon laser trabeculoplasty: often successful in pigmentary glaucoma; these patients are exceptions to the general rule that laser trabeculoplasty is less effective in younger patients.

Selective laser trabeculoplasty: repeatable alternative to argon laser trabeculoplasty.

Laser iridectomy: has been proposed to eliminate the backward bowing of the iris and consequent rubbing of the pigment epithelium on the lens zonules by eliminating the reverse pupillary block and equalizing the pressure in the anterior and posterior chambers; there are no long-term, large studies showing the benefit of this treatment, so it remains experimental at present.

Filtering surgery: indications are the same as for open-angle glaucoma (*see* Glaucoma, primary open-angle and normal-tension).

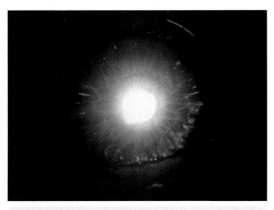

Pigmentary glaucoma showing typical iris transillumination pattern.

General references

Ball SF: Pigmentary glaucoma. In Yanoff M, Duker JS, editors: *Ophthalmology*, E-dition, St Louis, 2006, Elsevier.

Campbell DG: Pigmentary glaucoma: mechanism and role for laser iridotomy. *J Glaucoma* 3: 173-174, 1994.

Farrar SM, Shields MB: Current concepts in pigmentary glaucoma, *Surv Ophthalmol* 37: 233-252, 1993.

Wilensky JT: Diagnosis and treatment of pigmentary glaucoma. In *Focal points: clinical modules for ophthalmologists*, vol 15, module 9, San Francisco, 1987, American Academy of Ophthalmology.

DIAGNOSIS

Definition

A chronic and progressive form of optic neuropathy with a characteristic acquired loss of optic nerve fibers.

Synonyms

Common abbreviations include POAG (primary open-angle glaucoma) and NTG (normal-tension glaucoma).

Symptoms

- Most patients are asymptomatic and unaware of any vision problem.
- **Decreased vision:** patients with far-advanced disease at diagnosis may complain of decreased vision; some may be aware of defects in their field of vision earlier in the course of the disease; many who do not volunteer symptoms note a variety of visual problems, such as with night driving, fluctuating vision, with reading or close work, and going from brightly lit to dim environments.
- **Side effects of treatment:** a variety of complaints are related to effects of treatment.

Signs

Optic Disc Cupping and Loss of Retinal Nerve Fiber Layer

- Glaucoma produces a characteristic optic neuropathy in which there is loss of the neuroretinal rim of the optic disc with associated enlargement of the optic cup, an increase in the area of pallor of the disc, excavation of the neuroretinal rim, and exposure and backward bowing of the lamina cribrosa. This is accompanied by loss of the retinal nerve fiber layer (NFL). *See* figure.
- Two patterns of damage to the optic nerve and NFL are recognized: *diffuse* (concentric loss of neuroretinal rim, cup enlargement, thinning of retinal NFL) and *focal* (preferential loss of neuroretinal rim and cup enlargement in one area, marked defect in one area of NFL).

Visual Field Loss

- The most common form of visual field loss is the *nerve fiber bundle defect.* In its early stages the defect is characterized by the tendency to respect the horizontal midline, especially in the nasal portion of the visual field. Defects are generally located in the Bjerrum or arcuate area, which extends from 1 or 2 degrees from fixation to 20 degrees from fixation. Defects also tend to have an arcuate shape, being wider circumferentially than radially. The nerve fiber bundle defect is not specific for glaucoma and may be seen in many other optic nerve diseases.

Afferent Pupil Defect

- In any glaucoma with asymmetric damage to the optic nerve, an afferent pupil defect may be seen in the eye with the greater degree of cupping.

Elevated Intraocular Pressure

- Most patients with open-angle glaucoma have an intraocular pressure (IOP) >21 mm Hg at least some of the time. Different studies have shown that 10%-40% of patients with open-angle glaucoma do not have an elevated IOP; such patients are said to have *normal-tension glaucoma.* IOP in many glaucoma patients is highly variable and may show considerable diurnal fluctuation.

Differential diagnosis

Other forms of glaucoma
Chronic angle-closure glaucoma.
Chronic secondary open-angle glaucomas (e.g., pigmentary, exfoliative, posttraumatic).
Nonglaucomatous optic neuropathies
Compressive lesions of the optic nerve and chiasm.
Arteritic and nonarteritic forms of ischemic optic neuropathy.
Congenital anomalies of the optic nerve.
Degenerative optic neuropathies (e.g., optic disc drusen).

Cause

Unknown, but may be genetic, resulting from degenerative changes in the extracellular matrix of the trabecular meshwork, or from poor circulation that can produce chronic ischemia.

Epidemiology

- The prevalence of open-angle glaucoma varies with the population being studied. The Baltimore Eye Survey found a prevalence of ~1.0% in the adult white population and ~4.2% in the adult black population [1]. The prevalence increases greatly with age. Significant risk factors for the presence of open-angle glaucoma include IOP, race, age, family history, optic nerve cupping, and central corneal thickness.

Classification

- It is thought that open-angle glaucoma represents a final common pathway of several causative factors. Classifications have been proposed on the basis of the presence or absence of these factors, including normal-tension and high-tension glaucoma, vasospastic or nonvasospastic glaucoma, and focal ischemic or senile sclerotic glaucoma.

Pathology

- There is degeneration of the collagen of the trabecular beams, degeneration and loss of trabecular endothelial cells, and collapse of the intertrabecular spaces. There is a reduction in the pore density and number of giant vacuoles in the endothelium of Schlemm's canal. The optic nerve shows loss of nerve fibers, capillaries, and glial cells. There is thinning and backward bowing of the lamina cribrosa and undermining of the disc margin, producing the characteristic "bean pot" appearance.

Diagnosis continued on p. 164

TREATMENT

Diet and Lifestyle

- Recent studies have shown that regular aerobic exercise is associated with a long-term reduction in IOP. Patients in the appropriate physical condition should be encouraged to exercise.
- Some evidence indicates that smoking is associated with glaucomatous damage, and patients who smoke should be encouraged to quit.

General Treatment
Target Pressure

- Before beginning treatment, the clinician should establish a *target pressure,* a theoretical pressure level at which progression of the glaucomatous damage will no longer occur. There is no way to determine this precisely for each patient, but most clinicians establish an initial target pressure of 30%-50% below the pretreatment pressure level. Patients with more advanced disease or who appear to be progressing more rapidly require a lower target pressure. If the target pressure is not achieved with the initial therapy, additional therapeutic modalities are indicated.

Pharmacologic Treatment

- Treatment is usually initiated with medication. Some drugs lower IOP by enhancing the outflow of aqueous. Other drugs act by reducing the production of aqueous by the ciliary body. Most clinicians would try two medications, one from each group. If the combination of two drugs does not achieve the target pressure, or the clinician may add a third drug or recommend a laser or surgical procedure. The drugs available for treating glaucoma and their side effects are listed in Appendix A. The miotics and prostaglandin analogs enhance aqueous outflow. Epinephrine and dipivefrin appear to have dual action on both outflow and production. The other agents inhibit the formation of aqueous.

Nonpharmacologic Treatment
Argon Laser Trabeculoplasty

Using an argon laser, small-diameter laser burns are placed on the trabecular meshwork. This lowers the IOP in ~70%-80% of the patients treated. The mechanism by which laser trabeculoplasty lowers IOP is unknown. Laser trabeculoplasty is indicated when the target pressure cannot be achieved with medication. Although laser trabeculoplasty produces good initial results in most open-angle glaucoma patients, the effect seems to diminish with time; after 5 yr, less than half of all patients continue to show good IOP control.

Selective Laser Trabeculoplasty

Similar to argon laser trabeculoplasty (ALT) but is repeatable and results in less damage to the trabecular meshwork compared with ALT.

Treatment aims
To preserve vision by lowering IOP below the target pressure.

Prognosis
- Without treatment, open-angle glaucoma is a progressive disease and will produce some degree of visual disability in most patients. With proper treatment, it is estimated that <5% of open-angle glaucoma patients will become blind as a result of their disease.

Follow-up and management
- Open-angle glaucoma is a chronic, progressive, lifelong illness. Regular follow-up with optic-disc evaluation and visual field testing is required. The treatments for glaucoma have a high failure rate over time and often produce adverse effects. Once the target pressure has been achieved and the disease appears stabilized, patients should be seen every 3-6 mo, with detailed optic disc evaluation and perimetry every 6-12 mo. Patients with more advanced disease will require more frequent follow-up.

Treatment continued on p. 165

DIAGNOSIS—cont'd

Investigations

Imaging of the optic disc and NFL: stereo photography of the optic disc and red-free photography of the NFL should be performed to aid in the detection of glaucomatous damage and to provide a baseline record of the appearance of the optic disc at diagnosis. In some settings, computerized image analysis may be available.

Automated static perimetry: to detect and monitor visual field defects.

Serial tonometry: in some patients, especially those with lower IOP levels, serial tonometry or diurnal tension curves may be useful in defining the role of IOP and the effect of treatment.

Pachymetry: the Ocular Hypertensive Treatment Study showed that *central corneal thickness* (CCT) is a factor in the progression to primary open-angle glaucoma. Thinner CCT is a significant risk factor for progression. Goldmann's applanation tonometry assumes a CCT of 500 μm. The IOP is underestimated in thin corneas and overestimated in thick corneas.

Neuroimaging; carotid flow studies; systemic, vascular, and neurologic evaluation: these types of studies may be indicated in some patients with atypical features (e.g., low IOP levels); younger patients; and patients with rapidly progressive visual loss, greatly asymmetric disease, atypical patterns of visual field loss, or changes in the optic disc.

Pearls and Considerations

1. Glaucoma is a leading cause of irreversible blindness, second only to macular degeneration.
2. The Ocular Hypertension Treatment Study has demonstrated a reduced risk of glaucoma development in ocular hypertension patients who are started on preemptive IOP-lowering therapy.

Referral Information

Refer for glaucoma surgery as appropriate.

TREATMENT—cont'd

Filtering Surgery

Glaucoma filtering surgery creates a fistula from the anterior chamber to the subconjunctival space. This allows aqueous to flow out of the eye, lowering the IOP. Filtering surgery is indicated in patients whose glaucoma is progressive and in those who are at high risk for progression despite the use of medical and laser treatments. In most glaucoma patients who have not had prior surgery, glaucoma filtering surgery has a success rate of ~75%-90%. Risk factors for failure of filtering surgery include younger age, black African ancestry, previous ocular surgery, long-term use of glaucoma medications, and intraocular inflammation, membrane growth, or neovascularization. In these patients, filtering surgery may be modified by the use of antifibrotic agents (e.g., 5-fluorouracil, mitomycin-C) or an aqueous tube-shunt device (e.g., Molteno tube).

Complications

Blindness: the major complication of neglected open-angle glaucoma.

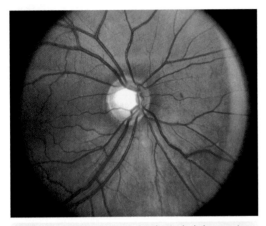

Primary open-angle glaucoma showing typical glaucomatous cupping of the optic nerve.

General references

Bell JA, Noecker RJ: Primary open angle glaucoma, 2006, www.emedicine.com.

Shields MB: Open-angle glaucomas: In *Textbook of glaucoma,* ed 4, Baltimore, 1998, Lippincott Williams & Wilkins, pp 153-176.

Thomas JV, Belcher CD III, Simmons RJ: *Glaucoma surgery,* St Louis, 1992, Mosby.

Werner EB: Normal-tension glaucoma. In Ritch R, Shields MB, Krupin T, editors: *The glaucomas,* ed 2, St Louis, 1996, Mosby, pp 769-797.

Wilson MR, Martone JF: Epidemiology of chronic open-angle glaucoma. In Ritch R, Shields MB, Krupin T, editors: *The glaucomas,* ed 2, St Louis, 1996, Mosby, pp 753-768.

Glaucoma, pseudoexfoliative   (365.52)

DIAGNOSIS

Definition
Elevated intraocular pressure (IOP) and optic neuropathy secondary to flakes of granular material on the inner surface of the anterior chamber.

Synonyms
Pseudoexfoliation glaucoma, pseudoexfoliation syndrome.

Symptoms
- Most patients are asymptomatic and unaware of any problem with their vision.
- **Loss of vision:** if the disease is far advanced when diagnosed, the patient may be aware of the loss of vision; many patients with pseudoexfoliation syndrome also develop cataracts and may present with loss of vision on that basis. *See also* Pseudoexfoliation of the lens (366.11).

Signs
Elevated IOP: usually significantly elevated and often extremely asymmetric; often very labile in pseudoexfoliative glaucoma.

Optic disc cupping: indistinguishable from other forms of open-angle glaucoma.

Visual field loss: visual field defects of the nerve fiber bundle are seen as in other forms of open-angle glaucoma (*see* Glaucoma, primary open-angle and normal-tension).

Deposit of whitish fibrillar material: deposition of a flaky, white material on the anterior lens capsule looks as though it is arising from the surface of the lens; typically there is a disc-shaped deposit centrally, a midperipheral clear zone, and additional material deposited on the peripheral portion of the lens; the clear zone corresponds to the area of the lens in contact with the pupillary margin of the iris; additional deposits of this whitish material may be seen on the pupillary margin, anterior iris stroma, corneal endothelium, and trabecular meshwork.

Pigment dispersion: some degree of pigment dispersion in the anterior segment is usually seen, with corneal endothelial pigment, pigment dotting of the anterior iris stroma, and heavy pigment in the trabecular meshwork (quite common); a pigment line is often seen anterior to Schwalbe's line on gonioscopy (Sampaolesi's line).

Iris transillumination: atrophy and transillumination defects of the peripupillary iris are often seen.

Shallow anterior chamber: the anterior chamber is shallower and the angle is narrower than average in many patients with pseudoexfoliation.

Investigations
- Special investigations other than those for open-angle glaucoma are not required (*see* Glaucoma, primary open-angle and normal-tension).

Complications
Subluxation of the lens: one of the characteristic changes in pseudoexfoliation syndrome is laxity and degeneration of the lens zonules; as a result, dehiscence of the zonules and spontaneous subluxation of the lens may occur.

Difficulties with cataract surgery: the weakness of the zonules increases the risk of capsule rupture and vitreous loss during cataract surgery; the pupil of patients with pseudoexfoliation often dilates poorly, making cataract surgery more difficult.

Pearls and Considerations
1. Pseudoexfoliation is rarely seen in patients under 50 yr of age.
2. Often presents unilaterally, but will eventually involve the fellow eye in up to 40% of cases.

Referral Information
Refer for glaucoma surgery as appropriate.

Differential diagnosis
True capsular delamination: usually the result of trauma, exposure to infrared radiation, uveitis, pigmentary glaucoma, or primary amyloidosis.

Cause
- The cause of pseudoexfoliation syndrome is unknown. The glaucoma is thought to result from obstruction of aqueous outflow by collection of the exfoliation material in the trabecular meshwork and by the effects of the excess pigment on the trabecular endothelial cells.

Epidemiology
- Pseudoexfoliation is common in certain ethnic groups and uncommon in others. The highest prevalences are reported in individuals of Scandinavian ancestry, particularly in Finland and Iceland. Pseudoexfoliation syndrome is often seen as an incidental finding in the absence of glaucoma. The frequency of the disease increases with age and is rare in younger individuals.
- About 10% of patients with pseudoexfoliation syndrome develop glaucoma.

Associated features
- Cataract is more common in patients with pseudoexfoliation syndrome than in the general population. Although shallow anterior chambers and narrow angles are more common in pseudoexfoliation syndrome, angle-closure glaucoma is unusual. Iris rigidity and ischemia are common findings and result in poor pupil dilation.

Pathology
- There is extensive atrophy and depigmentation of iris pigment epithelial cells. The pseudoexfoliation material is fibrillar and appears to be derived from basement membrane. In addition to being found on the anterior lens capsule, the material is widely deposited on all the structures of the anterior segment. It is also found in association with blood vessels in the iris, ciliary body, and conjunctiva. The material has been reported in the skin and even in the liver.

TREATMENT

Diet and Lifestyle

- No special precautions are necessary.

Pharmacologic Treatment

- Pharmacologic treatment is similar to that for open-angle glaucoma (*see* Glaucoma, primary open-angle and normal-tension). Although it is often less effective and labile, poorly controlled IOP often persists.

Nonpharmacologic Treatment

Argon laser trabeculoplasty: produces results similar to or better than those seen in open-angle glaucoma.

Selective laser trabeculoplasty: indications similar to those for open-angle glaucoma.

Filtering surgery: indications similar to those for open-angle glaucoma.

See Glaucoma, primary open-angle and normal-tension.

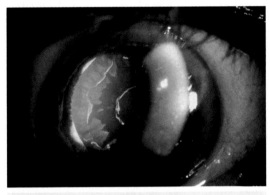

Pseudoexfoliative glaucoma showing deposition of white material on the anterior lens surface.

Treatment aims
To control IOP and preserve visual function.

Prognosis
- The prognosis is somewhat worse than with open-angle glaucoma because of the increased difficulty in controlling IOP. The high prevalence of cataract and the increased risk of complications after cataract surgery also contribute to a poorer visual prognosis.

Follow-up and management
- Patients should be followed with optic disc evaluation and perimetry at regular intervals, as in open-angle glaucoma. The frequency of follow-up will depend on the severity of the disease.

General references

Konstas AG, Jay JL, Marshall GE, Lee WR: Prevalence, diagnostic features and response to trabeculectomy in exfoliation glaucoma, *Ophthalmology* 100:619-627, 1993.

Lumme P, Laatikainen L: Exfoliation syndrome and cataract extraction, *Am J Ophthalmol* 116: 51-55, 1993.

Pons ME, Eliassi-Rad B: Glaucoma, pseudoexfoliation, 2006, www.emedicine.com.

Prince AM, Streeten BW, Ritch R, et al: Preclinical diagnosis of pseudoexfoliation syndrome, *Arch Ophthalmol* 105:1076-1082, 1987.

Ritch R: Exfoliation syndrome: the most common identifiable cause of open-angle glaucoma. *J Glaucoma* 3:176-178, 1994.

Threlkeld AB, Hertzmark E, Strum RT, et al: Comparative study of the efficacy of argon laser trabeculoplasty for exfoliation and primary open-angle glaucoma, *J Glaucoma* 5:311-316, 1996.

Glaucoma, pupillary-block angle-closure   (365.2)

DIAGNOSIS

Definition
An acute elevation in intraocular pressure (IOP) resulting from the iris pushing forward and decreasing or halting aqueous outflow.

Synonyms
None.

Symptoms
Blurred vision: *acute* (365.22) and *intermittent* (365.21) forms are characterized by rapid onset of blurred vision; *chronic* angle-closure glaucoma (365.23) is usually asymptomatic unless far advanced with severe visual field loss.

Colored haloes: occasionally a patient may note colored haloes around lights caused by the diffraction effect of the corneal edema.

Pain: *acute* angle-closure glaucoma is a very painful condition; the rapid increase in IOP is accompanied by significant inflammation and ischemia, both of which will produce pain; the pain may be so severe that it completely disables the patient and produces vomiting; *intermittent* angle-closure glaucoma is characterized by episodes of mild to moderate pain that the patient may describe as a "headache" and may not localize to the eye; *chronic* angle-closure glaucoma is typically painless.

Signs
Elevated intraocular pressure: marked elevation of IOP is typically seen in all forms of angle-closure glaucoma; because the disease often presents in only one eye, the pressure in the fellow eye may be normal.

Closed angle: on gonioscopy the angle will be closed, usually in all quadrants.

Dynamic indentation gonioscopy: should be performed to determine if oppositional versus synechial closure; indentation gonioscopy may help break the attack.

Hyperopia: most eyes with angle-closure glaucoma are hyperopic.

Corneal edema: in acute angle-closure glaucoma, the cornea is usually edematous because of the rapid increase in IOP; the appearance of the cornea has been described as "steamy," resembling a bathroom mirror after a hot shower.

Dilated pupil: the pupil in acute angle closure is usually fixed in the middilated position and typically appears vertically oval; the pupil may remain permanently dilated, and areas of iris stromal atrophy may develop; the pupil is usually normal in the intermittent and chronic forms.

Ocular inflammation: a marked degree of inflammation with hyperemia and anterior-chamber flare and cells typically is seen in *acute* angle-closure glaucoma; in *intermittent* angle-closure glaucoma, milder degrees of inflammation may be present; inflammation is not present in *chronic* angle-closure glaucoma.

Glaukomflecken: in severe cases of acute angle-closure glaucoma, small, white, comma-shaped opacities may be seen in the anterior subcapsular region of the lens (*see* figure).

Optic disc changes: in acute angle-closure glaucoma, the sudden increase in IOP may cause an ischemic optic neuropathy with disc edema and permanent loss of a portion of the visual field; after the acute phase, a flat optic atrophy may be seen; recurrent attacks of intermittent angle-closure and chronic angle-closure glaucoma are generally associated with more typical glaucomatous cupping of the optic disc.

Differential diagnosis
- Includes other forms of angle closure not thought to result from primary pupillary block:
  Plateau iris syndrome, ciliary block (malignant) glaucoma.
  Angle closure in association with retinopathy of prematurity.
  Phacomorphic glaucoma.
  Nanophthalmos.
- Also includes other forms of acute glaucoma that may or may not be caused by angle closure:
  Neovascular glaucoma.
  Uveitis.
  Posner-Schlossman syndrome.
  Phacolytic glaucoma.
  Schwartz-Matsuo syndrome.

Cause
- Eyes at risk for developing pupillary-block angle-closure glaucoma are smaller than normal. The area of contact between the pupillary margin and the anterior surface of the lens is greater than normal. This increases the resistance to aqueous flow from the posterior to the anterior chamber at the pupil. If this pupillary block is great enough, the aqueous pressure in the posterior chamber may exceed that in the anterior chamber enough to cause the peripheral iris to bow forward until it comes into contact with the trabecular meshwork, thereby obstructing the outflow of aqueous.

Epidemiology
- Most studies of Western populations have shown a prevalence of critically narrow angles of 0.5%-1.0%. The prevalence of angle-closure glaucoma is 0.1%-0.2%. The majority of patients with angle-closure glaucoma have the chronic forms. The acute form is somewhat less common.

Classification
Acute angle-closure glaucoma (365.22).
Intermittent (subacute) angle-closure glaucoma (365.21).
Chronic angle-closure glaucoma (365.23).

Diagnosis continued on p. 170

TREATMENT

Diet and Lifestyle
- No special precautions are necessary.

Pharmacologic Treatment
Acute Angle-Closure Glaucoma
- The first line of treatment is hyperosmotics. If the patient's general health will permit intravenous mannitol or oral isosorbide, either should be given to lower IOP as soon as possible. Aqueous suppressants (e.g., β-adrenergic blockers, α-adrenergic agonists, or carbonic anhydrase inhibitors) are also useful as initial treatment. If the patient is having severe pain, analgesics (including narcotics, if necessary) should be given. Once the IOP begins to decrease, a weak miotic (e.g., 1% or 2% pilocarpine) should be given to constrict the pupil and open the angle, which facilitates laser iridectomy. Pilocarpine should also be placed in the fellow eye at the time of diagnosis to prevent angle closure and to facilitate a prophylactic iridectomy.

Long-Term Treatment (All Forms)
- Many patients with angle-closure glaucoma will fail to achieve complete IOP control after laser iridectomy and may require long-term medical treatment. The agents and indications are similar to those for open-angle glaucoma (*see* Glaucoma, primary open-angle and normal-tension).

Treatment aims
To control IOP and preserve visual function.

Other treatments
- Dynamic indentation gonioscopy may occasionally open a closed angle and break an attack quickly. Chamber-deepening procedures, which involve hyperinflating the anterior chamber, may open an angle closed with synechiae and avoid the need for filtering surgery. Rarely, a laser iridectomy cannot be performed, and surgical iridectomy may be necessary.

Prognosis
- The prognosis depends on the duration of angle closure. In patients with acute attacks who are treated promptly, the angle usually can be opened, and long-term pharmacologic treatment is not required. In neglected acute attacks or advanced cases of chronic angle-closure glaucoma, long-term pharmacologic treatment or filtering surgery will usually be needed.

Follow-up and management
- Once the iridectomy has been completed and the IOP brought under control, the patient should be followed as any other chronic glaucoma patient, with regular optic disc evaluation and perimetry at intervals determined by the severity of the disease.

Treatment continued on p. 171

DIAGNOSIS—cont'd

Investigations

Gonioscopy of the fellow eye: the fellow eye of a patient with pupillary-block angle-closure glaucoma will almost always have an anatomically narrow angle (*see* Anatomically narrow angle).

Complications

Permanent corneal edema: severe cases may damage the corneal endothelium, resulting in permanent corneal edema.

Iris atrophy: permanent dilation of the pupil may result in troublesome glare and blurred vision.

Cataract: cataract formation is more common following an episode of acute angle-closure glaucoma.

Optic nerve damage: ischemic optic neuropathy or glaucomatous cupping may result in permanent loss of visual function.

Pearls and Considerations

Angle-closure glaucoma can result in bilateral blindness within 2-3 days of onset!

Referral Information

Refer immediately for peripheral iridotomy.

TREATMENT—cont'd

Nonpharmacologic Treatment

Laser iridectomy: the definitive treatment for pupillary block; should be performed as soon as the cornea is clear enough and as the patient's condition permits; there is no need to wait for the IOP to become normal before performing iridectomy; the fellow eye should be treated at the same sitting to prevent angle closure; by placing a hole in the iris, aqueous is allowed to flow freely from the posterior to the anterior chamber, thus eliminating pupillary block.

Filtering surgery: in many cases, iridectomy alone followed by pharmacologic treatment will not control IOP; the trabecular meshwork may be damaged, or the angle may be permanently closed with peripheral anterior synechiae; filtering surgery may then be necessary; the indications are much the same as for open-angle glaucoma (*see* Glaucoma, primary open-angle and normal-tension).

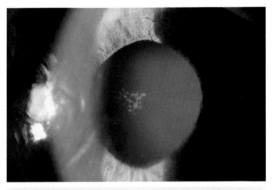

Acute angle-closure glaucoma showing the partially dilated pupil and white anterior lens opacities known as *glaukomflecken.*

General references

American Academy of Ophthalmology, Preferred Practice Pattern Committee: *Primary angle-closure glaucoma,* San Francisco, 1996, The Academy.

Erie JC, Hodge DO, Gray DT: The incidence of primary angle-closure glaucoma in Olmstead County, Minnesota, *Arch Ophthalmol* 115: 177-181, 1997.

Kim YY, Jung HR: Clarifying the nomenclature for primary angle closure glaucoma, *Surv Ophthalmol* 42:125-136, 1997.

Lowe RF: A history of primary angle closure glaucoma, *Surv Ophthalmol* 40:163-170, 1995.

Simmons RB, Montenegro MH, Simmons RJ: Primary angle closure glaucoma. In Tasman W et al, editors: *Duane's clinical ophthalmology* (CD-ROM), Baltimore, 2004, Lippincott Williams & Wilkins.

Glaucoma suspect: open angle with borderline findings (365.0 and 365.01)

DIAGNOSIS

Definition
A person who has one or more risk factors that may lead to the development of glaucoma.

Synonym
Preglaucoma.

Symptoms
- Patients will present with some feature that places them at greater risk for the development of glaucoma, but most are asymptomatic.

Signs
Glaucoma-like discs: patients have some features that suggest early glaucomatous change in the optic discs (e.g., asymmetry, early cup enlargement) but also have normal intraocular pressure (IOP) and visual fields.

Investigations
Complete eye examination with gonioscopy: to rule out the presence of any other form of glaucoma or another cause for the optic disc changes.

Intraocular pressure: should be measured on several occasions and at different times of the day to rule out the presence of early open-angle glaucoma.

Pachymetry: should be performed to determine central corneal thickness (CCT). Thinner corneas underestimate IOP, and thicker corneas overestimate IOP.

Perimetry: should be performed initially and at regular intervals to detect the development of an early visual field defect, indicating the development of definitive glaucomatous damage.

Optic disc and red-free photography of the retinal nerve fiber layer: should be performed to better detect any changes that may occur in the future; alternatively, computerized image analysis of the optic disc and nerve fiber layer may be performed.

Pearls and Considerations
Risk factors for glaucoma include age, race, family history, systemic health, elevated IOP, and enlarged or asymmetric cup-to-disc (C/D) ratio.

Referral Information
None; monitor these patients regularly for signs of progression to glaucoma.

Differential diagnosis

Primary open-angle glaucoma (in which visual field defects and elevated IOP have not been detected).

Early chronic angle-closure glaucoma.

- Other causes of optic neuropathy and congenital optic disc anomalies should be ruled out.

Classification

- The reason for the glaucoma suspicion should be documented.

Glaucoma suspect with glaucoma-like discs: implies normal IOP and visual fields.

Glaucoma suspect with ocular hypertension: implies normal visual field and optic discs.

Glaucoma suspect with historical risk factors (e.g., family history, black, high myopia).

TREATMENT

Diet and Lifestyle
- No special precautions are necessary.

Pharmacologic Treatment
- No pharmacologic treatment is recommended. Glaucoma suspects without definitive evidence of optic disc damage do not require treatment.

Nonpharmacologic Treatment
- No nonpharmacologic treatment is recommended.

Treatment aims
- To monitor for progression to glaucoma and begin appropriate treatment when indicated.

Prognosis
- The prognosis is good. Most patients with glaucoma-like discs do not develop glaucoma, although their risk is somewhat higher than in the general population.

Follow-up and management
- After obtaining visual fields and baseline photographs of the optic disc and nerve fiber layer, these patients should be followed annually.

General references

Airaksinen PJ, Tuulonen A, Werner EB: Clinical evaluation of the optic disc and retinal nerve fiber layer. In Ritch R, Shields MB, Krupin T, editors: *The glaucomas*, ed 2, St Louis, 1996, Mosby, pp 617-657.

Miglior M, Bozzini S, Ratiglia R: Glaucomatous and glaucoma-like optic neuropathy, *Metab Pediatr Syst Ophthalmol* 13:119-128, 1990.

Peigne G, Schwartz B, Takamoto T: Differences of retinal nerve fiber layer thickness between normal and glaucoma-like (physiologic cups) matched by optic disc area, *Acta Ophthalmol Scand* 71:451-457, 1993.

Schwartz B, Tomita G, Takamoto T: Glaucoma-like discs with subsequent increased ocular pressures, *Ophthalmology* 98:41-49, 1991.

Glaucomatocyclitic crisis (Posner-Schlossman syndrome)   (364.22)

DIAGNOSIS

Definition
An acute unilateral elevation in intraocular pressure (IOP) of uncertain pathogenesis.

Synonym
Posner-Schlossman syndrome.

Symptoms
Pain: glaucomatocyclitic crisis is a syndrome characterized by unilateral attacks of marked elevation of IOP and minimal to mild signs of an anterior uveitis; patients usually complain of a mild degree of ocular discomfort and photophobia.

Blurred vision, haloes: patients usually complain of some blurred vision and may describe colored haloes around lights.

Signs
Elevated intraocular pressure: during attacks, IOP typically is greatly elevated; pressures >40 mm Hg and even >60 mm Hg are not unusual.

Hyperemia: typically the eye is white during an attack, but a mild ciliary flush may be seen.

Corneal edema: corneal epithelial bedewing may be present.

Anterior-chamber reaction: flare and cells are characteristically absent during an attack; a rare cell may be seen; keratic precipitates are either absent or few in number, but very fine keratic precipitates may be seen, especially in the peripheral cornea and angle.

Heterochromia: iris stromal atrophy with hypochromia may be seen after recurrent attacks.

Gonioscopic findings: the angle is generally widely open; keratic precipitates may be visible gonioscopically in patients even though none are seen with the slit lamp.

Investigations
Optic disc imaging: the appearance of the optic disc should be well documented with photography or other imaging techniques to monitor the development of cupping.

Perimetry: as with any glaucoma, perimetry should be carried out at regular intervals to detect the development of visual field loss.

Complications
Persistent elevation of IOP: recurrent attacks may lead to persistent elevation of IOP and development of open-angle glaucoma.

Optic disc cupping and visual field loss: caused by recurrent attacks or persistent elevation of IOP.

Pearls and Considerations
Recurrences and elevated IOP are common.

Referral Information
Refer unresponsive patients for glaucoma surgery.

Differential diagnosis
- Any anterior uveitis associated with an elevated IOP may resemble glaucomatocyclitic crisis. Inflammatory signs in glaucomatocyclitic crisis are minimal or absent altogether. Typically, the hyperemia and anterior-chamber reaction increase after treatment for the elevated IOP. Most other types of uveitis will have more prominent signs of inflammation. Because of its unilateral nature and heterochromia, glaucomatocyclitic crisis may resemble Fuchs' heterochromic iridocyclitis; however, Fuchs' is characterized by constant signs of anterior-chamber reaction.

Cause
- The cause is unknown. The mechanism of the marked elevation in IOP is thought to be either an inflammatory response localized to the trabecular meshwork (trabeculitis) or the result of the release of chemical mediators (e.g., prostaglandins, cytokines) into the aqueous.

Epidemiology
- Most cases are spontaneous and occur in young adults 20-50 yr of age. A few familial cases have been described.

Pathology
- There are no reports of the histopathology of glaucomatocyclitic crisis.

TREATMENT

Diet and Lifestyle
- No special precautions are necessary.

Pharmacologic Treatment
Antiinflammatory Drugs
- Moderate doses of topical corticosteroids are usually very effective in controlling the inflammation and shortening the attack. In patients at risk for complications of topical steroids, systemic nonsteroidal antiinflammatory agents (e.g., indomethacin) have been effective.

Aqueous Suppressants
- α-Adrenergic agonists (e.g., apraclonidine, brimonidine) seem to be particularly effective, but β-blockers or carbonic anhydrase inhibitors may also be used. As with any inflammatory glaucoma, miotics and prostaglandin analogs should be avoided.

Nonpharmacologic Treatment
- Filtering surgery may be indicated in severe or recalcitrant cases, but this is rare. Laser trabeculoplasty is ineffective.

Treatment aims
To control inflammation and IOP to shorten the attack.
- There is no known treatment that will prevent attacks.

Prognosis
- Glaucomatocyclitic crisis is usually a self-limited disease. Attacks tend to diminish and disappear after age 50 yr.

Follow-up and management
- Patients should be advised to seek medical attention at the onset of an attack. Cooperative patients who understand their condition may be given medication to use at the onset of an attack if it is not possible to see a physician promptly. As with any glaucoma, regular follow-up and evaluation of the optic disc and visual field are essential.

General references
Krupin T, Feitl ME, Karalekas D: Glaucoma associated with uveitis. In Ritch R, Shields MB, Krupin T, editors: *The glaucomas*, ed 2, St Louis, 1996, Mosby, pp 1235-1237.
Posner A, Schlossman A: Syndrome of unilateral recurrent attacks of glaucoma with cyclitic symptoms, *Arch Ophthalmol* 39:517-528, 1948.
Wang RC, Rao NA: Idiopathic and other anterior uveitis syndromes. In Yanoff M, Duker JS, editors: *Ophthalmology*, E-dition, St Louis, 2006, Elsevier.

DIAGNOSIS

Definition

Orbital inflammation or increase in volume of the orbital tissue associated with thyroid disease that may lead to decreased ocular mobility, exposure keratitis, optic neuropathy, and exophthalmos.

Synonyms

Thyroid eye disease, Graves' ophthalmopathy.

Symptoms

Exophthalmos.
Diplopia.
Tearing and lacrimation.
Conjunctival hyperemia.
Eyelid retraction.
Spontaneous subluxation of globe.

Signs

Upper eyelid retraction: most reliable sign.
Eyelid lag: unreliable sign.
Swollen eyelids: fingerlike or jelly roll–like edema; diurnal improvement.
Lagophthalmos.
Decreased blinking (or increased if irritated).
Exophthalmos: eye is displaced in the direction of the tethered muscle.
Resistance of the globe to retrodisplacement.
Restricted motility: noncomitant strabismus that can be diurnally variable (*see* Fig.1).
Head-moving strategy: makes patients appear to have a visual field defect.
Inferior rectus muscle infiltration: develops 60%-70% of the time, creating (1) an elevation deficit that simulates a superior rectus muscle paresis; (2) the absence of a Bell's phenomenon, promoting greater corneal exposure; (3) elevated intraocular pressure (IOP) in attempted upgaze because of the inferior tethering of the globe; and (4) an inferiorly displaced globe because of an infiltrated inferior rectus muscle that restrains the globe.
Medial rectus muscle infiltration: occurs 25% of the time and creates an abduction deficit (pseudo–sixth-nerve palsy).
Superior rectus muscle infiltration: occurs in 10% of Graves' disease patients and creates a depression deficit simulating an inferior rectus palsy.
Dysthyroid optic neuropathy: occurs as the result of severe crowding of the orbital apex in 2%-5% of patients with Graves' ophthalmopathy; dysthyroid optic neuropathy has an insidious and acute onset; older diabetic men seem to be at greatest risk; there is greater risk in later-onset ophthalmopathy and with a globe that decompresses posteriorly with limitation of motility.
Red eye: occurs because of injection over the recti muscles, exposure from exophthalmos, and infrequent blinking; can lead to keratitis, ulcer, and corneal melt.
Frequency of rectus muscle involvement: inferior > medial > superior > lateral.

Differential diagnosis

Idiopathic orbital pseudotumor, lymphoid tumor, sarcoid, amyloidosis, Wegener's syndrome, optic nerve sheath and sphenoid wing meningiomas, carotid-cavernous fistula, orbital cellulitis, orbital cysts, neoplasms, vascular anomalies, eye prominence.

Cause

- Graves' ophthalmopathy occurs within 18 mo of the onset of hyperthyroidism.
- Graves' disease is a multisystem disorder of unknown cause characterized by hyperthyroidism, infiltrative ophthalmopathy, and infiltrative dermopathy.
- Graves' disease can occur in isolation without the hyperthyroidism.

Epidemiology

- Genetically preselected population with immunogenetic predisposition; HLA-DR3 and HLA-D8 have been identified as genetic markers.
- Ratio of female to male is 3.2:1.0. The mean age of onset for men and women is ~44 yr.

Immunology

- T lymphocytes fail to prevent proliferation of randomly mutating B lymphocytes. The B lymphocytes spawn autoantibodies that attack EOM fibers and connective tissue.
- Poorly functioning or absent T-suppressor lymphocytes allow influx of cytotoxic T lymphocytes, contributing to further destruction.

Pathology

- The EOMs are infiltrated by lymphocytes, plasma cells, and mast cells. Hydrophilic mucopolysaccharides and collagen formation create degenerative changes in the EOMs. Fibroblasts produce hydrophilic glycosaminoglycans that accumulate in the retroocular tissues. This contributes to the edema of the orbital connective tissue and EOMs.
- Late findings: fibrosis and fatty infiltration.

Diagnosis continued on p. 178

TREATMENT

Diet and Lifestyle

- Patients should stop smoking, sleep with head elevated, and apply cold compresses to relieve eyelid edema.

Pharmacologic Treatment

- Treatment of the underlying thyroid gland dysfunction will improve symptoms. The development, improvement, or worsening of Graves' disease is unrelated to the mode of therapy.

Artificial tear substitutes and ointments.

Steroids: prednisone, 30-120 mg.

Immunosuppressives: cyclosporine.

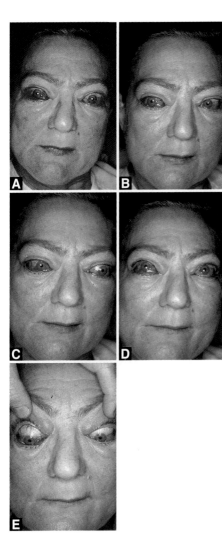

A

B

C

D

E

Figure 1 A, Woman with severe Graves' disease and almost complete limitation of bilateral eye movement. **B** and **C,** Restricted right and left gaze. **D** and **E,** Limited upgaze and downgaze. Note the typical injection over the medial and lateral rectus muscles, particularly visible in the right eye.

Treatment aims

To protect the cornea.

To monitor and prevent dysthyroid optic neuropathy.

To lessen or eliminate diplopia.

Prognosis

- Remission of the signs of Graves' ophthalmopathy is unpredictable.
- In Graves' disease, eyelid retraction may spontaneously remit in ~50% of patients.
- Exophthalmos tends to remain unchanged.
- There is a high incidence of spontaneous remission of diplopia.
- Dysthyroid optic neuropathy is unpredictable.

Follow-up and management

- Monitor for dysthyroid optic neuropathy.
- Routinely observe optic nerve function with the following:

Snellen acuity test.

Threshold visual field test.

Relative afferent pupillary test.

Contrast sensitivity test.

Ophthalmoscopy and fundus photos.

Motility measurements.

Treatment continued on p. 179

DIAGNOSIS—cont'd

Investigations

Palpebral fissure measurement, corneal evaluation, quantitation of motility and exophthalmos, retrodisplacement, optic nerve function.

Orbital magnetic resonance imaging (MRI) or computed tomography (CT): not every patient with Graves' disease requires orbital imaging.

Extraocular muscles (EOMs): EOM enlargement with sparing of tendons (*see* Fig. 2).

Serum thyroid-stimulating hormone (TSH), calculated free thyronine (T_4) index, thyroid-stimulating immunoglobulins, antithyroid antibodies, serum triiodothyronine (T_3), acetylcholine receptor antibody.

- A small percentage of patients fail to demonstrate any laboratory thyroid abnormality.
- 10% of patients with Graves' disease have hypothyroidism or autoimmune thyroiditis.
- Associated with myasthenia gravis.

Complications

Dysthyroid optic neuropathy.
Subluxation of globe.

Pearls and Considerations

CT scanning is more useful than MRI for viewing the bony landmarks when evaluating Graves' disease.

Referral Information

1. Refer to endocrinologist for treatment of the underlying disease.
2. Refer for surgical evaluation if orbital decompression is indicated.

TREATMENT—cont'd

Nonpharmacologic Treatment
Prism, patches, tape, eye exercises.
Sequence of surgical interventions:
1. Orbital decompression.
2. Ocular muscle surgery.
3. Adjustment of eyelid margin.
4. Blepharoplasty.
Retrobulbar radiation therapy (up to 2000 cGy).

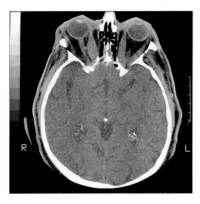

Figure 2 Magnetic resonance image of orbits in Graves' disease demonstrating enlargement of extraocular muscles with sparing of muscle tendons.

General references
Bartalena L, Marcocci C, Pinchera A: Orbital radiotherapy for Graves' ophthalmopathy, *J Clin Endocrinol Metab* 89(1):13-14, 2004.
Kusuhara T, Nakajima M, Imamura A: Ocular myasthenia gravis associated with euthyroid ophthalmology, *Muscle Nerve* 28(6):764-766, 2003.
Terris DJ, Levin P: Orbital decompression for Graves' disease, 2003, www.emedicine.com.
Wiersinga WM, Prummel MF: An evidence-based approach to the treatment of Graves' ophthalmopathy, *Endocrinol Metab Clin North Am* 29(2):297-319, vi-vii, 2000.
Yeh S, Foroozan R: Orbital apex syndrome, *Curr Opin Ophthalmol* 15(6):490-498, 2004.

Hypertension, ocular   (365.04)

DIAGNOSIS

Definition
Increased intraocular pressure (IOP) in the absence of any clinical evidence of nerve fiber layer (NFL) damage.

Synonyms
None; typically abbreviated OHT.

Symptoms
- Ocular hypertension (OHT) is a condition in which IOP is repeatedly >21 mm Hg, the anterior-chamber angle is open, and the optic disc, retinal NFL, and visual field are normal. Patients are asymptomatic.

Signs
Elevated intraocular pressure: IOP is >21 mm Hg on more than one measurement made at different times.

Investigations
Optic disc and NFL photography or imaging: elevated IOP is often associated with evidence of glaucomatous damage to the optic nerve and NFL. A normal optic disc must be documented to support the diagnosis of OHT.

Perimetry: the visual field must be shown to be normal.

Pachymetry: Goldmann's applanation tonometer was calibrated based on a central corneal thickness (CCT) of 500 μm. The IOP may be underestimated with thinner corneas and overestimated with thicker corneas. The Ocular Hypertension Treatment Study (OHTS), a multicenter clinical trial, showed that OHT patients have thicker-than-average CCT.

Complications
Glaucomatous damage to the optic nerve: elevated IOP is the principal risk factor for the development of glaucoma; patients with OHT have approximately a tenfold greater risk of developing glaucoma than the normal population.

Differential diagnosis
- The differential diagnosis includes other conditions in which elevated IOP may be seen without producing symptoms, including:

Open-angle glaucoma.

Chronic angle-closure glaucoma.

Certain secondary glaucomas (e.g., pigmentary glaucoma, pseudoexfoliative glaucoma, posttraumatic glaucoma).

Cause
- The cause is unknown, but the IOP is believed to be genetically controlled. Because IOP tends to increase with age in most populations, age-related changes in the trabecular meshwork may play a role.

Epidemiology
- 5%-10% of the adult population have OHT, with the percentage increasing with age. An estimated 1% of these patients per year develop evidence of glaucomatous damage to the optic nerve.
- Significant risk factors for the progression to glaucoma found in the OHTS were CCT, age, pattern standard deviation, cup-to-disc ratio, and IOP.
- Race and family history are other well-described risk factors.

TREATMENT

Diet and Lifestyle
- No special precautions are necessary.

Pharmacologic Treatment
For Lowering Intraocular Pressure (*see* Glaucoma, Primary Open-Angle and Normal-Tension)

The 5-year OHTS results have cleared some of the controversy concerning treatment of OHT. The study reported a reduction in progression of glaucoma in the treated group. The progression rate in the treated OHT patients was 4.4% versus 9.5% in the untreated group. Of note is the significance of CCT on risk of glaucoma progression. The risk of progression increases to 36% for untreated OHT with CCT <555 μm and IOP >25.75.

Nonpharmacologic Treatment
- Laser and surgical treatment is generally not indicated in OHT.

Treatment aims
- To reduce or eliminate the risk of developing glaucomatous damage; at present, the best way to achieve this goal is not known.

Prognosis
- ~10% of asymptomatic patients with open angles and elevated IOP show evidence of glaucomatous damage to the optic nerve; the others have OHT. Of these, long-term longitudinal studies show a good prognosis, with only 10%-20% of OHT patients developing glaucomatous damage over a 10-yr period.

Follow-up and management
- Because OHT patients are at risk for glaucoma and because it is impossible to predict which patients will develop damage, all OHT patients should be followed at regular intervals with careful optic disc evaluation and perimetry. Examination once or twice per year is probably adequate, with optic disc imaging and perimetry every 12-18 mo.

General references
American Academy of Ophthalmology, Preferred Practice Pattern Committee: *Primary open-angle suspect*, San Francisco, 1995, The Academy.

Gordon MO, Beiser JA, Brandt JD, et al: The Ocular Hypertension Treatment Study: baseline factors that predict the onset of primary open-angle glaucoma, *Arch Ophthalmol* 120(6):714-720, 829-830 (discussion), 2002.

Kass MA: The Ocular Hypertension Treatment Study, *J Glaucoma* 3:97-100, 1994.

Kass MA, Heuer DK, Higgenbotham EJ, et al: The Ocular Hypertension Treatment Study: a randomized trial determines that topical ocular hypotensive medication delays or prevents the onset of primary open-angle glaucoma, *Arch Ophthalmol* 120(6):701-713, 829-830 (discussion), 2002.

Shields MB: Glaucoma screening. In *Textbook of glaucoma*, ed 4, Baltimore, 1998, Lippincott Williams & Wilkins, pp 137-141.

Shields MB: Intraocular pressure and tonometry. In *Textbook of glaucoma*, ed 4, Baltimore, 1998, Lippincott Williams & Wilkins, pp 46-51.

Hypertensive retinopathy   (362.11)

DIAGNOSIS

Definition
Retinal complications of elevated systemic blood pressure.

Synonyms
None.

Symptoms
- Patients are asymptomatic in early stages.
- Later stages can have blurry or distorted vision.

Signs
Focal narrowing and straightening of retinal arterioles: *see* figure.
"Nicking of the retinal veins": arteriovenous crossing changes.
Increased light reflex and loss of transparency of blood column.
Arteriolar and venous tortuosity.
Cotton-wool spots.
Dot and blot hemorrhages.
Retinal edema.
Optic nerve edema.
Venous-venous collaterals [1].

Investigations
Blood pressure measurement.
Visual acuity testing.
Slit-lamp and dilated fundus examinations.
Fluorescein angiography: to look for evidence of impedance to blood flow, local areas of nonperfusion, and leakage from dilated capillaries.

Complications
Vascular occlusive disease (venous and arteriolar).
Macroaneurysm formation.
Optic neuropathy.
Optic nerve edema.
Blindness.

Pearls and Considerations
The Scheie Classification System identifies the following stages of hypertensive retinopathy:
Stage 0: normal.
Stage 1: broadening of the light reflex from the arteriole, with minimal or no arteriovenous compression.
Stage 2: light reflex changes and crossing changes are more prominent.
Stage 3: arterioles have a "copper wire" appearance, with more arteriovenous compression.
Stage 4: arterioles have a "silver wire" appearance, and arteriovenous crossing changes are most severe.

Referral Information
Refer to internist for evaluation, management, and control of hypertension.

Differential diagnosis
Congenital venous tortuosity.
Involutional sclerosis (atherosclerosis associated with aging).

Cause
Acute and/or chronic systemic hypertension.

Epidemiology
- 10%-15% of the adult population have hypertensive retinal changes.

Classification
Essential hypertensive retinal changes as described in Signs section.
Malignant hypertension (which includes the findings of essential hypertension plus exudative retinal detachment and optic nerve edema) [2].

Associated features
Heart failure.
Renal failure.
Stroke.
Peripheral vascular disease.

Pathology
- Retinal arterioles develop thickening of their walls as a result of intimal hyalinization, medial hypertrophy, and endothelial hypertrophy.

TREATMENT

Diet and Lifestyle
- Lose weight and exercise.
- Monitor sodium intake.

Pharmacologic Treatment
- Control blood pressure with medication supervised by the patient's primary care physician.

Nonpharmacologic Treatment
- No nonpharmacologic treatment is recommended.

Treatment aims
To normalize systemic blood pressure.

Prognosis
Good.

Follow-up and management
- Yearly dilated eye examinations to monitor blood vessel changes.

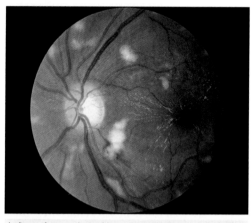

Left eye from patient with marked hypertension and grade III hypertensive retinopathy. Note cotton-wool spots (areas of axoplasmic flow backup) and macular star (exudates in Henle's outer plexiform layer of neural retina).

Key references
1. Leishman R: The eye in general vascular disease: hypertension and arteriosclerosis, *Br J Ophthalmol* 41:641-701, 1957.
2. Hayreh SS, Servais GE, Virdi PS, et al: Fundus lesions in malignant hypertension. III. Arterial blood pressure, biochemical, and fundus changes, *Ophthalmology* 93:45-59, 1986.

General reference
Murphy RP, Larn LA, Chew EY: Hypertension. In *Retina*, ed 4, E-dition, St Louis, 2006, Elsevier.

Hyphema   (361.41)

DIAGNOSIS

Definition
An accumulation of blood in the anterior chamber.

Synonyms
None.

Symptoms
Acute pain with injury and rebleeding: from acute glaucoma.
Photophobia.
Loss of vision or distortion of vision.

Signs
Tearing, squinting.
Injection of globe.
Blood in anterior chamber of eye.
Corneal opacity.

Investigations
Visual acuity.
Amount of blood in anterior chamber.
Status of cornea: presence of blood staining, other opacities or abrasions.
Status of lens: luxation, cataract.
Intraocular pressure with minimal globe manipulation.
Sickle cell hemoglobin status.
Fundus examination.

Complications
Glaucoma: from trabecular meshwork blockade by fresh red blood cells, crenated cells, ghost cells, and hemosiderin.
Corneal blood staining: from endothelial decompensation caused by inflammation, glaucoma, and red blood cell toxicity.
Amblyopia: in young child.
Cataract: from inflammation, glaucoma.
Central retinal artery occlusion: from glaucoma, especially in patients with sickle cell disease, trait, or hemoglobin SC.
Chronic: glaucoma associated with filtration-angle recession.
Vitreous hemorrhage.

Pearls and Considerations
1. Even a small hyphema can indicate major intraocular trauma.
2. Uncomplicated hyphemas will generally resolve in 5-6 days.

Referral Information
Hyphema patients should be hospitalized in most cases.

Cause
- Most cases result from trauma, but must consider spontaneous hyphemas caused by juvenile xanthogranuloma, retinoblastoma, or herpes zoster.

Epidemiology
- Traumatic hyphema is most common in children; mean age, 9 yr (in many series).
- Highest incidence of secondary rebleeding is at 3-4 days after trauma; rates vary from 0.4%-38.0% in patients receiving no systemic treatment.
- Highest rebleeding rates are reported in American urban populations, predominantly black; lowest in Scandinavian and Canadian series.
- Children and those taking aspirin are at increased risk for rebleeding.

Associated features
- Consider posterior globe rupture in patients with hypotony and total hyphema.
- Macular injury is the leading cause of any permanent vision loss.
- Glaucoma and corneal blood staining are most frequent reasons for surgical intervention.

Pathology
- Most traumatic hyphemas are caused by shearing rupture of the ciliary muscle after blunt contusion.
- Secondary bleeding may be caused by fibrinolysis and clot retraction or bleeding of fragile new capillaries.
- Corneal blood staining is an impregnation of the corneal stroma by hemoglobin and hemosiderin.

TREATMENT

Diet and Lifestyle
- No special precautions are necessary.

Pharmacologic Treatment
- Most physicians will treat hyphemas with cycloplegia (often atropine) and antiinflammatory drops (either steroids or nonsteroidal formulations).

Standard dosage	Aminocaproic acid, 100 mg/kg PO every 4 hr; maximum, 30 g/day.
Side effects	Nausea and vomiting (common), hypotension, syncope, acute renal failure, thrombotic complications (rare).
Contraindications	Because of side effects, many physicians use this drug only in patients from populations with high rebleeding rates (e.g., blacks).
Special points	Aminocaproic acid shown to reduce rebleeding rate in adults; from studies done in populations with known high rebleeding rates.

- Glaucoma is usually treated with drugs that decrease aqueous secretion or, acutely, with osmotic agents.

Nonpharmacologic Treatment
- Many physicians will place patients on bed rest with head of bed elevated 30 degrees and with bathroom privileges. The traumatized eye should be shielded. Routine bilateral patching, sedation, and strict bed rest are rarely performed today.
- Most patients will require hospitalization, but cooperative patients with small hyphemas may be managed at home with daily visits to the ophthalmologist.

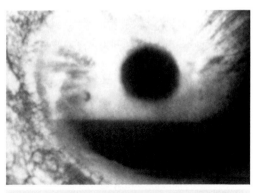

Hyphema of 30% in inserted eye.

Treatment aims
To resolve the hyphema.
To clear the cornea and lens.
To achieve normal intraocular pressure (IOP) and visual acuity.

Other treatments
- Surgical lavage of the hyphema may be necessary if IOP remains elevated, the cornea decompensates, or the hyphema does not resolve.
- There is danger to the optic nerve if IOP remains >50 mm for >5 days, >45 mm for >1 wk, or >35 mm for >2 wk. In patients with sickle cell trait or disease, or hemoglobin SC, lavage should be considered if IOP with treatment is >24 mm for >24 hr.
- There is danger of corneal blood staining if IOP is >25-30 mm for more than 6 days in an eye with more than half the anterior chamber filled with blood.

Prognosis
- Prognosis depends on the size of the initial hyphema; whether rebleeding has occurred; the presence of glaucoma; and damage to the cornea, lens, or macula.
- Most hyphemas of less than half the anterior chamber resolve without sequelae in a few days and without surgical intervention.

Follow-up and management
- Daily bedside visits of hospitalized patients are recommended, including evaluation of visual acuity, corneal clarity, amount of hyphema, and IOP if glaucoma concerns exist.
- Long-term follow-up up is mandatory in patients with traumatic angle recession, because ~1% per year will develop glaucoma.

General reference
Shepard J, Williams PB: Hyphema, 2005, www.emedicine.com.
Wilson FM: Traumatic hyphema: pathogenesis and management, *Ophthalmology* 687:910-919, 1980.

Internuclear ophthalmoplegia   (378.86)

DIAGNOSIS

Definition

A lesion of the medial longitudinal fasciculus (MLF) resulting in paresis of adduction and dissociated nystagmus.

Synonyms

None; abbreviated INO.

Symptoms

Blurred vision.
Double vision (vertical and horizontal).
Oscillopsia.

Signs (*see* Fig. 2)

Adduction deficit that varies from the absence of adduction to a mild decrease in the velocity of adduction without any limitation in the extent of movement: a "slowness" of adduction is seen more often than abducting nystagmus of the fellow eye; internuclear ophthalmoplegia (INO) is named "right" or "left" by the adduction deficit; the lesion is located on the same side as the adduction deficit; to "flush out" the adduction deficit, the patient must make large-amplitude horizontal saccades or be tested with optokinetic tape.

Abducting nystagmus with an inward drift with an outward corrective saccade that may be hypermetric, hypometric, or orthometric: the nystagmus intensity will decrease if the patient fixates with the eye with nystagmus.

Hypertropic eye: on the side of the adduction deficit, representing ocular skew torsion.

Convergence failure: suggests that the lesion involves the MLF in the midbrain; this is labeled an "anterior" INO.

Intact convergence: implies that the lesion has involved the MLF more caudally in the pons, sparing the medial rectus subnucleus; this is termed a "posterior" INO.

Investigations

Magnetic resonance imaging (MRI): with attention to the brainstem.
Anti-Ach Ab; Tensilon (edrophonium) test: to rule out myasthenia gravis.

Classification

- Variations of INO include *binocular* (BINO), "wall-eye" (WEBINO), and the "one-and-a-half" syndrome (1&1/2).
- BINO is an INO in each eye, i.e., bilateral adduction deficits with bilateral abducting nystagmus (*see* Fig. 1).
- WEBINO is a BINO with a manifest exotropia in primary position; the eye opposite the side of the lesion is deviated outward.
- 1&1/2 is gaze palsy in one direction and INO in the opposite direction; PPRF or cranial nerve (CN) VI nucleus and ipsilateral MLF lesions.
- Midbrain lesion (more rostral disease): Cogan's anterior INO convergence is affected because of CN III nuclei involvement.

Differential diagnosis

Inferior-division third-nerve palsy.
Orbital disease.
End-position nystagmus.
Myasthenia gravis (pseudo-INO).

Cause

- Unilateral disease (INO) is caused more often by brainstem infarction and observed more frequently in older males. The onset is apoplectic and associated with an ocular skew torsion sign in ~50% of cases.
- Bilateral disease (BINO) is likely caused by demyelinating disease, is more common in younger patients, and has an equal gender incidence. It has a more progressive onset.
- Convergence is present in 80% of both INO and BINO patients.
- Less common causes include:

Arnold-Chiari malformation with associated hydrocephalus and syringobulbia.
Meningoencephalitis.
Tuberculous meningitis.
Paraneoplastic encephalomyelitis.
Human immunodeficiency virus (HIV)–related cytomegalovirus (CMV) encephalitis.
Head trauma.
Drug intoxications.
Systemic lupus erythematosus.
Migraine.
Syphilis.
Supratentorial arteriovenous malformation.
Intracranial tumors.
Nutritional, degenerative, and metabolic disorders.

Pathology

Damage to MLF.

- Explanations for the abducting nystagmus include:
1. Increased convergence tone.
2. Disinhibition of the medial rectus muscle on the opposite side of the lesion.
3. Interruption of descending internuclear fibers that project to the fourth-nerve nucleus.
4. Gaze-evoked nystagmus.
5. Adaptation to the contralateral medial rectus muscle weakness.

Diagnosis continued on p. 188

TREATMENT

Diet and Lifestyle
- No special precautions are necessary.

Pharmacologic Treatment
- No pharmacologic treatment is recommended.

Treatment aims
To diagnose the underlying disease.

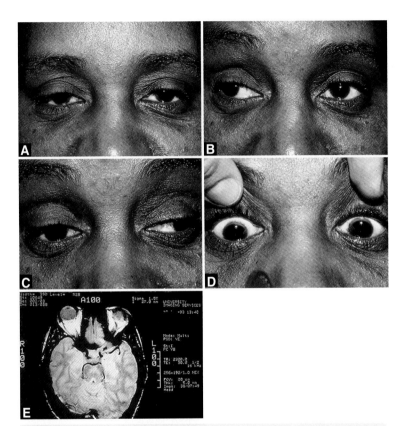

Figure 1 **A**, Woman with multiple sclerosis who has binocular internuclear ophthalmoplegia (BINO) in primary position. **B**, In right gaze, she has a left adduction deficit. **C**, In left gaze, she has a right adduction deficit. She has both right-eye and left-eye abducting nystagmus. **D**, Convergence is defective, suggesting that the lesion is anterior or in the midbrain. **E**, Corresponding T2-weighted axial MRI scan through the midbrain with high signal in the medial longitudinal fasciculus.

Treatment continued on p. 189

187

DIAGNOSIS—cont'd

Pearls and Considerations
1. INO can be unilateral or bilateral
2. The most common cause of INO (especially bilateral) in young adults is multiple sclerosis.

Referral Information
Refer for extensive systemic workup to rule out brain tumors, demyelinating disease, and other systemic etiologies.

TREATMENT—cont'd

Nonpharmacologic Treatment

- Prisms and patches are sometimes helpful.

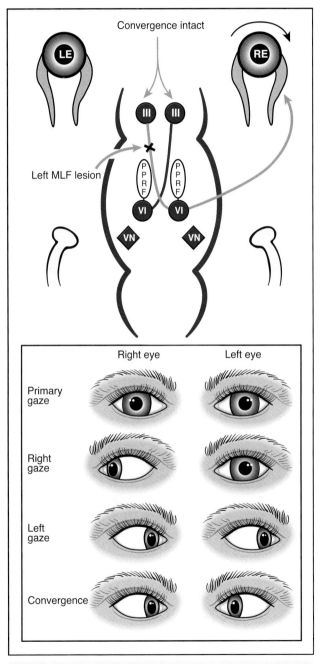

Figure 2 Brainstem diagram and ocular motility manifestations of the left MLF lesion. (*From Klein L, Bajandas FJ: Neuro-ophthalmology review manual, ed 5,* Thorofare, NJ, Slack.)

General references

Gray M, Forbes RB, Morrow JI: Primary isolated brainstem injury producing internuclear ophthalmoplegia, *Br J Neurosurg* 15(5):432-434, 2001.

Keane JR: Internuclear ophthalmoplegia: unusual causes in 114 of 410 patients, *Arch Neurol* 62(5):714-717, 2005.

Leigh RJ, Daroff RB, Troost BT: Supranuclear disorders of eye movements. In Tasman W et al, editors: *Duane's clinical ophthalmology* (CD-ROM), Philadelphia, 2004, Lippincott Williams & Wilkins.

Levin A, Arnold A: *Neuro-ophthalmology,* New York, 2005, Thieme Medical Publishers.

DIAGNOSIS

Definition
Inflammation of the uveal tract.

Synonyms
Iritis, uveitis, pars planitis.

Symptoms
Pain.
Redness.
Photophobia.
Increased lacrimation.
Blurry vision.
- Pain, decreased vision, and redness may be minimal in subacute cases.

Signs
Acute
Ciliary injection of the conjunctiva (hyperemia around the limbus).
Fine to large keratic precipitates (granulomatous) and fibrin dusting of the corneal endothelium.
Anterior chamber shows many cells, variable flare, and in rare cases, a hypopyon.
Dilated iris vessels and, rarely, a hyphema.
Posterior synechiae (adhesion of the pupillary iris to the lens).
Iris nodules.
Anterior vitreous cells.
Cystoid macular edema and, rarely, a disc edema.
Low intraocular pressure: usually, but may be elevated.

Chronic
Variable conjunctival redness as well as anterior-chamber reaction.

Investigations
Histories: onset and duration of symptoms, systems review (especially of arthritic, gastrointestinal, and genitourinary disorders), insect bite, rash, sexual, drug, family back disorders (e.g., ankylosing spondylitis).
Visual acuity testing.
Slit-lamp examination.
Intraocular pressure.
Dilated fundus examination.
- If uveitis is bilateral, granulomatous, or recurrent, then consider workup: complete blood count, erythrocyte sedimentation rate, antinuclear antibody, rapid plasma reagin, fluorescent treponemal antibody absorption, purified protein derivative (tuberculin) with anergy panel. Obtain a chest radiograph and consider HLA-B27.

Complications
Cataract.
Glaucoma.
Corneal edema.
Cystoid macular edema.

Pearls and Considerations
1. Upon second presentation of idiopathic iridocyclitis, patients should be referred for full systemic workup.
2. Anterior chamber cells and flare are best observed at the slit lamp with a bright conic section and room lights very dim.

Differential diagnosis
Rhegmatogenous retinal detachment (pigment cells in the anterior chamber).
Leukemia.
Retinoblastoma: in children.
Intraocular foreign body.
Malignant melanoma.
Juvenile xanthogranuloma.

Cause
Idiopathic: most common.
HLA-B27–positive iridocyclitis.
Juvenile rheumatoid arthritis.
Fuchs' heterochromic iridocyclitis.
Herpes simplex keratouveitis.
Syphilis.
Traumatic, sarcoid, and tuberculosis iridocyclitis.

Classification
Acute: signs and symptoms appear suddenly and last for up to 6 wk.
Chronic: onset is gradual and inflammation lasts longer than 6 wk.
Granulomatous: insidious onset; chronic course; eye nearly white; iris nodules and large keratic precipitates (mutton fat) present; posterior segment is commonly involved.
Nongranulomatous: acute onset; shorter course; red eye and intense flare present; no iris nodules.
Infectious: viruses, bacteria, rickettsiae, fungi, protozoa, parasites.
Noninfectious: exogenous (trauma, chemical injury), endogenous (immunologic types 1-4 hypersensitivities).

Associated features
Iris heterochromia, corneal band keratopathy.

Immunology
Mostly type III hypersensitivity reaction but also type II.

Pathology
Neutrophils, eosinophils, and lymphocytes in the anterior chamber and on the corneal endothelial and iris surfaces: large keratic precipitates and iris nodules are granulomas.

TREATMENT

Diet and Lifestyle

- No special precautions are necessary.

Pharmacologic Treatment

Cycloplegia

Standard dosage   Cyclopentolate 1%-2%, 3 times daily for mild to moderate inflammation;

Atropine 1%, 2-3 times daily for moderate to severe inflammation.

Prednisolone acetate 1%, every 1-6 h.

Special points   Consider subtenons injection of steroid or systemic steroid, if patient unresponsive to topical therapy.

Treat secondary glaucoma with topical antiglaucoma medication.

If an infectious cause is determined, then the specific management should be added to the above regimen.

Consider a rheumatology consult.

Nonpharmacologic Treatment

Glaucoma surgery (e.g., tube-shunt devices): to control intraocular pressure.

Cataract surgery: usually not undertaken until the eye rests for at least 6 mo.

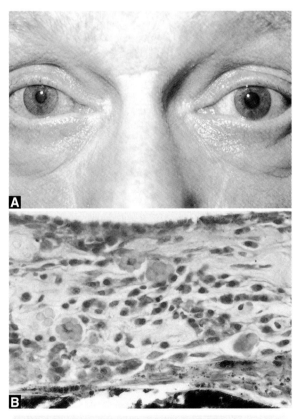

A, Ciliary injection and constricted right pupil caused by chronic endogenous uveitis ("acute" iritis). **B**, Iris shows chronic nongranulomatous inflammation with lymphocytes, plasma cells, and Russell bodies (large, pink, globular structures).

Treatment aims

To lessen or obviate inflammatory response in the anterior chamber and anterior vitreous.

Other treatments

- Other immunosuppressive therapy may be necessary to control inflammation.

Prognosis

- Prognosis is usually good with therapy.
- Patients with juvenile rheumatoid arthritis and Fuchs' heterochromic iridocyclitis have a high complication rate with cataract surgery.
- Patients with sarcoid, tuberculosis, and syphilis do well with appropriate therapy.

Follow-up and management

- Patients should be followed every 1 to 7 days in the acute phase and every 1 to 6 mo when stable. Complete ocular examination should be performed at each visit.
- If the anterior-chamber reaction is improving, then the steroid should be tapered slowly for a 3-wk period. In some cases, chronic low-dose steroids may be needed to prevent recurrence.

General references

Albert DM, Jakobiec FA, editors: *Principles and practice of ophthalmology,* vol 1, Philadelphia, 1994, Saunders.

American Academy of Ophthalmology: *Basic and clinical science,* section 8, San Francisco, 2006-2007, American Academy of Ophthalmology.

Kotaniemi K, Savolainen A, Karma A, et al: Recent advances in uveitis of juvenile idiopathic arthritis, *Surv Ophthalmol* 48:489, 2003 (major review).

Teyssot N, Cassoux N, Lehoang P, et al: Fuchs heterochromic cyclitis and ocular toxocariasis, *Am J Ophthalmol* 139:915, 2005

Wright K: *Textbook of ophthalmology,* Baltimore, 1997, Williams & Wilkins.

Iris atrophy, essential or progressive (iridocorneal-endothelial syndrome) (364.51)

DIAGNOSIS

Definition
Decompensation or breakdown of the iris tissue.

Synonyms
None; abbreviated ICE (iridocorneal-endothelial) syndrome.

Symptoms
Distortion of the pupil: patients are usually asymptomatic, but the patient or a family member may notice the distortion of the pupil.

Decreased vision: if there is associated corneal edema or if the glaucoma is far advanced, the patient may complain of decreased vision in the involved eye.

Pain: rare, but may occur in cases of severe corneal decompensation with bullous keratopathy; may be caused by angle closure.

Age at onset: usually in young or middle-aged adults (20-50 yr).

Signs
Corneal changes: the corneal endothelium assumes a characteristic "beaten metal" appearance that can be seen with the slit lamp; corneal edema may be present.

Iris atrophy and nodules: iris changes may be atrophic or nodular; in the atrophic form, displacement of the pupil *(corectopia)* and atrophic defects in the iris stroma and pigment epithelium *(polycoria)* may be seen; in the nodular type, pigmented, pedunculated nodules are seen on the iris surface; the disease is usually unilateral.

Elevated intraocular pressure (IOP): approximately half of patients with (ICE syndrome develop glaucoma; IOP is usually extremely elevated; significant optic nerve cupping and visual field loss are seen, depending on the duration of the elevated IOP; the glaucoma is more severe in the iris atrophy and iris nevus syndrome variations.

Anterior-chamber-angle closure: gonioscopy may reveal angle closure by peripheral anterior synechiae (PAS) without pupillary block; the PAS extend beyond Schwalbe's line. In earlier cases, all or some of the angle may be open.

Investigations
Complete eye examination: including gonioscopy.

Photography: photographic documentation of the anterior segment as well as the optic nerve is useful to monitor the progression of the disease.

Perimetry: should be performed at regular intervals.

Complications
Glaucoma and corneal edema: the glaucoma may be very difficult to control, resulting in permanent vision loss in the affected eye; persistent corneal edema may require corneal transplantation.

Referral Information
Refer for glaucoma surgery and penetrating keratoplasty as appropriate.

Differential diagnosis
Corneal endothelial disorders (e.g., posterior polymorphous corneal dystrophy, Fuchs' endothelial dystrophy).
Acquired iris abnormalities (e.g., herpesvirus infections, iritis, previous episodes of acute glaucoma and iris melanoma).
Hereditary iris conditions (e.g., Axenfeld-Rieger syndrome).

Cause
- The cause is unknown. The lack of family history, adult onset, and unilaterality of most cases would suggest an acquired cause. Some speculate that the cause is infectious, possibly herpes simplex virus or Epstein-Barr virus.

Epidemiology
- ICE syndrome is rare, and most cases are sporadic.
- The disease is more often seen in women.

Classification
- *Essential iris atrophy* is used for cases in which the iris atrophy predominates.
- *Chandler's syndrome* is used for cases in which corneal changes predominate and iris atrophy is minimal.
- *Cogan-Reese syndrome*, also called the *iris nevus syndrome*, is used to describe cases in which iris nodules are the predominant feature.

Pathology
- Corneal changes are characterized by an abnormal endothelial cell membrane that proliferates onto the iris surface and over the anterior-chamber angle. The membrane interferes with the function of the trabecular meshwork, resulting in glaucoma. As the membrane contracts, it pulls the peripheral iris into the angle, forming PAS.
- Atrophic changes are seen in the iris with loss of both stroma and pigment endothelium, resulting in distortion, displacement of the pupil, and full-thickness holes in the iris. In the nodular type, pigmented lesions resembling nevi are seen over the anterior surface of the iris.

Iris atrophy, essential or progressive (iridocorneal-endothelial syndrome)   (364.51)

TREATMENT

Diet and Lifestyle
- No precautions are necessary.

Pharmacologic Treatment
- Miotics are generally ineffective in treating the glaucoma associated with ICE syndrome. Aqueous suppressants and prostaglandin analogs are often successful in the early stages of the disease; as the disease progresses, however, medical treatment is less likely to achieve control of IOP.
- Hypertonic saline solutions can aid in the control of the corneal edema.

Nonpharmacologic Treatment
Laser: laser trabeculoplasty is of no benefit in the glaucoma associated with ICE syndrome; because the angle closure is not caused by pupillary block, laser iridectomy is likewise of no benefit.

Filtering surgery: filtering surgery or the use of aqueous shunt devices is often successful, but late failures are common because of endothelialization of the fistula. Yttrium-aluminum-garnet (YAG) laser can be used to cut the endothelial cell membrane and reopen the fistula.

Cyclodestructive procedures: when IOP cannot be controlled with medical or surgical treatment, a cyclodestructive procedure may be used.

Corneal transplantation: in patients with corneal edema that causes reduced vision, corneal transplantation may help to restore vision, although success rates are lower in ICE syndrome than in other causes of corneal edema.

Treatment aims
To preserve vision by controlling IOP.

Prognosis
- The prognosis is poor.
- ICE syndrome is the result of a proliferation of an abnormal cellular membrane inside the anterior chamber; there is no treatment that halts this process. As the proliferation continues, the glaucoma becomes more severe and resistant to standard treatments. Severe and permanent loss of vision in the affected eye is a common outcome.

Follow-up and management
- Patients should be followed at regular intervals to monitor the progression of the disease; IOP and the appearance of the cornea and optic disc should be recorded at each visit.
- Visual fields should be tested frequently, depending on the severity of the glaucoma.
- Although there is no cure and the ultimate prognosis is poor, useful vision may often be preserved for a long time with careful follow-up and treatment.

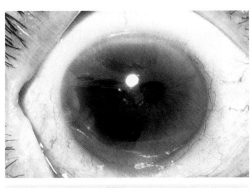

Iridocorneal-endothelial (ICE) syndrome showing distortion and displacement of the pupil as well as large areas of iris atrophy.

General references

Eagle RC Jr, Font RL, Yanoff M, Fine BS: Proliferative endotheliopathy with iris abnormalities in the iridocorneal endothelial syndrome, *Arch Ophthalmol* 97:2104-2111, 1979.

Glaucoma and the iridocorneal endothelial syndrome, *Arch Ophthalmol* 110:346-350, 1992.

Ritch R, Wilson MR, Samples J: Management of iridocorneal endothelial syndrome, *J Glaucoma* 3:154-159, 1994.

Shields MB: Progressive iris atrophy, Chandler's syndrome, and the iris nevus (Cogan-Reese) syndrome: a spectrum of disease, *Surv Ophthalmol* 24:3-20, 1979.

Keratitis   (370.9)

DIAGNOSIS

Definition
Inflammation of the cornea.

Synonyms
Keratoconjunctivitis, keratopathy.

Symptoms
Redness.
Ocular pain.
Decreased vision.
Photophobia.
Discharge.

Signs
Corneal infiltrate/ulcer: if infectious keratitis (*see* Fig. 1).
Ring infiltrate: seen in acanthamebiasis, topical anesthetic abuse.
Hypopyon: more common in infectious keratitis.
Corneal edema.
Dendrites, pseudodendrites: if epithelial involvement in herpes simplex virus (HSV) or herpes zoster virus (HZV); may be early sign of *Acanthamoeba* infection (*see* Fig. 2).
Periorbital rash: seen with HZV keratitis; occasionally seen with HSV keratitis.
Epithelial defect.

Investigations
Corneal cultures: bacterial and fungal cultures on all patients, consider additional cultures (Löwenstein-Jensen, nonnutrient agar with *Escherichia coli* overlay) if atypical organism suspected or history of LASIK.
• Consider cultures of contact lenses or contact lens case.
Viral cultures: may be performed to support diagnosis of HSV, but this is typically a clinical diagnosis.
Corneal biopsy: consider if keratitis continues to progress, highly suspect infectious organisms, but routine cultures negative.

Differential diagnosis
Bacterial keratitis.
Fungal keratitis.
Herpes simplex keratitis.
Herpes zoster keratitis.
Acanthamoeba.
Sterile corneal infiltrate.
Topical anesthetic abuse.
Atypical mycobacteria.

Cause
• *Pseudomonas* most common cause of bacterial keratitis in contact lens wearers; main risk factor is sleeping with contact lenses.
• Fungal keratitis seen after outdoor or dirty ocular trauma or in patients with chronic ocular surface disease.
• *Acanthamoeba* most often seen in contact lens wearers with homemade or tap water cleaning solutions or those wearing contact lenses while swimming, fishing, or using hot tub.
• Atypical mycobacteria recognized etiology of infectious keratitis following LASIK.

Diagnosis continued on p. 196

TREATMENT

Diet and Lifestyle

Prevent corneal ulcers by avoiding sleeping in contact lenses.

Clean contact lenses daily; use enzyme weekly.

Consider daily disposable soft contact lenses as alternative.

Pharmacologic Treatment

Infectious Keratitis

Standard dosage

If bacterial keratitis: fortified antibiotics, broad spectrum. Typical combination includes fortified cefazolin (50 mg/ml) or fortified vancomycin (25 mg/ml) and fortified tobramycin (15 mg/ml) or fortified gentamicin (15 mg/ml). After giving a loading dose of drops every 5-15 min, use every 1 hr, around the clock initially. For smaller infiltrates, consider topical gatifloxacin or moxifloxacin every hour daily in place of fortified antibiotics.

Special points: fortified antibiotics need to be made by hospital or compounding pharmacy and usually have a limited shelf life of a few days to 2 wk.

If fungal ulcer: topical natamycin 5% (especially for filamentous fungi), or amphotericin B 0.15% (especially for molds, candida) every hour; consider topical voriconazole as well.

If hypopyon or significant anterior-chamber reaction: cycloplegia. Atropine 1%, 3 times daily if hypopyon; scopolamine 0.25% or Cyclogel 1%-2%, 2 or 3 times daily for mild to moderate anterior-chamber inflammation.

Herpes Simplex Keratitis

Standard dosage:

For epithelial/dendritic disease: trifluridine every 2 hr. Can also use oral antivirals (e.g., acyclovir, 400 mg 5 times daily) in place of topical agents.

For stromal keratitis: topical steroids (prednisolone acetate 1%) 4 times daily. Need to give antiviral prophylaxis, either with trifluridine (4 times daily) or oral antiviral (acyclovir, 400 mg twice daily). Also consider cycloplegia (Cyclogel 1%-2% or scopolamine 0.25%, 2 or 3 times daily).

Treatment aims

Eradicate infection or inflammation of cornea with minimal scarring.

Other treatments

- If visually significant scar remains after treatment of keratitis, consider rigid, gas-permeable contact lenses. If unable to tolerate contact lens or vision poor despite contact lens, consider corneal transplantation.

Prognosis

- Prognosis depends on severity and location of keratitis.
- Small, peripheral corneal ulcers may heal without visual sequelae, whereas large, central infectious ulcers may require corneal transplantation for visual rehabilitation.
- HSV is a chronic condition with possible reactivation of disease.

Follow-up and management

- Patients with ulcers seen on daily basis until infection is under control. Topical antibiotics can then be tapered slowly.
- HSV and HZV patients can be seen 1 wk after initial visit, and every 2-6 wk thereafter depending on response to medications.

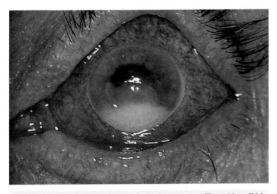

Figure 1 Central corneal ulcer with hypopyon. *(From Yanoff M, Fine BS: Ocular pathology, ed 5, Mosby, St Louis, 2002.)*

Treatment continued on p. 197

DIAGNOSIS—cont'd

Complications
Corneal scarring.
Corneal perforation.
Elevated intraocular pressure: most common with HZV.
Recurrent keratitis: especially with HSV.

Pearls and Considerations
Usually avoid steroids acutely, especially if fungal infection or HSV epithelial keratitis.

Referral Information
Consider referral if ulcer progresses despite treatment, or if perforation appears likely or occurs.

TREATMENT—cont'd

Herpes Zoster Keratitis

Pseudodendrites or superficial punctate keratitis (SPK): frequent lubrication with preservative-free artifical tears every 1 to 2 hr. May benefit from topical steroids as well (prednisolone acetate 1%, 4 times daily).

Stromal keratitis: topical steroids (prednisolone acetate 1%, initially every 2-4 hr); steroids must be tapered very slowly over months to years.

Nonpharmacologic Treatment

- No contact lens wear.
- For herpes simplex epithelial keratitis, consider debridement of dendrites.

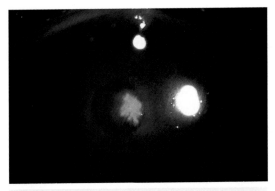

Figure 2 Herpes simplex dendrite staining with fluorescein. *(From Yanoff M, Fine BS: Ocular pathology, ed 5, Mosby, St Louis, 2002.)*

General references

American Academy of Ophthalmology: *Basic and clinical science,* section 8, San Francisco, 2006-2007, The Academy.

Smolin G, Thoft RA: *The cornea: scientific foundation and clinical practice,* Boston, 2004, Little, Brown.

Tasman W, Jaeger E, editors: *Duane's clinical ophthalmology,* vol 4, Philadelphia, 2005, Lippincott-Raven.

Yanoff M, Fine B: *Ocular pathology: a color atlas,* Philadelphia, 1988, Lippincott.

Keratoconus   (371.60)

DIAGNOSIS

Definition
Noninflammatory, usually bilateral protrusion of the cornea.

Synonym
Conical cornea.

Symptoms
Progressive decrease in vision.
Sudden onset of pain, redness, tearing, and blurred vision in acute hydrops.

Signs
Central corneal ectasia with thinning (*see* Fig. 1).
Irregular corneal reflex on retinoscopy.
Vogt's striae: parallel tension lines in posterior corneal stroma.
Fleisher ring: iron line outlining protruding cone (*see* Fig. 2).
Munson's sign: bulging of eyelid in downward gaze.
Hydrops: acute break in Descemet's membrane causing significant edema and opacification of cornea.

Investigations
Slit-lamp examination.
Retinoscopy: water-drop or scissors reflex.
Refraction.
Computed corneal topography: irregular astigmatism with inferior steepening.
Keratometry: irregular mires and steepening.

Complications
Hydrops: *see* Signs.

Pearls and Considerations
Consider keratoconus in young patients who present with decreased vision and an otherwise normal examination; examine closely for signs.

Referral Information
Refer to contact lens specialist for rigid gas-permeable contact lenses. If no improvement in vision or unable to tolerate, consider referral for surgical management.

Differential diagnosis
Pellucid marginal degeneration.
Keratoglobus.

Cause
- Unclear; may be related to chronic eye rubbing.
- Associated with Down syndrome, atopic disease, and mitral valve prolapse.

TREATMENT

Diet and Lifestyle
No special precautions are necessary.

Pharmacologic Treatment
For Acute Hydrops
Standard dosage   Scopolamine 0.25%, 2 or 3 times daily.

Sodium chloride 5%, drops or ointment, 4 times daily.

Nonpharmacologic Treatment
- Patients counseled to refrain from eye rubbing.
- Mild cases may be treated with glasses or soft contact lenses.
- Moderate to advanced cases require rigid, gas-permeable contact lenses.
- Intrastromal corneal rings may be used as an alternative to contact lenses.
- Corneal transplantation, either penetrating keratoplasty or deep anterior lamellar keratoplasty, performed when patients are intolerant of contact lenses or cannot achieve adequate vision with contact lenses.

Treatment aims
To optimize visual acuity.

Prognosis
Prognosis for good visual acuity is excellent.

Follow-up and management
- Every 6-12 mo for patients doing well with glasses or contact lenses.
- Patients with hydrops should be seen every 1-4 wk until resolved.

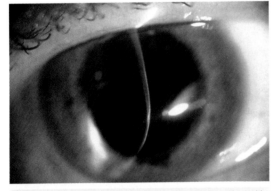

Figure 1   Central corneal thickening and ectasia in patient with keratoconus.

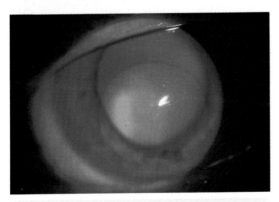

Figure 2   Fleisher ring seen with cobalt-blue light.

General references
American Academy of Ophthalmology: *Basic and clinical science,* section 8, San Francisco, 2006-2007, The Academy.
Smolin G, Thoft RA: *The cornea: scientific foundation and clinical practice,* Boston, 2004, Little, Brown.
Tasman W, Jaeger E, editors: *Duane's clinical ophthalmology,* vol 4, Philadelphia, 2005, Lippincott-Raven.
Yanoff M, Fine B: *Ocular pathology: a color atlas,* Philadelphia, 1988, Lippincott.

Lacrimal drainage inflammation (375.3)

DIAGNOSIS

Definition
Infection or inflammation of the lacrimal excretory system.

Synonym
Dacryocystitis.

Symptoms
Tearing.
Mucous discharge.
Pain.
Lump in medial canthal area.
- Episodes develop suddenly.

Signs
Mass in medial canthal area: with erythema extending along the inferior orbital area (*see* figure).
Mucus reflux through the canaliculi: resulting from pressure on the sac.

Investigations
External ocular examination.
Evaluation of extent of erythema and tenderness: for possible cellulitis.
Pressure on sac: to see if reflux can be elicited.
Examination of nasal passages: for possible rhinitis, septal deviation, or mass.
General eye examination evaluating vision, motility, etc.: to rule out evidence of orbital cellulitis.
Sinus radiographs, computed tomography scan: to rule out an underlying cause.
Schirmer testing.
Dacryocystography.

Complications
If left untreated, can lead to **chronic obstructive problems** with marked tearing.
May result in **fistula formation** to skin if drainage occurs externally.
May lead to **orbital cellulitis.**

Pearls and Considerations
1. May be acute, subacute, or chronic.
2. 60% of cases are recurrent.
3. Often characterized by a palpable, painful mass at the inner canthus.

Referral Information
No referrals are necessary.

Differential diagnosis
Sinusitis.
Cellulitis.
Canaliculitis.

Cause
- Cause is believed to be an anatomic abnormality that results in stasis of tear flow. The restriction of flow results in inflammation of the lacrimal passages, caused by an increase in the number of normal bacterial tear flora that accumulate in the blocked lacrimal sac. Causes of the anatomic abnormality include impatency, stone, trauma, sinus inflammation or infection, and stenosis of ostium.
- Rarely, systemic diseases have been associated, including sarcoidosis, tuberculosis, and collagen vascular disease.

Epidemiology
- Common incidence is in two age groups: <2 yr and >40 yr.
- In adult forms, there is a female predominance.

Classification
Acute dacryocystitis: sudden onset, increased symptoms.
Chronic dacryocystitis: indolent chronic course.
Congenital dacryocystitis: usually caused by incomplete canalization at the valve of Hasner.

Immunology
- Although no immunologic factors are involved in the causes of lacrimal tract infections, the potency of the immune protection system may explain the relative rarity of the condition.
- High quantities of immunoglobulin A (IgA) are found in tears; also, IgA, IgD, and IgE are found in the conjunctivae that line the lacrimal system.

Pathology
- Most believe that the agents responsible are *Staphylococcus aureus, S. epidermidis, Streptococcus* sp., and *Haemophilus* sp. (in young children).

TREATMENT

Diet and Lifestyle
- No special precautions are necessary.

Pharmacologic Treatment
Systemic antibiotics: either IV or PO, depending on extent of infection.
Analgesics: for pain control.
- Avoid antipyretics in order to assess whether patient becomes febrile.

Nonpharmacologic Treatment
Acute dacryocystitis: digital decompression, if possible.
Chronic dacryocystitis: digital decompression of sac, but definitive treatment requires surgical intervention with dacryocystorhinostomy.
Congenital dacryocystitis: massage of sac with digital decompression: if resolution fails to occur over a short treatment period; lacrimal system should be probed because success rates of probing fall dramatically >1 yr of age.

Treatment aims
To resolve pain and the infectious process through prevention of complications (e.g., cellulitis, fistula formation, chronic tearing).

Prognosis
- Congenital obstructions meet with good success if treated before 1 yr of age with probing. Many will open spontaneously over the first several months of life.
- Acute and chronic obstructions may require surgical manipulation, but such surgeries reach high levels of success for ultimate patency and relief of symptoms.

Follow-up and management
As needed to ensure adequate control of infection and subsequent restoration of system patency to prevent persistent epiphora (tearing).

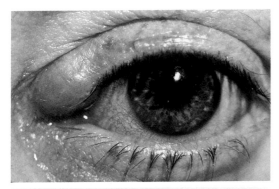

Focal edema and erythema in area of left upper medial canthus in patient with *Leptothrix* canaliculitis.

General references
Tse D: Lacrimal system. In Roy F, editor: *Ocular differential diagnosis*, Baltimore, 1997, Lippincott Williams & Wilkins, pp 127-145.
Hornblss A et al: *Oculoplastic, orbital, and reconstructive surgery*, vol 2, Baltimore, 1990, Lippincott Williams & Wilkins.
Meyer D, Linberg J: Acute dacryocystitis. In *Oculoplastic and orbital emergencies*, Norwalk, Conn, 1990, Appleton & Lange, pp 29-43.
Tasman W, Jaeger E, editors: *Duane's clinical ophthalmology*, vol 4, Philadelphia, 2005, Lippincott-Raven.

Lattice degeneration   (362.63)

DIAGNOSIS

Definition
A thinning of the peripheral retina characterized by local round, oval, or linear patches of pigmented or nonpigmented thinning.

Synonym
Snail-track degeneration.

Symptoms
- Patients are asymptomatic.

Signs
Round, oval, or elongated areas of retinal thinning: with sharp borders usually located between the ora serrata and the equator; common locations are found from the 11 to 1 o'clock positions and between the 5 and 7 o'clock positions; retinal thinning found in the inferotemporal quadrant is the most common (*see* figure).
- Lattice often has white lines, which represent sheathed vessels. Small, round atrophic retinal holes may be found within the lattice degeneration or adjacent to these areas.

Investigations
Visual acuity testing.
Biomicroscopic examination.
Dilated fundus examination.

Complications
Retinal tears: may occur with posterior vitreous detachments or trauma, leading to retinal detachment.
- The vitreous is more firmly attached to the edges of the lattice; thus, when the vitreous separates, the retina may tear at the edge of an area of lattice.

Pearls and Considerations
Lattice degeneration must be differentiated from other forms of peripheral retinal degenerations because other forms do not predispose the patient to retinal detachment as does lattice degeneration.

Referral Information
Refer to retinal specialist if secondary detachment or tear occurs.

Differential diagnosis
Peripheral pigmentation.
Cystoid degeneration.

Cause
- Lattice degeneration is more common in myopic patients.
- There may be an inheritance pattern of autosomal dominance.

Epidemiology
- 7% of the population will have lattice degeneration.
- Lattice degeneration tends to be bilateral in 45% of patients.
- The disease is equally distributed between the two genders.
- There is no racial predilection.
- In ~30% of eyes with a rhegmatogenous retinal detachment, this is secondary to lattice degeneration.

Classification
Peripheral retinal degeneration.

Associated features
May be seen in patients with pigment dispersion syndrome.

Pathology
- There is a lack of internal limiting membrane, overlying vitreous liquefaction, vitreous condensation, and exaggerated vitreoretinal adherence at the borders of these lesions.
- There may be associated retinal pigment abnormalities (e.g., focal pigment loss, pigment migration into retina and around retinal vessels).
- Trypsin digest reveals loss of capillaries and decreased number of endothelial cells.
- There is also glial proliferation at the interface between the retina and formed vitreous.

TREATMENT

Diet and Lifestyle
- Safety glasses are recommended for sports-related activity for individuals with large patches of lattice degeneration.
- In patients with a history of retinal detachment and lattice degeneration in their fellow eye, high-impact sports are not recommended.

Pharmacologic Treatment
- No pharmacologic treatment is recommended.

Nonpharmacologic Treatment
- Prophylactic laser surgery or cryotherapy is indicated in patients with retinal breaks secondary to vitreoretinal traction or with a history of retinal detachment in their fellow eye. Prophylactic laser therapy is not indicated for the lattice with atrophic holes, which is asymptomatic.
- Controversy remains over whether prophylactic laser surgery should be performed in the fellow eye in patients with a history of retinal detachment; despite laser therapy, retinal tears can still develop at the edge of the laser scars.

Treatment aims
To educate patients on signs and symptoms of retinal detachment.

Prognosis
- Depends on degree of vitreoretinal adhesion, pigment changes, and associated round retinal holes.
- Overall, the incidence of retinal detachment is still quite low.

Follow-up and management
Annual dilated eye examinations.
- Patients need to be educated on the signs and symptoms of a retinal detachment (flashes, floaters, peripheral shadows, and loss of vision) and taught that this is an ocular emergency.

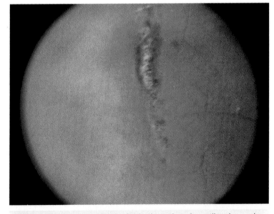

Elongated oval area of retinal thinning, sharply outlined margins with increased pigmentation, and white, sclerosed vessels traversing the area.

General references
Edwards AO, Robertson JE: Hereditary vitreoretinal degenerations. In *Retina*, ed 4, E-dition, St Louis, 2006, Elsevier.
Kroll AJ, Patel SC: Retinal breaks. In Albert DM, Jakobiec FA, editors: *Principles and practice of ophthalmology*, vol 2, Philadelphia, 1994, Saunders, pp 1057-1061.
Wesley P, Liebman J, Walsh JB, Rich R: Lattice degeneration of the retina and pigment dispersion syndrome, *Am J Ophthalmol* 114:539-543, 1992.

Leber's hereditary optic neuropathy   (377.39)

DIAGNOSIS

Definition
A condition found primarily in young men resulting in dyschromatopsia and bilateral reduction in visual acuity.

Synonyms
None; often abbreviated LHON.

Symptoms
Acute, rapid, irreversible, painless central vision loss: usually in one eye, followed by second eye in days to weeks.
"Mist" or "fog" obscuring vision.
Mild dyschromatopsia.
- Vision loss acute to subacute with stabilization in <4 mo.

Signs
Acuity loss: can be asymmetric; most Snellen acuities are worse than 20/200 but range from 20/20 to no light perception.
Color vision: significantly affected.
Central or cecocentral scotoma: 25-30 degrees of absolute scotoma surrounded by a relative scotoma.
Hyperemic nerve: during the acute phase of visual loss; late in course of diagnosis, pale.
Dilated and tortuous vessels.
Retinal and optic disc hemorrhages.
Retinal striations.
Obscurations of the disc margin.
Circumpapillary telangiectatic microangiopathy.
Peripapillary edema of the nerve fiber layer.
Acquired cupping of the optic disc.
Arteriolar attenuation.

Investigations
D-15 and Farnsworth Munsell 100-hue test.
Electrocardiography.
Magnetic resonance imaging.
Flourescein angiography.
Molecular genetic test.

Pearls and Considerations
- Absence of dye leakage from the disc or papillary region on fluorescein angiography.
- LHON is in the differential diagnosis of acute, painless loss of vision in a young patient.

Referral Information
Genetic testing is available for relatives.

Differential diagnosis
Toxic nutritional optic neuropathy.
Optic neuritis (papillitis).
Acute disseminated encephalomyelitis.

Cause
Mitochondrial DNA point mutations: three DNA mutations (11778, 3460, and 14484) account for ~90%-95% of cases of LHON.

Epidemiology
- Dominance in men is 80%-90%.
- Occurrence rate in woman at risk is 4%-32%.
- Onset of visual loss occurs at ages 15-35 yr. However, patient age can range from 5-80 yr.
- Singleton cases constitute 57%-90% of reported cases.

Associated features
- The 11778 mitochondrial DNA mutation has associated cardiac conduction abnormalities.
- The 3460 mitochondrial DNA mutation has the highest association with the cardiac preexcitation syndromes (Wolff-Parkinson-White and Lown-Ganong-Levine).
- The controversial 15257 mitochondrial DNA mutation may have a maculopathy resembling Stargardt's disease.

TREATMENT

Diet and Lifestyle
- Patients should avoid tobacco and excessive alcohol use.

Pharmacologic Treatment
- Treatment with the following pharmacologic agents remains controversial:
  Coenzyme Q10.
  Succinate.
  Vitamin K_1.
  Vitamin K_3.
  Vitamin C.
  Thiamine.
  Vitamin B_2.
  Idebenone.

Nonpharmacologic Treatment
Low-vision aids.

Treatment aims
To maximize usable vision.

Prognosis
- In most patients with LHON, the visual loss is usually permanent.
- Patients <20 yr of age have a better prognosis, with final acuities of better than 20/80.
- LHON patients with the 11778 mitochondrial DNA mutation have only a 4% chance of spontaneous recovery.
- LHON patients with the 14484 mitochondrial DNA mutation have 37%-65% spontaneous recovery.
- Improvement usually occurs gradually over 6-12 mo. There are reports of significant visual recovery years after onset of visual loss.
- Recurrence of LHON is unlikely.

General references
Howell N: LHON and other optic nerve atrophies: the mitochondrial connection, *Dev Ophthalmol* 37:94-108, 2003.
Johns DR, Colby KA: Treatment of Leber's hereditary optic neuropathy: theory to practice, *Semin Ophthalmol* 17(1):33-38, 2002.
Man PY, Turnbull DM, Chinnery PF: Leber hereditary optic neuropathy, *J Med Genet* 39(3): 162-169, 2002.
Mroczek-Tonska K, Kisiel B, Piechota J, Bartnik E: Leber hereditary optic neuropathy: a disease with a known molecular basis but a mysterious mechanism of pathology, *J Appl Genet* 44(4):529-538, 2003.
Newman NJ: Hereditary optic neuropathies. In Miller NR, Newman NJ, editors: *Walsh and Hoyt's clinical neuro-ophthalmology*, Baltimore, 1998, Williams & Wilkins.
Newman NJ: Hereditary optic neuropathies, *Eye* 18(11):1144-1160, 2004.
Sadun AA, Gurkan S: Hereditary, nutritional and toxic optic atrophies. In *Retina*, ed 4, E-dition, St Louis, 2006, Elsevier.

DIAGNOSIS

Definition
A white pupillary reflex.

Synonym
Cat's eye reflex.

Symptoms
Decreased visual acuity: in most patients.

Signs
White pupillary reflex: may arise from the cornea, lens, vitreous, or retina of the involved eye(s) (*see* figure).

Investigations
History: age at onset, presence of prematurity, family history of retinoblastoma or other cause, contact with puppies or kittens.

Complete eye examination: with special attention to corneal diameter, lens, vitreous, and retina.

Ultrasound: to detect calcification in retinoblastoma and retinal detachment in *retinopathy of prematurity* (ROP), toxocariasis, and *persistent hypertrophic primary vitreous* (PHPV).

Fluorescein angiography: to test for Coats' disease, retinoblastoma.

Serum enzyme-linked immunosorbent assay: to test for toxocariasis.

Magnetic resonance imaging of the orbit and brain: to detect retinoblastoma.

Restriction fragment length polymorphisms: to detect gene for Norrie disease.

Complications
- **Retinal detachment:** occurs in patients with PHPV, ROP, retinoblastoma, toxocariasis, choroidal coloboma, or Coats' disease.
- **Amblyopia:** if patient presents before 5 yr of age.
- **Local and distant metastases, death:** occurs in patients with retinoblastoma.
- **Glaucoma:** occurs in patients with PHPV or ROP.
- **Norrie disease:** bilateral retinal detachments at an early age; progressive sensorineural hearing loss, mental retardation.

Differential Diagnosis/Cause
Retinoblastoma: usually occurs in otherwise-normal eye as one or more white lesions in the inner retina; vitreous metastases and extension through sclera may occur; iris neovascularization and tumor hypopyon occur rarely; age of onset usually 12-18 mo; autosomal dominant transmission (hereditary cases usually bilateral).

Toxocariasis: usually unilateral, presenting at ~7 yr of age; forms include isolated white retinal mass, pars planitis, acute vitritis, vitreous traction, and retinal detachment; no systemic eosinophilia.

PHPV: congenital developmental anomaly with microphthalmos, shallow anterior chamber, elongated ciliary body processes invading the posterior lens and causing cataract, and iris vascular engorgement; retina may contain tufts of dysplastic tissue.

ROP: usually bilateral and symmetric; found in infants with history of prematurity, low birth weight, supplemental oxygen; peripheral retinal neovascularization with traction bands from lens to retina, leading to retinal detachment in severe cases.

Coats' disease: usually unilateral disease of males, presenting at ~7 yr of age; peripheral retinal microaneurysms leak lipid into and below the retina, which may cause retinal detachment.

Norrie disease: bilateral total retinal detachments at birth or shortly after in males, with vitreoretinal hemorrhage, retrolental mass, cataract, glaucoma, optic nerve atrophy, phthisis.

Incontinentia pigmenti: obliterative arteritis beginning in retinal periphery and moving toward nerve; cataracts associated; characteristic pigmented skin lesions in bathing suit distribution.

Congenital cataract, choroidal coloboma, myelinated nerve fibers, congenital retinal schisis.

Epidemiology
Retinoblastoma: incidence is ~1:20,000 live births; 94% of cases are sporadic (somatic mutations, unilateral); 6% are familial (germinal mutations, autosomal dominant inheritance, usually bilateral); no gender or race predilection; gene isolated to 13q14 locus; some patients will have 13q- deletion.

PHPV: not hereditary; no gender or race predilection.

ROP: not hereditary; no gender predilection; may have characteristic of racial disease.

Coats' disease: not hereditary; no race predilection; 90% of those affected are men.

Norrie disease: X-linked recessive; gene isolated to DXS7 locus on Xp 11; no race predilection.

Incontinentia pigmenti: X-linked dominant; lethal in males; only noted in females; no race predilection.

Pathology
Retinoblastoma: sheets of small basophilic cells, with frequent calcification in the areas removed from retinal vessels; may grow toward the vitreous, through the sclera, or both; exits the eye through the vortex veins, down the optic nerve, and from aqueous veins.

PHPV: enlarged ciliary body process invades the lens; traction bands from the lens to retina.

ROP: retinal neovascularization at junction of vascular and avascular retina attaches to lens and causes retinal detachment; engorgement and tortuosity of posterior pole retinal vessels and iris vessels.

Coats' disease: miliary aneurysms of peripheral retinal vessels; intraretinal and subretinal lipid deposition in fovea and periphery.

Norrie disease: dysplastic, detached retina with absent photoreceptos; retinal gliosis.

Incontinentia pigmenti: occlusive retinal vasculitis with detachment, optic nerve atrophy.

Toxocariasis: retinal nematode with zonular inflammatory surround of eosinophils, granulomatous cells.

Choroidal coloboma: absent retinal pigment epithelium, choriocapillaris, outer retina; inner retina is thin, acellular.

Congenital retinal schisis: splitting of retinal nerve fiber layer.

Diagnosis continued on p. 208

TREATMENT

Diet and Lifestyle

- Infants are at risk of acquiring toxocariasis if they ingest ova of *Toxocara canis* or *T. catis*. This usually occurs through contact with the ova in puppy feces or on puppy fur.

Pharmacologic Treatment

- No pharmacologic treatment is recommended.

Nonpharmacologic Treatment

Retinoblastoma: enucleation, external proton beam radiation, scleral plaque placement, systemic drugs as indicated in each case.

Coats' disease: photocoagulation of abnormal vessels.

Toxocariasis: topical or systemic steroids.

PHPV: lensectomy, removal of fibrous tissue invading lens.

ROP: photocoagulation or cryotherapy to avascular retina, repair of retinal detachment, management of amblyopia, strabismus, glaucoma as indicated.

Treatment aims

Retinoblastoma: to preserve vision, life.

Coats' disease: to destroy abnormal retinal vessels and resolve foveal lipid.

Toxocariasis: to control intraocular inflammation.

PHPV: to improve visual acuity; prevent phthisis.

Prognosis

Retinoblastoma: ~70% of globes can be salvaged with some useful vision; <5% of children will die of metastatic tumor; patients with hereditary retinoblastoma (germinal mutation) have a 26% chance of dying from second cancer in 40 yr.

Toxocariasis: eyes require enucleation; vision compromised in most patients.

Coats' disease: significant recovery of visual acuity, if treated early.

PHPV: few eyes will develop good visual acuity even after lensectomy; some will develop glaucoma, require enucleation.

Norrie disease: all children bilaterally blind.

Incontinentia pigmenti: varies greatly, and many children maintain useful vision; some will be bilaterally blind.

Treatment continued on p. 209

DIAGNOSIS—cont'd

Pearls and Considerations

Leukokoria is the presenting symptom in 90% of retinoblastoma cases and is considered the classic clinical presentation for retinoblastoma.

Referral Information

Varied; dependent on cause of the condition.

TREATMENT—cont'd

Norrie disease: no known treatment.
Incontinentia pigmenti: no known treatment.
Choroidal coloboma: no known treatment; repair of secondary retinal detachment.
Congenital retinal schisis: no treatment needed, unless retinal detachment occurs.

Follow-up and Management
Varies with cause of leukokoria.

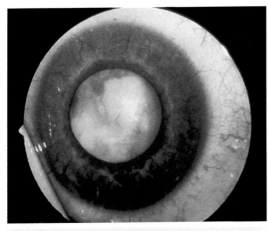

White pupillary reflex in patient with retinoblastoma.

General references

Catalano RA: Incontinentia pigmenti, *Am J Ophthalmol* 110:696-703, 1990.

Eagle RC: Retinoblastoma and simulating lesions. In Tasman W et al, editors: *Duane's clinical ophthalmology* (CD-ROM), Philadelphia, 2004, Lippincott, Williams & Wilkins.

Goldberg MF, Mafee M: Computed tomography for diagnosis of persistent hyperplastic primary vitreous (PHPV), *Ophthalmology* 90:442-450, 1983.

Haik BK: Advanced Coats' disease, *Trans Am Ophthalmol Soc* 89:371-380, 1991.

Holmes LB: Norrie's disease: an X-linked syndrome of retinal malformations, mental retardation, and deafness, *N Engl J Med* 284:367-374, 1971.

Jain IS, Mohan K, Jain S: Retinoblastoma: modes of presentation, *J Ocul Ther Surg* 4:83-87, 1985.

Patz A: Observations on the retinopathy of prematurity, *Am J Ophthalmol* 100:164-172, 1985.

Sang DN, Albert DM: Retinoblastoma: clinical and histopathologic features, *Hum Pathol* 13: 133-136, 1982.

Watzke RC, Oaks JA, Folk JC: *Toxocara canis* infection of the eye: correlation of clinical observations with developing pathology in the primate model, *Arch Ophthalmol* 102:282-288, 1984.

DIAGNOSIS

Definition

1. *Nonexudative* form: an inherited retinal condition typified by drusen, retinal pigment epithelium (RPE) changes, and visual disturbances.
2. *Exudative* form: an advanced form in which choroidal neovascular membranes develop under the RPE and leak fluid and blood, ultimately leading to a blinding, disciform scar.

Synonyms

None; typically abbreviated ARMD; nonexudative form often referred to as "dry" and exudative form as "wet."

Symptoms

Metamorphopsia (distortion).
Blurry vision.
Scotomas (small areas of vision missing).

Signs

Decreased vision.
Abnormal Amsler grid.
Subretinal and intraretinal hemorrhage, fluid, and lipid exudation secondary to choroidal neovascularization (CNV): *see* Figs. 1 and 2.
Pigment alteration in the macula.

Investigations

Careful history to determine the duration of symptoms.
Visual acuity testing.
Amsler grid testing: look for areas of distortion, doubling of lines, and areas missing; the Amsler grid tests the central 20 degrees of visual field.
Slit-lamp examination.
Dilated fundus examination: pay careful attention to the macula, best viewed with a Goldmann fundus lens.
Fluorescein angiography (FA): used to determine whether there is the presence of CNV, RPE detachment, or tear; if CNV is seen on FA, it is important to categorize the leakage pattern as "well defined" or "occult," as well as to define the location, to determine whether the patient is eligible for extrafoveal laser treatment; *see* Fig. 3.
Indocyanine angiography: may be used as a secondary test if FA shows poorly defined leakage or if the area in question is obscured by blood.
Optical coherence tomography (OCT): used to determine anatomic distortions of the retina, RPE, and choriocapillaris. Best method of determining intraretinal edema, thickness, and scarring. Useful in determining response to anti-VEGF therapy.

Differential diagnosis

Parafoveal telangiectasia.
Macroaneurysm secondary to hypertension.
Chronic central serous retinopathy.
Macular granuloma.
Idiopathic CNV: secondary CNV caused by ocular histoplasmosis, trauma with choroidal rupture, angioid streaks, and multifocal choroiditis.

Cause

Dry ARMD: Thickening of Bruch's membrane.
Drusen deposits.
RPE atrophy.
Wet ARMD: Growth of choroidal neovascular vessels with leakage and bleeding into neurosensory retina.

Epidemiology

- Leading cause of visual loss and blindness in people aged >60 yr.
- More than 1.6 million Americans older than age 60 have advanced ARMD.
- ARMD is far more prevalent among white than among black people.

Classification

Dry ARMD: occurs in the majority of individuals affected by ARMD. Patients develop drusen and then pigment alteration in the macula (coalescence of drusen leads to areas of pigment atrophy). The smaller areas of atrophy coalesce with time. Patients develop gradual loss of vision with distortion and scotomas.
Wet ARMD: ~10% of patients develop choroidal neovascularization characterized by serous or hemorrhagic detachment of the macula and RPE. Eventually, if untreated, subretinal fibrosis occurs, leading to a disciform scar.

Pathology

Drusen: round, discrete, yellowish sub-RPE deposits of eosinophilic extracellular material (periodic acid–Schiff positive).
Basal-laminar drusen: represent focal thickening of the RPE basement membrane and the inner collagenous layer of Bruch's membrane.
Choroidal neovascular membranes: blood vessel growth from the choroid into the subretinal space with fibroblasts.

Diagnosis continued on p. 212

TREATMENT

Diet and Lifestyle

- Age Related Eye Disease Study (AREDS) vitamins reduced the rate of exudative ARMD by about 25% over a 6-yr period. The specific amounts of antioxidants and zinc used in the study were 500 mg vitamin C, 400 IU vitamin E, 25,000 IU vitamin A, 80 mg zinc oxide, and 2 mg cupric oxide (latter added to prevent zinc-induced anemia) [1].
- All patients with exudative disease in one eye and all patients with nonexudative ARMD should take an AREDS vitamin formula. It is not clear whether there is any benefit to the eye once exudative disease has started. Vitamins are used to prevent conversion of dry ARMD to wet ARMD.
- Patients should be counseled to stop smoking, because smoking doubles the risk of developing wet ARMD.

Treatment aims
To improve vision.

Other treatments
Low-vision aids.

Prognosis
- Eventual decline to legal blindness is common, if not treated.
- Incidence of CNV in the fellow eye is 5%-14% per year.

Follow-up and management
- All patients need to be instructed to test their vision daily with an Amsler grid, looking for blurry vision or areas of distortion or missing vision. If these changes develop, patients will need to be treated as an emergency and should contact their ophthalmologist immediately.

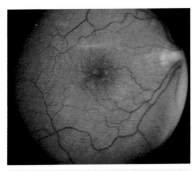

Figure 1   Drusen in the macula.

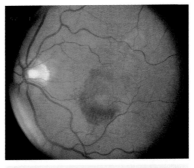

Figure 2   Choroidal neovascularization with drusen, subretinal fluid, and hemorrhage.

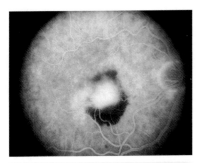

Figure 3   Fluorescein angiogram of the same patient in Fig. 2, showing central poorly defined leakage with a surrounding area of hypofluorescence caused by blockage from blood.

Treatment continued on p. 213

DIAGNOSIS—cont'd

Complications
Decreased vision.

Vitreous hemorrhage: secondary release of subretinal blood into the vitreous cavity.

Optical coherence tomography (OCT): used in determining retinal thickness and response to treatment. Resolution of edema is now documented better with OCT than with FA (*see* Figs. 4 and 5).

Pearls and Considerations
1. According to international classification guidelines, ARMD cannot be diagnosed in patients <50 yr old.
2. RPE atrophy that progresses to larger areas is termed *geographic atrophy*.
3. ARMD is the leading cause of blindness in patients >50 yr of age in the United States.
4. Although ARMD is an accepted genetic disorder, smoking has been demonstrated to double a patient's risk for the disease.
5. AREDS formula vitamins come in both smokers' and nonsmokers' formulations. The smokers' formulations are β-carotene free.

Referral Information
Monitor dry form, and refer for immediate retinal treatment when progression to the exudative form is suspected.

TREATMENT—cont'd

Pharmacologic Treatment

- The treatment of choice has now become serial intravitreal injections of anti-VEGF-A (vascular endothelial growth factor type A) medications. Currently there is one selective VEGF-A inhibitor (pegaptanib [Macugen]) [2] and two pan-isoform VEGF-A inhibitors (bevacizumab [Avastin] and ranibizumab [Lucentis]) [3]. The goal of therapy is to improve, not just stabilize, vision. Ranibizumab and pegaptanib are FDA approved for use in the treatment of ARMD; bevacizumab [4] is FDA approved for colon cancer so its use in the eye is off-label. The most impressive visual results are seen with bevacizumab and ranibizumab so these two medications are now the most commonly used forms of therapy. If patients are treated soon after the onset of exudative disease, they may be able to carry on activities of daily living and lead productive lives.

Nonpharmacologic Treatment

- Thermal laser is currently reserved for the small minority of patients with extrafoveal well-defined lesions (i.e., patients in whom the lesion is far enough away from the center of the macula not to induce scotomas or threaten the fovea with treatment).
- Photodynamic therapy was the mainstay of therapy for subfoveal lesions until the advent of anti-VEGF medications. Because it only results in visual improvement approximately 10% of the time, photodynamic therapy is now used infrequently as the initial treatment of choice.

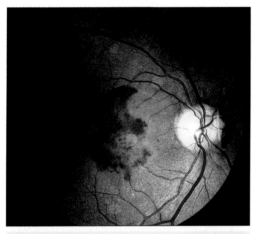

Figure 4   Classic subfoveal choroidal neovascular membrane with surrounding intraretinal hemorrhage.

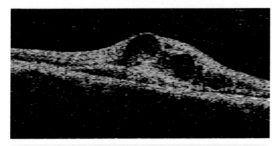

Figure 5   OCT of same patient in Fig. 4 demonstrates intraretinal growth of choroidal neovascular membrane with associated intraretinal cystic fluid and thickening of neurosensory retina.

Key references
1. Age-Related Eye Disease Study Research Group: A randomized, placebo-controlled, clinical trial of high-dose supplementation with vitamins C and E, beta carotene, and zinc for age-related macular degeneration and vision loss: AREDS Report No. 8, *Arch Ophthalmol* 119:1417-1436, 2001.
2. Gragoudas ES, Adamis AP, Cunningham ET Jr, et al, for the VEGF Inhibition Study in Ocular Neovascularization Clinical Trial Group: Pegaptanib for neovascular age-related macular degeneration, *N Engl J Med* 351:2805-2816, 2004.
3. Rosenfeld PJ, Brown DM, Heier JS, et al: Ranibizumab for neovascular age-related macular degeneration, *N Engl J Med* 355:1419-1431, 2006.
4. Avery RL, Pieramici DJ, Rabena MD, et al: Intravitreal bevacizumab (Avastin) for neovascular age-related macular degeneration, *Ophthalmol* 113:363-372.e5, 2006.

Macular edema, cystoid (postoperative)   (362.53)

DIAGNOSIS

Definition
Fluid-filled spaces within the retinal layers of the macula.

Synonyms
None; typically abbreviated CME.

Symptoms
Gradual, painless loss of central vision: usually starting within 1 mo after eye surgery.
Ocular irritability.

Signs
Ruptured anterior hyloid face.
Vitreous incarceration in the wound.
Iris incarceration in the wound.
Poor pupillary dilation.
Peaked pupil secondary to adherent vitreous.
- Fovea may be normal in appearance.
- Obvious intraretinal cysts are often see clinically. In chronic cases, alteration in the pigment layer may occur.

Investigations
Careful slit-lamp examination: look for evidence of vitreous in the wound or anterior chamber and for a rent in the lens capsule.
Close inspection of the fovea: a contact lens may show the changes better than a handheld lens.
Fluorescein angiography: shows early symmetric leakage from the perifoveal capillaries; the pattern of leakage is classically "petalloid" in shape (*see* Fig.1); the degree of leakage does not necessarily correspond to the level of visual acuity; there may also be evidence of leakage without clinical evidence of edema.
Optical coherence tomography: shows intraretinal cystoid spaces. Neurosensory retina is thickened. There is loss of the normal foveal indentation.

Complications
Permanent visual loss: most cases, however, usually resolve spontaneously within a few weeks to months.

Pearls and Considerations
Cataract extraction is the most common cause of, although any intraocular surgery can produce CME.

Referral Information
Optometrists comanaging postcataract patients should refer a patient immediately to the performing surgeon on suspicion of CME.

Differential diagnosis
Hypotony maculopathy.
Preexisting macular degeneration.
Edema associated with other conditions, e.g., diabetes, vein occlusion, hypertension, retinal telangiectasia uveitis, macular pucker, and epinephrine use in aphakia.

Cause
- Most often occurs after uncomplicated cataract surgery.
- Less common after extracapsular surgery than intracapsular surgery.
- Iris-supported intraocular lenses are associated with a high incidence of CME.
- More common in patients with vitreous loss or disruption of the anterior hyloidal face.

Epidemiology
- 1% of post–cataract surgery patients have clinical evidence of CME [1].
- 10%-20% of patients will have angiographic evidence of CME, but most are asymptomatic [2].

Associated features
- CME is more common in older patients.
- If one eye develops CME, the other is thought to be at risk.

Pathology
Accumulation of watery, proteinaceous material within the inner and outer plexiform layers; the edema can greatly distort the neural elements; loss of photoreceptors occurs in chronic cases [3].

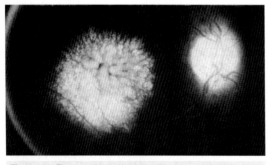

Figure 1 Fluorescein angiogram showing petalloid leakage pattern in the macula with hyperfluorescent leakage off the optic nerve (Irvine-Gass syndrome).

TREATMENT

Diet and Lifestyle
- No special precautions are necessary.

Pharmacologic Treatment
- Topical cyclooxygenase inhibitors such as ketorolac tromethamine (Acular) have been shown to reduce angiographic evidence of CME but may not improve vision.
- Continued topical prednisolone acetate 1% 4 times daily may decrease inflammation, which may be contributing to the edema.
- Oral acetazolamide (250 mg/day) and/or posterior subtenons injection of steroids have shown limited success.
- Intravitreal injection of triamcinolone can produce a dramatic improvement in vision and reduction in fluid as measured by OCT.

Nonpharmacologic Treatment
- Pars plana vitrectomy has occasionally been effective in patients with chronic CME with vision of 20/80 or less of at least 2-3 months' duration [4].
- Neodymium:yttrium-aluminum-garnet (Nd:YAG) vitreolysis of strands adherent to the cataract wound has shown a positive effect in resolving CME.

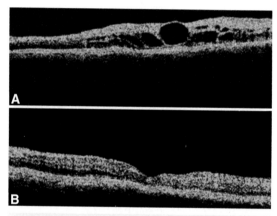

A, OCT shows cystoid macular edema preintraocular steroid injection. **B**, Postinjection. Edema fluid resolved.

Treatment aims
Decrease inflammation.
Lysis of vitreous adhesions.
Restore vision.

Prognosis
- Good, because most cases resolve spontaneously over weeks to months.

Follow-up and management
- Each treatment attempted should be given at least 3-4 wk to show an effect before altering therapy.

Key references
1. Tolentino FI, Schepens CL: Edema of the posterior pole after cataract extraction: a biomicroscopic study, *Arch Ophthalmol* 78:781 1965.
2. Wright PL, Wilkinson CP, Balyeat HD, et al: Angiographic cystoid macular edema after posterior chamber lens implantation, *Arch Ophthalmol* 106:740-744, 1988.
3. Blair NP, Kim SH: Cystoid macular edema after ocular surgery. In Albert DM, Jakobiec FA, editors: *Principles and practice of ophthalmology*, Philadelphia, 1994, Saunders, pp 898-904.
4. Fung WE: Vitrectomy for chronic aphakic cystoid macular edema: results of a national collaborative, prospective, randomized investigation, *Ophthalmology* 92:1102-1111, 1985.

Macular hole, idiopathic   (362.83)

DIAGNOSIS

Definition
A discontinuity in the foveal retina from the internal limiting membrane to the outer photoreceptor layer.

Synonyms
None.

Symptoms
Decreased vision: to the 20/200 range; patients may not appreciate the visual loss until they cover their other eye.

Visual distortion.

Signs
Central scotoma: abnormal Amsler grid.

Full-thickness hole: in the fovea, ranging in size from 200-400 μm.

Halo of fluid: often present (*see* Fig. 1)

Yellow deposits in the base of the hole: *see* Fig. 1.

Small, overlying retinal operculum.

Macular pucker.

Investigations
Careful history: to determine previous trauma or eye surgery.

Visual acuity.

Amsler grid testing.

Slit-lamp examination.

Dilated fundus examination.

Watkze-Allen test: interruption of the vertical slit beam of light or "pinching" of the light beam implies an interruption in retinal tissue because of the hole.

Fluorescein angiography: will show a round, hyperfluorescent spot in the center of the fovea from secondary changes in the retinal pigment epithelium (RPE).

Optical coherence tomography: better than fluorescein. Will show tenting of neurosensory retina (a cyst) or a full-thickness defect in the neurosensory retina (a hole; see Fig. 2).

Complications
Retinal detachment: rare.

Pearls and Considerations
1. Although most macular holes are idiopathic, they can also be related to trauma, laser treatment, cystoid macular edema, retinal vascular disease, retinal pucker, or hypertensive retinopathy. Patients presenting with macular hole should have these underlying conditions ruled out.
2. Up to 10% of patients may develop a cyst or a hole in the fellow eye.

Referral Information
Refer to retinal specialist for surgical intervention.

Differential diagnosis
Pseudohole with an associated epimacular membrane: usually the vision is better.
Pseudohole associated with severe macular edema.

Cause
Unknown.

Epidemiology
- Occurs primarily in women in their 6th decade of life.
- Bilateral in 10% of cases.
- 5%-15% of cases caused by trauma.

Classification
Stage IA: yellow spot in the center of the fovea with loss of foveal depression.
Stage IB: transition from stage IA to a small, yellow halo in the fovea. Cyst seen on OCT.
Stage 2: full-thickness macular hole <200 μm in size; it may begin eccentrically. Best seen with OCT.
Stage 3: full-thickness macular hole >200 μm in size; usually includes a cuff of fluid, yellow deposits in the base, overlying operculum, and cystoid edema. Can be seen clinically quite readily.
Stage 4: full-thickness macular hole with posterior vitreous detachment [1].

Associated features
May be associated with vitreoretinal traction or partial separation of the posterior vitreous.

Pathology
- Full-thickness retinal defect: in the fovea with rounded edges; the edges may be detached from the RPE because of subretinal fluid.
- Cystoid spaces: may be seen in the retina.
- Overlying epiretinal membrane.
- Variable photoreceptor atrophy.
- Yellow deposits in the hole: represent xanthophyll-laden macrophages.

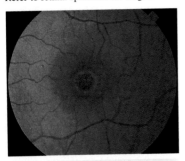

Figure 1   Stage 3 macular hole with a rim of fluid and yellow deposits in the base of the hole.

TREATMENT

Diet and Lifestyle
- No precautions are necessary.

Pharmacologic Treatment
- No pharmacologic treatment is recommended.

Nonpharmacologic Treatment
Pars plana vitrectomy, separation of the posterior vitreous from the surface of the retina, peeling of the internal limiting membrane, and fluid-gas exchange with face-down positioning for at least 5 days.
- Surgical intervention for stage 1 macular holes was no better than natural history [2].
- Surgical intervention for stages 2-4 macular holes resulted in significantly better vision at 6 months after surgery compared with natural history [3].

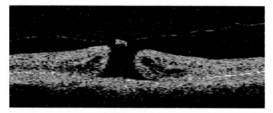

Figure 2 OCT demonstrating full-thickness macular hole with operculum in overlying posterior vitreous.

Treatment aims
To seal the macular hole.
To improve vision by at least two lines of Snellen acuity with surgery.

Prognosis
- ~80% of patients with stage 2 macular holes will progress to stage 3 or 4 holes within 6 mo with considerable loss of vision.
- Most patients with successful closure of the macular hole with surgery will have significantly better vision at 6 mo compared with natural history.
- There is a significant risk of cataract formation after vitrectomy for macular holes.

Follow-up and management
Amsler grid testing of the fellow eye to detect early stage 1 or 2 holes.

Key references
1. Gass JD: Idiopathic senile macular hole: its early stages and pathogenesis, *Arch Ophthalmol* 106:629-639, 1988.
2. De Bustros S: Vitrectomy for prevention of macular holes: results of a randomized multi-centered clinical trial, *Ophthalmology* 101:1055-1066, 1994.
3. Kim JW, Freeman WR, Azen SP, et al: Prospective randomized trial of vitrectomy or observation for stage 2 macular holes, *Am J Ophthalmol* 121:605-614, 1996.

General references
Hughes BM, Valero SO: Macular hole, 2006, www.emedicine.com.
Sjardaa RN, Thompson JT: Macular hole. In *Retina*, ed 4, E-dition, St Louis, 2006, Elsevier.

Macular pucker and idiopathic preretinal macular fibrosis   (362.56)

DIAGNOSIS

Definition
Wrinkling of the retinal surface secondary to traction from an epiretinal membrane.

Synonyms
Surface-wrinkling retinopathy, cellophane retinopathy, epiretinal membrane.

Symptoms
Blurry vision.
Distorted vision (metamorphopsia).

Signs
Wrinkling of macular surface.
Fibrosis of the retina in the macula.
Displacement of the fovea: from tractional forces.
Posterior vitreous detachment: seen in 90% of cases.

Investigations
Visual acuity.
Amsler grid testing.
Dilated slit-lamp and fundus examinations: a characteristic abnormal sheen to the retinal surface in the macular area suggests a membrane; sometimes obvious stria and superficial fibrosis are present; this may be more obvious with the green-filtered light on slit-lamp examination of the retina.
Fluorescein angiography (FA): shows distortion of retinal vasculature caused by areas of traction from the membrane. Late phases may show cystoid edema (CME).
Optical coherence tomography (OCT): often shows areas of adherence of vitreoretinal interface. Sometimes, if only horizontal traction, will only show thickening of internal limiting membrane with associated intraretinal thickening and loss of foveal depression.

Complications
Decreased vision.
Distorted vision.

Pearls and Considerations
1. Macular pucker can be a complication of retinal reattachment surgery.
2. Amsler grid is the most useful take-home tool for patients to monitor their level of visual involvement.

Referral Information
Refer to retinal specialist for surgical peel as appropriate for symptomatic patients.

Differential diagnosis
Macular hole.

Cause
- Abnormal proliferation of glial cells on the retinal surface can be seen after retinal cryotherapy, retinal laser, trauma, vitreous hemorrhage, and ocular surgery.

Epidemiology
- Disease usually occurs bilaterally.
- 75% of eyes retain good vision of 20/50 or better.

Pathology
- Some have suggested that migration of glial cells from the retina through the internal limiting membrane may be a natural component of aging [1]. Most membranes are probably composed of a variety of cells capable of developing myofibroblastic properties that are responsible for contraction [2].

TREATMENT

Diet and Lifestyle
- No precautions are necessary.

Pharmacologic Treatment
- No pharmacologic treatment is recommended.

Nonpharmacologic Treatment
- If the vision drops below 20/40 and the patient is bothered by decreased or distorted vision, surgical peeling of the membrane can be performed. There is a small risk of recurrence after vitrectomy [3].

Treatment aims
To improve vision.
To decrease distortion.

Prognosis
Good, because most cases of macular pucker do not progress, and vision remains better then 20/40.

Follow-up and management
- Yearly dilated eye examinations.
- Amsler grid testing at home by the patient to detect increasing distortion.

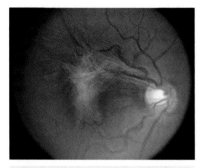

Figure 1 Extensive preretinal fibrosis.

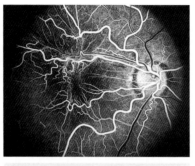

Figure 2 Fluorescein angiogram of the patient in Fig. 1, showing dislocation of the fovea superiorly and straightening of retinal vessels.

Key references
1. Sidd RJ, Fine SL, Owens SL, et al: Idiopathic preretinal gliosis, *Am J Ophthalmol* 94:44-48, 1982.
2. Wallow IH, Stevens TS, Greaser ML, et al: Actin filaments in contracting preretinal membranes, *Arch Ophthalmol* 102:1370-1375, 1984.
3. Michels RG: Vitrectomy for macular pucker, *Ophthalmology* 91:1384-1388, 1984.

General references
Green WR, Sebag J: Vitreoretinal interface. In *Retina*, ed 4, E-dition, St Louis, 2006, Elsevier.

Marcus Gunn (jaw-winking) syndrome   (374.73)

DIAGNOSIS

Definition
A congenital ptosis that includes winking of the affected eyelid with jaw movement.

Synonyms
Marcus Gunn phenomenon, Gunn's syndrome, Gunn phenomenon.

Symptoms
Esthetic deformity: in many patients.
Ptosis: in some patients may lead to chin-up head posture to maintain comfortable single binocular vision.

Signs
Affected upper lid elevates when mandible is depressed or moved to opposite side (external pterygoid muscle contracts): less often, affected upper lid elevates when patient clenches teeth (internal pterygoid muscle).
Ptosis: in many patients when mandible is closed (6% of patients with congenital ptosis have this syndrome); *see* Figs. 1 and 2.
Lid synkinesis: most noticeable in infancy when patient sucking bottle, in older children when chewing food or gum.
• Syndrome may be unilateral or bilateral and may be extremely asymmetric if bilateral.

Investigations
• Ask older child to chew gum or move mandible from side to side.
• Ask parent to provide bottle to younger child.
• Measure ptosis in primary position with mandible closed, and measure total extent of lid excursion as mandible moves from side to side.
• Document presence of chin-up head posture as patient views targets and mobilizes in space.

Complications
Amblyopia: if ptosis goes untreated and anisometropia is present.
Neck deformity: if child maintains a chin-up head posture.
Lagophthalmos: in downgaze after sling procedure.
Destruction of normal lid function in nonaffected eye: if bilateral levator ablation and sling procedures are performed.

Pearls and Considerations
Marcus Gunn (jaw-winking) phenomenon is present from birth and often noticed early by parents during breast or bottle feeding.

Referral Information
Only necessary in cases of severe ptosis; refer these patients to an oculoplastic specialist for ptosis surgery.

Differential diagnosis
• Aberrant regeneration of the third cranial nerve may lead to varying lid positions as the globe moves, but lid position is not dependent on mandible position, and patients often have strabismus and pupillary involvement.
Cyclic oculomotor spasm: during spastic phase, the pupil constricts, the eye adducts, and the ptotic lid elevates; during paralytic phase, the pupil dilates, the eye abducts, and the lid is ptotic; congenital, persists through life; more common in female patients; and usually unilateral.
Inverse Marcus Gunn phenomenon: ptotic lid elevates with opening of mouth (very rare).

Cause
• Congenital miswiring of levator muscle by branch of trigeminal nerve usually directed to the external pterygoid muscle; acquired cases have been described.

Epidemiology
• No known gender or race predilection.
• Rarely inherited as an autosomal dominant condition.

Associated features
• Combination of ptosis and synkinetic lid and mandible movement.
• May have chin-up head posture from ptosis.

Pathology
• Aberrant innervation of the levator with branch of trigeminal nerve usually destined for the external pterygoid muscle; other possibilities have been suggested when other jaw muscles are involved.

TREATMENT

Diet and Lifestyle
No special precautions are necessary.

Pharmacologic Treatment
No pharmacologic treatment is recommended.

Nonpharmacologic Treatment
Surgery is indicated for patients with significant ptosis or significant lid synkinesis with mandibular movement. The most effective treatment is disinsertion of the levator muscle in both eyes and suspension of both lids in a symmetric, nonptotic position; acceptable results can be obtained by disinsertion of only the involved levator when combined with suspension of both lids. Levator resection alone simply moves the lid synkinesis to a higher position, but may be effective if the lid synkinesis is very mild.

Treatment aims
To achieve symmetric lid position with no lid synkinesis.

Other treatments
- Many children learn to minimize mastication movements or close both eyes while eating.
- Biofeedback has been attempted but with minimal success.
- Metal lid supports can be fitted to spectacles to obviate ptosis.

Prognosis
- Good results can be obtained with levator tendon disinsertions and sling procedures, but the patient must accept lagophthalmos in downgaze after surgery.
- The condition becomes less conspicuous with age and sometimes disappears.

Follow-up and management
- Corneal protection after sling procedures requires lubrication for a few months at bedtime and, in some patients, at other times during the day. Children tolerate corneal exposure better than adults.

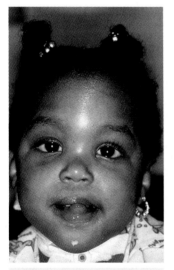

Figure 1 Lids in visual and symmetric position when mandible is in midline.

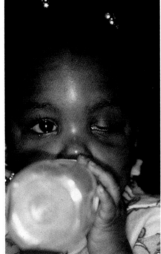

Figure 2 Right upper lid ptosis when patient sucks bottle and mandible moves to right side.

General references
Beard C, editor: *Ptosis*, ed 3, St Louis, 1980, Mosby.
Blaydon SM: Marcus Gunn jaw winking syndrome, 2006, www.emedicine.com.
Callahan A: Surgical correction of the blepharophimosis syndrome, *Trans Am Acad Ophthalmol Otolaryngol* 77:687–690, 1973.
Doucet TW, Crawford JS: The quantification, natural course, and surgical results in 57 eyes with Marcus Gunn (jaw-winking) syndrome, *Am J Ophthalmol* 92:702-707, 1981.

Mechanical strabismus (378.63): blowout fracture (802.6) and Graves' dysthyroid orbitopathy (242)

DIAGNOSIS

Definition
A deficit in ocular motility secondary to mechanical forces limiting extraocular muscle function.

Blowout fracture refers to break in the bony orbital floor without involvement of the bony rim.

Synonyms
None.

Symptoms
Diplopia and visual confusion: in strabismic gaze positions.

Dyscosmetic head postures (head tilts or turns): in some patients.

Loss of visual field, visual acuity, and color vision discrimination: in some patients with Graves' dysthyroid orbitopathy (GDO).

Pain from ulcers related to corneal exposure: in some patients with GDO.

Signs
Blowout Fracture

Enophthalmos, limitation of ductions (usually elevation with floor fracture, abduction with medial orbital wall fracture; *see* Fig. 1), **infraorbital hypesthesia.**

GDO

Lid retraction (*see* Fig. 2), **lid or conjunctival swelling and chemosis, duction limitations** (usually elevation or abduction), **exophthalmos, lagophthalmos, corneal exposure** (with resultant scarring, infection, or erosion).

Investigations
Blowout Fracture

History, visual acuity test, alignment in all gaze positions, ductions and versions, measurement of enophthalmos.

Magnetic resonance imaging or computed tomography: to document location and extent of fracture, entrapment of orbital tissue in maxillary or ethmoid sinuses, and sinus opacity from inflammation or infection.

Dilated anterior-segment and fundus examination: to rule out retinal, vitreous damage or intraocular foreign body.

Clinical photographs.

GDO

History of thyroid disease, visual acuity and visual field tests, color vision evaluation, ductions and versions, measurement of exophthalmos and lid retraction.

Magnetic resonance imaging: to document enlargement of extraocular muscles (EOMs) and encroachment of muscles around optic nerve.

Dilated fundus examination: to evaluate optic nerve, retinal vasculature.

Measurement of serum thyroid hormone: total or free thyroxine (T_4), total or free triiodothyronine (T_3).

Serum thyroid-stimulating hormone (TSH).

Autoantibody tests: antithyroid peroxidase, antithyroglobulin antibodies, anti-TSH receptor antibodies.

Differential diagnosis
Blowout fracture

Brown syndrome, fibrosis syndromes, enophthalmos (caused by breast carcinoma metastatic to the orbit).

GDO

Proptosis: caused by orbital masses, craniofacial anomalies, neurofibromatosis type 1 (pulsatile).

Lid retraction: congenital, or caused by overcorrection during ptosis surgery, aberrant regeneration of third cranial nerve, or topical α-adrenergic drugs.

Enlarged EOMs: caused by orbital myositis, orbital cellulitis; rarely a primary anomaly.

Cause
Blowout fracture

Usually caused by axial blunt trauma.

GDO

Presumably an autoimmune disease.

Epidemiology
Blowout fracture

Common in sports with small, hard projectiles (e.g., squash, tennis, baseball).

GDO

- 20% of patients with GDO will be clinically euthyroid, and all laboratory tests will be negative; ~40% of this population will eventually become hyperthyroid.

Classification
Blowout fracture (378.62).
GDO (378.63).

Associated features
Blowout fracture

Hyphema, ruptured globe, vitreous hemorrhage, retinal break or detachment, iris or retinal dialysis, uveltis, retinal hemorrhage, macular edema or hole.

GDO

Hyperthyroidism or hypothyroidism, Cogan lid-twitch sign (retraction of lid after rapid downward eye movement), bruit over eye or eyelid, upper-lid lag on downgaze, increased intraocular pressure on attempted upgaze, resistance to globe retropulsion, pretibial myxedema, diffuse goiter.

Diagnosis continued on p. 224

TREATMENT

Diet and Lifestyle
Blowout Fracture
- Protective eyewear during racquet sports and baseball will decrease incidence.

GDO
- Treatment of hyperthyroidism may exacerbate GDO signs and symptoms.
- Cigarette smoking significantly increases the risk of ophthalmopathy in Graves' disease.

Pharmacologic Treatment
For Blowout Fracture
Oral antibiotics to prevent or treat sinus infection, orbital cellulitis.

Nasal antihistamines, decongestants.

As required for uveitis, ocular complications.

For GDO
Judicious treatment of hypothyroidism or hyperthyroidism.

Systemic prednisone may decrease orbital, lid, and muscle swelling in acute cases.

Topical lubricants for exposed cornea.

Treatment aims
Blowout fracture

To reduce tissue entrapment and enophthalmos.

To achieve normal globe movement with no strabismus and comfortable single binocular vision without head posture.

GDO

To achieve normal visual acuity, visual fields, and color vision discrimination.

To achieve normal globe movement with no strabismus and comfortable single binocular vision without head posture.

To ensure patient has no exophthalmos.

Prognosis
Blowout fracture
- Repair is usually successful, but patient may have residual vertical diplopia in upgaze or downgaze. Infraorbital hypesthesia often persists.

GDO
- Most patients have one acute episode with smoldering course; may spontaneously resolve without sequelae.
- Severely enlarged muscles may require two- or three-wall orbital decompression. Most significantly affected patients will have limited ductions and diplopia in some gaze positions after strabismus surgery and decompression.

Follow-up and management
Blowout fracture
- If enophthalmos is not severe, conservative management for 10 days is recommended.
- If motility restriction persists and is significant to patient, surgical intervention at ~10 days after trauma is warranted.

GDO
- Many patients require management with an endocrinologist because of unstable thyroid status.
- Follow-up is dictated by clinical status and severity of optic nerve encroachment by muscles.

Treatment continued on p. 225

Mechanical strabismus (378.63): blowout fracture (802.6) and Graves' dysthyroid orbitopathy (242)

DIAGNOSIS—cont'd

Complications

Blowout Fracture

Permanent duction limitation: with head posture, strabismus in primary position.

Infraorbital hypesthesia, enophthalmos.

GDO

Corneal exposure: with resultant melting, scarring, or infection.

Optic nerve compression: with loss of visual acuity, visual field, and color perception and discrimination.

Head posture, diplopia: in primary position and reading position.

Dyscosmetic lid retraction, exophthalmos, and chemosis of lids or conjunctivae.

Pearls and Considerations

Trapdoor entrapment of the EOMs refers to entrapment of the orbital contents in which the broken bone has snapped back into place after initial injury. This condition compromises blood supply to the affected structures and requires surgical intervention within 24 hr.

Referral Information

Refer to appropriate subspecialist based on etiology of disease (e.g., endocrinologist, head and neck surgeon).

TREATMENT—cont'd

Nonpharmacologic Treatment
For Blowout Fracture

Surgical reduction of fracture with placement of rigid substance to bridge bony defect; release of entrapped orbital contents; strabismus surgery for residual strabismus; procedures include recession of tight muscles, using adjustable sutures when possible.

For GDO

Orbital decompression for optic nerve compression, profound exorbitism with corneal exposure, limited globe movement; lateral, medial tarsorrhapies for corneal protection; strabismus surgery for residual strabismus, limitation of ductions; procedures include recessions on tight muscles, using adjustable sutures when possible; resections are avoided; levator muscle and lower-lid retractor lengthening for lid retraction.

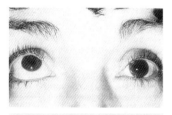

Figure 1   Limitation of upgaze in left eye after blowout fracture.

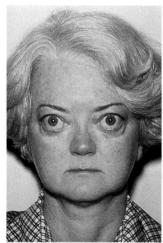

Figure 2   Lid retraction and exorbitism in patient with Graves' disease.

General reference
Fells P: Thyroid-associated eye disease: clinical management, Lancet 338:29, 1991.

DIAGNOSIS

Definition
Deficit in ocular motility secondary to mechanical forces limiting extraocular muscle function.

Synonyms
None.

Symptoms
Diplopia and visual confusion: in strabismic gaze positions.
Dyscosmetic head postures (head tilts or turns): in some patients.
Ptosis: in some patients who have fibrosis syndromes.

Signs
Brown Syndrome
Limitation of elevation in adduction: possible depression in adduction, Y-pattern exotropia, head turn away from involved eye, head tilt to same side as affected eye (*see* figure).

Fibrosis Syndromes
Limitation of ductions with chin-up head posture: may be generalized with fixed globe, or limited to certain muscle groups, usually including inferior recti.

"Heavy Eye" Syndrome
Hypotropia and esotropia: in a myopic eye: may adopt head tilt toward side of affected eye.

Investigations
Family history.
Complete motility examination in all gaze positions: patients who have mechanical strabismus will have ductions as limited as versions in pathologic gaze positions.
Dilated fundus examination: in patients who have "heavy eye" syndrome to look for staphyloma.
Magnetic resonance imaging: in patients with difficult motility patterns.
Forced-duction testing: will disclose tightness to elevation in adduction in patients who have Brown syndrome, tightness to elevation in patients who have "heavy eye" syndrome, and generalized tightness in patients who have fibrosis syndromes.

Complications
Amblyopia: in some patients who abandon head posturing.
Permanent neck deformity: from chronic head turns or tilts.

Classification
Brown syndrome (378.61).
Fibrosis syndromes (378.60).
"Heavy eye" syndrome (378.60).

Associated Features
Brown syndrome: as above; also, widening of lid fissure with attempted globe elevation in adduction; may have positive head-tilt test, but usually suggests ipsilateral palsy of inferior rectus not consistent with ductions and versions.
Fibrosis syndromes: often associated with pseudoptosis and true ptosis and chin-up head posture.
"Heavy eye" syndrome: associated with unilateral high myopia, often with staphyloma.

Pearls and Considerations
Topic too broad for specific recommendations.

Referral Information
Refer to appropriate subspecialist based on etiology of disease (e.g., endocrinologist, head and neck surgeon).

Differential diagnosis
Brown syndrome
Inferior oblique palsy: usually associated with A-pattern and superior oblique overaction, positive head tilt test; duction "up and in" better than version.
Blowout orbital fracture: history of trauma, enophthalmos.
Fibrosis syndromes
Partial third-nerve palsy: not inherited; usually unilateral; may involve pupillary sphincter.
Blowout fracture.
"Heavy eye" syndrome
Esotropia and hypotropia from fusion break.

Cause
Brown syndrome
Congenital: short superior oblique tendon.
Acquired: superior oblique tuck encircling element for retinal detachment repair, trauma, or inflammation of trochlea.
Fibrosis syndromes
Congenital: inherited as autosomal dominant in many families.
"Heavy eye" syndrome
Inferior misdirection of lateral rectus around equator of enlarged globe: with resultant limitation of elevation and abduction.

Epidemiology
Brown syndrome
- 60% of patients are female; 60% occur in left eye; bilateral cases rare.
- Identical twins are reported with left eye affected in one twin, right eye in the other; not inherited; shows no predilection for race or gender.
Fibrosis syndromes
- Usually bilateral but may be asymmetric.
- Congenital, often inherited as autosomal dominant; no race or gender predilection.
"Heavy eye" syndrome
- No eye, gender, or race predilection; not inherited; associated with unilateral high myopia.

TREATMENT

Diet and Lifestyle
- Many patients will adopt a head posture to maintain comfortable single binocular vision.
- Patients with fibrosis syndromes must adopt head posture to view straight ahead.

Pharmacologic Treatment
- No pharmacologic treatment is recommended.

Nonpharmacologic Treatment
For Brown Syndrome
- Strabismus surgery is indicated in the ~40% of patients who will adopt a head posture to view straight ahead with comfortable single binocular vision. Procedures include tenotomy (sparing intermuscular septum) and lengthening superior oblique tendon with plastic strips.

For Fibrosis Syndromes
- Strabismus surgery is indicated to permit patients to view in primary position without adopting a head posture. Large recessions are performed, using adjustable suture techniques when possible.

For "Heavy Eye" Syndrome
- Strabismus surgery is indicated to align the eyes and recover comfortable single binocular vision. Procedures include many different techniques, but information limited on most effective approach. Some surgeons advocate recession of inferior and medial recti, using adjustable suture techniques when possible.

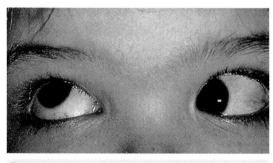

Brown syndrome in left eye with limitation of evaluation of left eye in adduction.

Treatment aims
Brown syndrome
To achieve straight eyes in primary position without the adoption of a head posture.
To achieve full elevation in adduction.
Fibrosis syndromes
To achieve straight eyes in primary position without the adoption of a head posture; full ductions and versions are rarely obtainable.
"Heavy eye" syndrome
To achieve straight eyes in primary position with comfortable single binocular vision.

Prognosis
Brown syndrome
- Modern surgical techniques permit attainment of postoperative alignment without head posture in most patients.
Fibrosis syndromes
- Most patients can attain improved ductions and versions after strabismus surgery.
"Heavy eye" syndrome
- Surgical experience is too limited to predict final outcomes.

Follow-up and management
Individualized.

General references
Brown HW: True and simulated superior oblique tendon sheath syndromes, *Doc Ophthalmol* 34:123-128, 1973.
Harley RD, Rodrigues MM, Crawford JS: Congenital fibrosis of the extraocular muscles, *Trans Am Ophthalmol Soc* 76:197-201, 1978.
Hansen E: Congenital fibrosis of the extraocular muscles, *Acta Ophthalmol* 46:469-479, 1968.
Krzizok TH, Kaufmann H, Traupe H: Elucidation of restrictive motility in high myopia by magnetic resonance imaging, *Arch Ophthalmol* 115:1019-1026, 1997.
Wang FM, Wertenbaker C, Behrens MM, et al: Acquired Brown's syndrome in children with juvenile rheumatoid arthritis, *Ophthalmology* 91:23-31, 1984.

Microhyphema   (364.41)

DIAGNOSIS

Definition
A small bleed in the anterior chamber of the eye (typically too small to settle or layer).

Synonyms
None.

Symptoms
Blurry vision.
Pain.
Photophobia: after blunt trauma.

Signs
Hyphema: blood in the anterior chamber with layering and/or clot.
Microhyphema: blood in the anterior chamber without layering.
Pupil may not be visualized: because of significant layering of blood.
Intraocular pressure (IOP): may be elevated.

Investigations
History: type of injury, onset of visual loss, sickle cell disease (IOP may be elevated; in black patients, obtain a sickle prep to rule out sickle cell disease).
Careful examination of the ocular adnexal structures, including eyelids: for laceration and the bony orbit.
Pupil examination: for a relative afferent pupillary defect (may be detected with visualization of one pupil)
Slit-lamp examination: need to rule out ruptured globe (peaked pupil, subconjunctival hemorrhage 360 degrees or localized subconjunctival hematoma, low IOP, hyperdeep or shallow anterior chamber, vitreous hemorrhage).
Dilated fundus examination: if no view, perform a β-scan ultrasound.

Complications
Elevated IOP.
Rebleeding with corneal blood staining.
Optic neuropathy.

Pearls and Considerations
1. Even a microhyphema can indicate major intraocular trauma.
2. Uncomplicated microhyphemas will generally resolve in 5-6 days.

Referral Information
Patients with microhyphema may be hospitalized.

Differential diagnosis
Intraocular foreign body.

Cause
- Usually related to blunt trauma.
- May occur spontaneously in patients with rubeosis iridis, blood-clotting abnormalities, juvenile xanthogranuloma, or leukemia.

Associated Features
- Angle recession and other injuries to angle structures.

TREATMENT

Diet and Lifestyle
Protective eyewear while participating in contact sports or operating machinery.

Pharmacologic Treatment
- Most patients with microhyphemas can be treated as outpatients. Consider admission for children, noncompliant patients, patients at high risk for recurrent bleeds, and patients with other source of ocular injuries. Enforce strict bed rest with head of bed elevated 30 degrees. A shield should be worn over involved eye at all times.

Standard dosage	Atropine 1% drops, 3 or 4 times daily.
	Topical steroid (e.g., prednisolone acetate 1%), 4-6 times daily.
Contraindications	No aspirin products should be administered.
	Avoid acetazolamide in patients with sickle cell disease.
Special points	If IOP is elevated, start antiglaucoma medication (e.g., timolol 0.5% twice daily).

Nonpharmacologic Treatment
- Anterior-chamber washout is indicated if:
1. IOP remains elevated despite maximal pharmacologic therapy.
2. Corneal-stromal blood staining develops.
3. The entire anterior chamber becomes filled with blood.

Treatment aims
To prevent rebleed.
To control IOP.
To prevent corneal blood staining and optic neuropathy.

Prognosis
Good, if no rebleeding occurs.

Follow-up and management
- Daily follow-up is needed with visual acuity check, IOP measurement, and slit-lamp examination if patients present with high IOP on initial visit. Otherwise, patients with microhyphema can be seen on third day after trauma, then again in 2 wk.
- A shield on the affected eye or glasses must be worn at all times for 2 wk.
- Advise the patient to refrain from strenuous physical activities for 2 wk from the injury date. Once the hyphema resolves beyond the 5th or 6th day, follow patient every 2-3 days, then 3-4 wk later for gonioscopy and dilated examination with scleral depression, tapering finally to every 6 mo to 1 yr to check for the development of angle-recession glaucoma.

General references
Albert DM, Jakobiec FA, editors: *Principles and practice of ophthalmology*, vol I, Philadelphia, 1994, Saunders.
American Academy of Ophthalmology: *Basic and clinical science*, section 8, San Francisco, 1994-1995, The Academy.
Shepard J, Williams PB: Hyphema, 2005, www.emedicine.com.
Wilson FM: Traumatic hyphema: pathogenesis and management, *Ophthalmology* 687:910-919, 1980.
Wright K: *Textbook of ophthalmology*, Baltimore, 1997, Lippincott Williams & Wilkins.

Monofixation syndrome (378.34)

DIAGNOSIS

Definition
A form of subnormal binocular vision characterized by central suppression scotoma, small-angle strabismus, and peripheral fusion.

Synonyms
Microtropia, microstrabismus; typically abbreviated MFS.

Symptoms
- Patients are usually asymptomatic unless they have a large phoria and develop asthenopic symptoms.

Signs
Esotropia or exotropia ≤8 prism diopters and/or hypertropia ≤4 prism diopters with possible superimposed phoria: most patients will not have a cosmetic deformity or even noticeable strabismus.

Investigations
- The diagnosis is usually confirmed by sensory testing, demonstrating peripheral fusion without central fusion.

Normal fusional vergence amplitudes.

Stereopsis from nil to 67 arc seconds.

Facultative central scotoma of about 3 degrees under binocular viewing conditions.

Positive 4–prism diopter base-out test: holding the prism before the nonfixing eye will not lead to eye movement because the image is merely moved within the foveal scotoma.

Cover test: may show larger deviation on alternate cover test than on cover-uncover test; MFS is the only form of strabismus in which this occurs.

Complications
Amblyopia
- Patients who have MFS are at risk for the development of amblyopia if they do not alternate fixation between the eyes. Age of onset is <5 years.
- 66% of patients with MFS are amblyopic, including:
  33% of patients with early-onset strabismus and postoperative MFS.
  66% of patients with acquired esotropia and MFS.
  75% of patients with MFS with no known cause.
  90% of patients with strabismus and anisometropia with MFS.
  100% of patients with no history of strabismus but anisometropia and MFS.

Other
- Some MFS patients will decompensate and develop a larger tropia with suppression and anomalous retinal correspondence; seems to occur more frequently in those with exotropia than esotropia.

Pearls and Considerations
Adults with mild amblyopia, subnormal stereovision, or subtle differences in binocular visual acuity may have undiagnosed MFS.

Referral Information
No referral required.

Differential diagnosis
- Patients who have small deviations may have no binocular vision; sensory testing is essential.
- Some authors separate MFS from "microtropia," "monofixational phoria," etc. These terms represent emphasis on one part of the presentation of some patients with MFS.

Causes
Occurs spontaneously, often in patients who have anisometropia.

After strabismus surgery for early-onset esotropia or exotropia.

After strabismus surgery for intermittent exotropia (risk, 1%).

After reversal of amblyopia in patients with aligned eyes.

After reversal of constant, acquired strabismus.

Organic foveal lesions (e.g., toxoplasmosis) in one eye.

Associated features
- Sensory status does not fit strict definitions of "normal" or "abnormal" retinal correspondence. Sensory testing is more consistent with normal because patients with MFS have normal fusional version amplitudes and some stereoptic ability.

TREATMENT

Diet and Lifestyle
• No special precautions are necessary.

Pharmacologic Treatment
• No pharmacologic treatment is recommended.

Nonpharmacologic Treatment
• Treatment is indicated only if the patient develops a larger angle of strabismus or is symptomatic from a large phoria.
• Amblyopia should be treated in typical fashion.
• Overzealous occlusion may lead to constant, large-angle strabismus in a few patients.

Treatment aims
• Sensory status is the same whether the patient has a small tropia or no tropia, so no treatment is indicated for the small tropia in many patients with MFS.
• No known treatment will render patients with *bifixational* MFS (possessing central fusion).
• Patients with large phorias may require treatment if symptomatic; this may include glasses, prisms, surgery, or fusional training exercises.

Prognosis
• Esotropic patients who have MFS tend to have a stable alignment.
• Exotropic patients tend to decompensate into larger exotropia.

Follow-up and management
• Amblyopia should be treated as usual.
• Follow-up is individualized.

General references
Arthur BW, Smith JT, Scott WE: Long-term stability of alignment in the monofixation syndrome, *J Pediatr Ophthalmol Strabismus* 26:224-229, 1989.
Gupta BK: Monofixation syndrome, 2005, www.emedicine.com.
Jampolsky A: Characteristics of suppression in strabismus, *Arch Ophthalmol* 54:683-686, 1955.
Parks MM: Stereoacuity as an indicator of bifixation. In Knapp P, editor: *Strabismus Symposium*, New York, 1968, Karger.
Parks MM: The monofixation syndrome. In Dabezies O, editor: *Strabismus*, St Louis, 1971, Mosby, pp 131-135.

DIAGNOSIS

Definition
A disorder of the neuromuscular junction caused by an autoimmune attack on the acetylcholine (ACh) receptors at the neuromuscular junction.

Synonyms
None; myasthenia gravis also known as Erb-Goldflam disease.

Symptoms
Diplopia, ptosis, "flattened smile" (lips elevate but fail to retract), nasal speech, respiration weakness.

Signs
Medial rectus weakness, gaze nystagmus, convergence insufficiency, pupil-sparing pseudo–third-nerve palsy, pseudo–fourth-nerve palsy, pseudo–sixth-nerve palsy, pseudo–gaze palsy, isolated extraocular muscle (EOM) weakness, double-elevator palsy, hypermetric saccades (if gaze restricted), hypometric saccades (if gaze unrestricted), fatigue (on rapid following, in sustained lateral gaze, on optokinetic nystagmus), ptosis (alternating, unilateral or bilateral), diurnal eyelid fatigue, ptosis that worsens in bright sunlight, eyelid opposite ptotic lid is retracted, posttetanic facilitation (may cause eyelid to be elevated), peek sign on attempted eyelid closure, weakness of orbicularis oculi, Cogan's eyelid twitch (in ~10% of patients).

Investigations
- Examination includes applying an ice pack to the ptotic eyelid for 2 min to assess ptosis improvement. Observe whether patients appear to be involuntarily "peeking" out of their eyelids when they close their eyes. Assess for weakness of orbicularis oculi muscle. Observe whether the eyelid overshoots the eye as the patient looks from a downgaze to the primary position (lid twitch). Ask the patient to look upward and suppress blinking (one eyelid is mechanically held while observing whether the fellow eyelid curtains).
- Appraise improvement of the ptosis or diplopia after sleep.

Serum ACh receptor antibody: positive in ~50% of patients with ocular myasthenia; 87% with generalized myasthenia.

Edrophonium (Tensilon) test: false negatives and positives occur; false negatives occur 18% of the time in ocular myasthenic and 29% in generalized myasthenic patients.

Neostigmine (Prostigmin) test.

Repetitive nerve stimulation.

Single-fiber electromyography: if necessary; abnormal in 67% of patients with ocular myasthenia when examining the extensor digitorum brevis muscle; abnormal in 86% of patients when the facial muscle was also studied.

Computed tomography of the mediastinum.

Pulmonary function studies.

Antinuclear antibody, rheumatoid factor, thyroid function tests, antithyroid antibodies, postprandial blood glucose, complete blood count.

Differential diagnosis
Graves' orbitopathy.
Botulism.
Chronic progressive external ophthalmoplegia.
Oculopharyngeal dystrophy.
Miller-Fisher variant of Guillain-Barré syndrome.
Myotonic dystrophy.
Cavernous sinus syndrome.
Decompensated phoria.
Progressive supranuclear gaze palsy.

Cause
- Reduction of available ACh receptors at neuromuscular junctions; caused by autoimmune attack with destruction (distortion of postsynaptic membrane geometry) and antagonism (blockade) at the available receptor sites.

Epidemiology
- Incidence rate is 1:20,000 to 0.4:1 million per year.
- Prevalence rate is 1:8000-200,000.
- Disease occurs from infancy to the senium.
- Peak incidence is in second and third decades of life, affecting mostly women. Another peak in incidence occurs in sixth and seventh decades, affecting mostly men.
- There is no racial or geographic predilection.

Classification
- Ocular myasthenia gravis is a nonprogressive form involving only ocular motility problems and eyelid weakness.

Associated features
Bulbar signs: include chewing, eating, and swallowing and breathing.
Flaccid dysarthria: characterized by hypernasality, decreased articulation, dysphonia, and decreased loudness.
Associated immunologic disorder: diabetes mellitus, thyroid disease, systemic lupus erythematosus, rheumatoid arthritis; increased incidence of malignancies; occur in 23% of patients.
Thymomas: in 10% of patients, particularly older men; 50% of patients with thymomas have myasthenia gravis.

Diagnosis continued on p. 234

TREATMENT

Diet and Lifestyle

- 33% of patients with myasthenia experience the first symptoms after an emotional upset.
- 66% of myasthenic patients note aggravation of established symptoms by psychologic factors.

Pharmacologic Treatment

Anticholinesterases: pyridostigmine, neostigmine, ambenonium.
Propantheline: for adverse gastrointestinal side effects of anticholinesterase medication.
Corticosteroids (e.g., prednisone).
Immunosuppressives: azathioprine, cyclosporine.

Treatment aims
To eliminate the diplopia and ptosis.
To improve systemic weakness.

Other treatments
Prisms and glasses for diplopia: rarely successful.
Patches.
Eyelid tape: for ptosis.
Ptosis crutch: if available.
Strabismus and ptosis surgery: contraindicated.

Prognosis
- 85% of patients who present with ocular myasthenia gravis convert to generalized myasthenia.
- Approximately 90% of ocular myasthenic patients who convert to generalized myasthenia do so within 12 mo.
- Diplopia and ptosis are often resistant to systemic therapy.

Treatment continued on p. 235

DIAGNOSIS—cont'd

Complications

Myasthenic crisis: acute respiratory distress or bulbar symptoms.

Cholinergic crisis: overmedication with cholinesterase inhibitor leading to increased ACh accounting for increased salivation, lacrimation, sweating, vomiting, diarrhea, abdominal cramps, urgent or frequent urination, bronchial asthma, and pupillary miosis.

Thymoma.

- The following may exacerbate myasthenia gravis: hyperthyroidism, hypothyroidism, occult infection, aminoglycoside antibiotics, D-penicillamine, intravenous contrast dye, phenothiazines, β-blockers, quinine, and antiarrhythmic agents.

Pearls and Considerations

1. Ptosis and diplopia will eventually be present in 90% of myasthenia gravis patients.
2. Pupils react normally in ocular myasthenia patients.

Referral Information

If previously undiagnosed, refer to primary care physician for additional workup and treatment as indicated.

TREATMENT—cont'd

Nonpharmacologic Treatment
Plasmapheresis (plasma exchange).
Thymectomy.

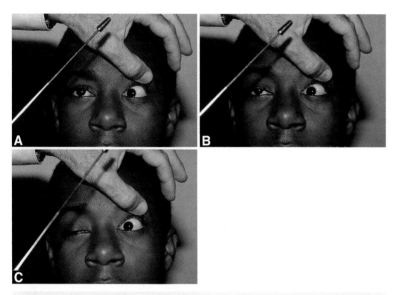

A, This child, age 10 yr, presented with a right ptosis. His left eyelid is elevated by the examiner while he stares up without blinking. **B,** Twenty seconds later, the right eyelid begins to "curtain." **C,** His eyelid position at 40 seconds demonstrates the eyelid fatigue consistent with myasthenia gravis.

General references

Barton JJ, Fouladvand M: Ocular aspects of myasthenia gravis, *Semin Neurol* 20(1):7-20, 2000.

Elrod RD, Weinberg DA: Ocular myasthenia gravis, *Ophthalmol Clin North Am* 17(3):275-309, 2004.

Evoli A, Batocchi AP, Minisci C, et al: Therapeutic options in ocular myasthenia gravis, *Neuromusc Disord* 11(2):208-216, 2001.

Freidman DI: Disorders of the neuromuscular junction. In Yanoff M, Duker JS, editors: *Ophthalmology*, E-dition, St Louis, 2006, Elsevier.

Nasolacrimal duct obstruction, congenital   (375.22)

DIAGNOSIS

Definition
Blockage of the lacrimal outflow drainage system resulting from a defect present since birth.

Synonyms
None.

Symptoms
Dysesthetic appearance of wet eyes; epiphora.
Decreased visual acuity: caused by viewing through tear lake.
Constant wiping of eyes.
Skin excoriation below eyes.
Increased risk of viral and bacterial infection of conjunctiva, lacrimal system, and orbit.

Signs
Elevated conjunctival tear meniscus.
Epiphora: tearing; worse in windy, cold weather.
Injected conjunctivae.
Mucus and pus in palpebral fissures.
Conjunctivitis: bacterial or viral.
Excoriation of skin of lower lids and cheeks: from constant moisture.
Proptosis from orbital cellulitis: rare.

Investigations
Dye-disappearance test: instill fluorescein in conjunctivae, investigate with cobalt-blue light; fluorescein should clear tear film 2-5 min after instillation.
Jones test 1: retrieval of dye from the nose after above; proves system is open.
Jones test 2: irrigate dye from conjunctiva, anesthetize cornea; cannulate sac and irrigate; retrieval of dye from nose proves dye reached lacrimal sac; difficult in children.
Sinus radiography: shows bony abnormalities.
Microscintigraphy: ^{99}Tc instilled in conjunctiva; serial photographs made with microcollimator over time; useful for evaluating efficiency of lacrimal pump.
Diagnostic probing: discloses areas of obstruction and narrowing.
Dacryocystography: water-soluble contrast material (Renografin-C) irrigated into canaliculi and films taken; both tear drainage systems can be simultaneously evaluated.
Nuclear magnetic resonance scanning: reserved for unusual cases (e.g., posttraumatic obstruction, craniofacial anomalies).

Complications
- Untreated nasolacrimal system obstruction (NSO) can lead to recurrent conjunctivitis, orbital cellulitis, dacryocystitis, permanent stricture of the system, and development of facial fistulae.

Pearls and Considerations
Probing cures 95% of congenital NSOs.

Referral Information
Refer to pediatric ophthalmologist for assessment; probing and additional surgical intervention as needed.

Differential diagnosis
Viral and bacterial conjunctivitis.
Corneal abrasion or foreign body.
Congenital glaucoma: look for enlarged, cloudy cornea with horizontal breaks in Descemet's membrane.
Uveitis.

Cause
- In children, membrane is usually obstructing the lacrimal duct outflow under inferior turbinate. Other causes include punctal and canalicular atresia, absence of lacrimal duct segment, and compression of system by nasal hemangioma.
- In adults, obstruction is often caused by trauma. Canaliculitis results from actinomycosis and acquired, punctal, or canalicular stenosis.

Epidemiology
- Perhaps 10% of children are born with NSO, but spontaneous opening usually occurs within a few weeks of birth.
- At 2 mo of age, 3% of children will be symptomatic.
- At 3 mo, 80% will resolve by 1 yr.
- At 6 mo, 70% will resolve by 1 yr.
- At 9 mo, 50% will resolve by 1 yr.

Associated features
Trauma to the nasal canthus.
Craniofacial anomalies.
Nasal hemangiomas.

Pathology
- Pathology depends on cause of obstruction. Most children will have membrane at lower end of lacrimal duct or atresia of part of the tear drainage system. Most adults will have traumatic destruction of part of system, tumor infiltration, or bacterial inflammations of sac or duct.

TREATMENT

Diet and Lifestyle

- No special precautions are necessary.

Pharmacologic Treatment

- Broad-spectrum antibiotics prophylactically control bacterial load in lacrimal sac and conjunctiva; however, no evidence suggests that they lead to opening of system.

Nonpharmacologic Treatment

Removal of pus and mucus from conjunctivae as needed.

Lacrimal sac massage: to empty sac contents onto conjunctiva, performed once or twice daily; however, no evidence suggests that massage downward promotes opening of obstructions in the lacrimal duct.

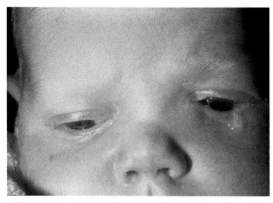

Acute dacryocystitis in left eye of infant.

Treatment aims
To achieve patent nasolacrimal system with normal function.
To prevent infection in nasolacrimal system.

Other treatments
Balloon dilation of the nasolacrimal system has shown promise in children who have difficult probing history; some surgeons perform as a first procedure.
Irrigation and probing of tearing children at ~1 yr of age, or sooner if recurrent conjunctivitis, orbital cellulitis, or dacryocystitis occurs; perform twice, with infracturing of the inferior nasal turbinate if repeated; usually performed in an operating room, may be performed in an office.
Intubation of system: with Silastic tube stents that remain for 6 mo to 1 yr.
Dacryocystorhinostomy: if Silastic intubation fails.
Conjunctivodacryocystorhinostomy: in patients without patent canaliculi.

Prognosis
- Initial irrigation and probing succeeds in 95% of patients at ≤13 mo of age, 75% at 13-24 mo, and 33% at >24 mo.

Follow-up and management
- Silastic tubes often require general anesthesia for removal.

General references
Bashour M: Nasolacrimal duct, congenital anomalies, 2005, www.emedicine.com.

Druse F. Hand SI, Ellis FD, Helveston EM: Silicone intubation in children with nasolacrimal obstruction, *J Pediatr Ophthalmol Strabismus* 17:389-393, 1982.

Hornblass A, Ingis TM: Lacrimal function tests, *Arch Ophthalmol* 97:1654-1658, 1979.

Kushner BJ:Congenital nasolacrimal system obstruction, *Arch Ophthalmol* 100:597-601, 1982.

MacEwen CJ, Young JD: The fluorescein disappearance test: an evaluation of its use in infants, *J Pediatr Ophthalmol Strabismus* 28:302-328, 1991.

Massaro BM, Gonnering RS, Harris GJ: Endonasal lacrimal dacryostorhinostomy: a new approach to nasolacrmial duct obstruction, *Arch Opthalmol* 108:1172-1176, 1990.

Nystagmus, congenital   (379.51)

DIAGNOSIS

Definition
A high-frequency, horizontal beating movement of the eyes that begins in the first few months of life.

Synonyms
None.

Symptoms
Decreased visual acuity: with lower acuity at distance than at near.

Cosmetic deformity: from unsteady eye movements or head posturing to maximize visual acuity.

Signs
Binocular uniplanar (usually horizontal) rhythmic eye movements that maintain same plane in all gaze positions: may have latent component.

- Patients may have associated head oscillations and may have null point removed from primary position, which creates a head posture.

Investigations
Family history.

Visual acuity at distance and near: monocular and binocular.

Head posturing at distance and near: head turn or tilt, chin up or down.

Description of eye movement in all gaze positions.

Complete eye examination: with special attention to iris transillumination, optic nerve hypoplasia or atrophy, perimacular depigmentation, aniridia, foveal aplasia, decreased skin or choroidal pigmentation, severely decreased or absent color vision discrimination.

Ocular movement recordings.

Electroretinography: absent cone response in patients who have congenital cone dystrophy.

Complications
- Typical binocular visual acuity is ~20/200 at distance and 20/30 at near.

Aniridia: 40% of patients will develop glaucoma from filtration-angle obstruction by iris root; peripheral corneal pannus may rarely compromise visual acuity.

Congenital cone dystrophy: photophobia.

Optic nerve hypoplasia: midline cerebral deformities, hypopituitarism.

Achromatopsia (rod monochromatism): severely decreased or absent color vision discrimination; photophobia.

Associated Features
Congenital cone dystrophy: bull's eye maculopathy with dropout of the retinal pigment epithelium around the macula; photophobia.

Achromatopsia: all colors interpreted as shades of gray.

Aniridia: grossly absent iris, progressive corneal pannus, glaucoma (40% of patients), optic nerve hypoplasia (40%), foveal aplasia with aberrant posterior-pole vasculature.

Wilms tumor associated with sporadic aniridia: ~1.5% of patients with Wilms tumor have sporadic aniridia; ~33% of patients who have sporadic aniridia will develop Wilms tumor.

Albinism: increased chiasmal decussation of optic nerves, decreased choroidal and dermal pigmentation (oculocutaneous albinism) or choroidal pigmentation (ocular albinism), iris transillumination, photophobia, dermal macromelanosomes (ocular albinism).

Optic nerve hypoplasia: agenesis of corpus callosum, absence of septum pellucidum, hypopituitarism.

Differential diagnosis
- *Acquired nystagmus:* null point with head posturing less common; *oscillopsia* (subjective sense of environmental movement) occurs only when nystagmus is acquired; patients who have acquired nystagmus will note eye movement when they view themselves in a mirror; nystagmus plane tends to vary in different gaze positions.
- *Nystagmoid eye movements:* generally seen in patients who have poor acuity; random nonrhythmic movements, often differing in waveform between the eyes.
- *Spasmus nutans:* nystagmus is never present at birth; acquired at ~4-6 mo of age; nystagmus waveform of small amplitude, high frequency, and often asymmetric; associated with head posture, titubations of head.
- *Periodic alternating nystagmus:* may be congenital or acquired; shifting null point drives side-to-side head posturing.

Cause
- The cause is not truly understood when the globes are anatomically normal; may represent inaccuracy in the eye's positional feedback loop ("leaky integrator"). Most patients who have congenital nystagmus have decreased visual acuity at distance.
- Patients who have aniridia have increased chiasmal decussation, which may contribute to unsteady eye movements.

Epidemiology
- Congenital nystagmus simplex has no race or gender predilection and is not inherited.
- Congenital cone dystrophy: autosomal dominant.
- Aniridia: sporadic, autosomal dominant.
- Albinism: ocular albinism is usually an X-linked recessive trait; oculocutaneous albinism is usually an autosomal recessive trait (*see* Albinism).
- Achromatopsia: complete form is inherited as an autosomal recessive trait; incomplete form may be inherited as an X-linked recessive trait.

Diagnosis continued on p. 240

TREATMENT

Diet and Lifestyle

- Many patients who have congenital nystagmus have photophobia and benefit from sunglasses and wide-brimmed hats.
- Patients with albinism have increased incidence of skin cancer and must wear ultraviolet-ray protective lotion when outdoors.

Pharmacologic Treatment

- Baclofen and Tegretol benefit some patients with periodic alternating nystagmus.

Nonpharmacologic Treatment

- Surgery is the mainstay of treatment for patients who have significant reproducible head postures caused by eccentric null points.

Kestenbaum procedure: generally requires surgery on muscles in both eyes; may be used for patients with horizontal, vertical, or oblique null points; often improves visual acuity.

Creation of exotropia with medial rectus recessions in both eyes: stimulation of convergence may dampen nystagmus.

Recession of four horizontal rectus muscles in patients who have horizontal null point: usually does not improve visual acuity, but patients find viewing target easier; perhaps eyes spend more time in primary position.

Associated Diseases

Congenital cone dystrophy, optic nerve hypoplasia, aniridia, albinism, bilateral macular lesions, kernicterus, achromatopsia, midline anomalies of central nervous system, cerebellar or brainstem hypoplasia.

Treatment aims

To obviate head posture at distance and at near.

To improve visual acuity at distance and near.

To improve visual comfort when viewing targets.

Other treatments

Biofeedback: can decrease amplitude and frequency of nystagmus, but does not improve visual acuity.

Prisms: base in same direction as head posture; often impractical because large prisms must be used; base-out prisms over each eye to create divergence if no head posture; stimulated convergence may dampen nystagmus.

Retrobulbar injection of botulinum toxin: temporarily decreases amplitude and frequency of nystagmus; increases visual acuity in one eye.

Prognosis

- Nystagmus amplitude and frequencey improve with age, but visual acuity usually does not.

Follow-up and management

- Patients who have spasmus nutans must have intracranial scanning to rule out chiasmatic and hypothalamic gliomas.
- Patients who have sporadic aniridia must have abdominal scanning and examination to rule out Wilms tumor. They should be examined every few months to rule out filtration-angle obstruction and glaucoma.

Treatment continued on p. 241

DIAGNOSIS—cont'd

Pearls and Considerations

1. Congenital nystagmus is often associated with ocular albinism.
2. When associated with visual disorders, congenital nystagmus is called *sensory defect nystagmus;* when it is not, it is called *motor defect nystagmus*.
3. The *null point* of nystagmus is a point in the horizontal visual field where the intensity of the nystagmus is low and visual acuity is best.

Referral Information

No referral necessary.

TREATMENT—cont'd

Pathology

Congenital cone dystrophy: aberrant retinal cone receptors.

Optic nerve hypoplasia: missing ganglion cell fibers in all amounts.

Achromatopsia: aberrant retinal cone receptors.

Aniridia: remnant of iris root usually detectable on gonioscopy; optic nerve hypoplasia typically found; often a large vessel crosses the usual macular location, absent foveal depression.

Albinism: absent ocular pigment in oculocutaneous form; ocular albinos have macromelanosomes in the iris and retinal pigment epithelia and in the skin.

General references

Abadi RV, Whittle J: The nature of head postures in congenital nystagmus, *Arch Ophthalmol* 109:216-220, 1991.

Dell'Osso LF, Flynn JT: Congenital nystagmus surgery: a quantitative evaluation of the effects, *Arch Ophthalmol* 97:462-468, 1979.

Yee RD: Nystagmus and saccadic intrusions and oscillations. In Yanoff M, Duker JS, editors: *Ophthalmology*, E-dition, St Louis, 2006, Elsevier.

Zubcov AA, Stark N, Weber A, et al: Improvement of visual acuity after surgery for nystagmus, *Ophthalmology* 100:1488, 1993.

DIAGNOSIS

Definition
Insufficient function of the oblique ocular muscles.

Synonyms
None; dissociated vertical deviation usually abbreviated DVD.

Symptoms
Oblique Muscle Dysfunctions

Diplopia and visual confusion: in patients who cannot suppress.

DVD

- Patients are usually asymptomatic because they have limited or no binocular vision during DVD movement.

Signs
Oblique Muscle Dysfunctions

Inferior oblique overaction: overelevation in adduction (*see* Fig. 1).
Inferior oblique underaction: underelevation in adduction.
Superior oblique overaction: overdepression in adduction.
Superior oblique underaction: underdepression in adduction.

DVD

Elevation, abduction, and extorsion: in nonfixing eye; present in primary position, abduction as well; movement is slow, not rapid version as inferior oblique overaction; not associated with V pattern; dependent on ambient illumination.

Investigations
Oblique Muscle Dysfunctions

Prism and alternate cover tests: measure in all gaze positions.
Head-tilt test: to uncover causal cyclovertical muscle palsy.
Subjective and objective tests: to reveal ocular torsion.

DVD

Prism and alternate cover tests: measure in all gaze positions; the endpoint may be difficult to determine (*see* Fig. 2).

Complications
Cosmetic deformity, loss of comfortable single binocular vision.

Adoption of head posture: to avoid gaze positions in which diplopia or imperfect binocular vision occurs; patients who have chronic postures may develop permanent neck muscle contracture.
Amblyopia: in patients <5½ yr of age.

Differential diagnosis
Oblique muscle dysfunctions

- Primary dysfunctions must be separated from secondary ones.
Primary: head-tilt test negative; no diplopia or visual confusion; no admission to torsion on subjective testing; objective evidence of fundus torsion.
Secondary: head-tilt test positive; may have diplopia or visual confusion; may admit to torsion on subjective testing; objective evidence of fundus torsion.
Inferior oblique overaction: DVD; aberrant regeneration of third cranial nerve; tether effect in Duane syndrome; rectus muscle rotation in patients who have craniosynostosis.
Inferior oblique underaction: Brown syndrome; blowout fracture; Graves' dysthyroid orbitopathy.
DVD
Inferior oblique overaction: in patients who have a mostly vertical movement.
Intermittent exotropia: in patients who have a mostly abducting movement.

Cause
Oblique muscle dysfunctions
Primary: cause unknown; perhaps from mismatch between coronal location of trochlea and inferior oblique origin ("sagittallization").
Secondary:

- Inferior oblique overaction often caused by ipsilateral superior oblique palsy, contralateral superior rectus palsy.
- Superior oblique overaction often caused by ipsilateral inferior oblique palsy, contralateral inferior rectus palsy.
DVD
Cause unknown; speculated to result from loss of superior oblique muscle tone in patients who have deficient fusional ability.

Epidemiology
Oblique muscle dysfunctions
Inferior oblique overaction: noted in 72% of patients who have early-onset esotropia, 35% of those who have accommodative esotropia and intermittent exotropia.
DVD
Noted in 75% of patients who have early-onset esotropia, 15% of those who have accommodative esotropia, 10% of those who have intermittent exotropia.

Diagnosis continued on p. 244

TREATMENT

Diet and Lifestyle
• No special precautions are necessary.

Pharmacologic Treatment
• No pharmacologic treatment is recommended.

Nonpharmacologic Treatment
Oblique Muscle Dysfunctions

Strabismus surgery: for patients who have cosmetically or functionally significant overaction or underaction.

Inferior oblique recession, anteriorization, myectomy: for inferior oblique overaction.

Treatment aims
Oblique muscle dysfunctions
Straight eyes in all gaze positions with no alphabet pattern.
Comfortable single binocular vision in all gaze positions.
DVD
Decreased amplitude and frequency of strabismus with improved cosmesis.

Prognosis
Oblique muscle dysfunctions
• Occasionally, untreated oblique muscle dysfunction spontaneously improves, but usually it is stable or becomes more pronounced.
• Strabismus surgery is usually successful.
DVD
• DVD is usually stable with time or becomes more pronounced if untreated; rarely improves spontaneously.
• Strabismus surgery is rarely curative, but usually decreases frequency and amplitude of eye movement.

Follow-up and management
Individualized according to clinical situation.

Treatment continued on p. 245

Oblique muscle dysfunctions and dissociated vertical deviation (378.31)

DIAGNOSIS—cont'd

Associated Features
Oblique Muscle Dysfunctions

Abduction movement of eye in extreme elevation or depression: in patients who have overacting oblique muscles.

Deficiency of movement of eye in extreme elevation or depression: in patients who have underacting muscles.

Alphabet patterns: V or Y pattern in patients who have inferior oblique overaction or superior oblique underaction; A pattern in patients who have superior oblique overaction or inferior oblique underaction; X pattern in patients who have all oblique muscles overacting; ♦ pattern in those who have all oblique muscles underacting.

DVD

- Some patients will present with a mostly elevating movement; others mainly abducting; a few mostly torsional; usually latent, but can be manifest with constant hypertropia and exotropia; very few patients will have globe depression with loss of fusion.

Pearls and Considerations
1. DVD will be present in all positions of gaze.
2. DVD does not have an associated A or V pattern.

Referral Information
Refer for strabismus surgery.

TREATMENT—cont'd

Superior oblique tuck: for inferior oblique underaction.
Superior oblique tendon recession, lengthening, tenotomy: for superior oblique overaction.
Superior oblique tendon tuck, Harada-Ito procedure: for superior oblique underaction.

DVD
Cause unknown; speculated to be remnant of primitive "righting reflex."

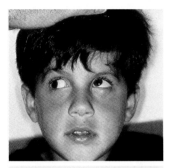

Figure 1 Overelevation in adduction in left eye of patient with inferior oblique overaction.

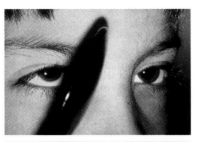

Figure 2 Dissociated vertical deviation (DVD) in primary gaze of right eye. The cover over the right eye dissociates the eyes.

General references

Diamond GR: Esotropia. In Yanoff M, Duker JS, editors: *Ophthalmology*, E-dition, St Louis, 2006, Elsevier.

Gobin MH: Sagitallization of the oblique muscles as a possible cause for the "A", "V", and "X" phenomena, *Br J Ophthalmol* 52:13, 1968.

MacDonald AL, Pratt-Johnson JA: The suppression patterns and sensory adaptations to dissociated vertical divergent strabismus, *Can J Ophthalmol* 9:113, 1974.

Sprague JB, Moore S, Eggers HM, Knapp P: Dissociated vertical deviation: with the Faden operation of Cuppers, *Arch Ophthalmol* 98:465, 1980.

Wilson ME, Parks MM: Primary inferior oblique overaction in congenital esotropia, accommodative esotropia, and intermittent exotropia, *Ophthalmology* 96:7, 1989.

Oculosympathetic paresis (Horner's syndrome)   (337.9)

DIAGNOSIS

Definition
A condition arising from interruption of sympathetic innervation to the eye and presenting with miosis, partial ptosis, and loss of hemifacial sweating.

Synonyms
Horner-Bernard syndrome; Horner's ptosis; oculosympathetic paresis usually abbreviated OSP.

Symptoms
Ptosis of 2-3 mm: can be variable.
Inverse ptosis of 1-2 mm: creating the illusion of enophthalmos.
Miosis.
Anhidrosis: occasionally helpful when the patient is questioned about perspiration or skin temperature during exercise.
- *Horner's syndrome* refers to the triad of ptosis, miosis, and anhidrosis.
- *OSP* can be applied to ptosis and miosis.
- Neck pain (history of neck trauma or manipulation, e.g., by chiropractor) [1].

Signs
Subtle ptosis: without the loss of the eyelid crease.
Miosis creating an anisocoria: greater in dim than bright illumination.
- Less helpful signs include an increased amplitude of accommodation, transient decrease in intraocular pressure, and change in tear viscosity.

Investigations
- In darkness, a paretic dilator will dilate the pupil at a slower rate than a normal pupil, called "dilation lag." Therefore, look for an anisocoria that is greater at 4-5 sec than at 10-12 sec into darkness.

Cocaine Ophthalmic Solution
- Cocaine ophthalmic solution of 4%-10% is used as a supersensitivity test. (This test is less effective in darkly pigmented patients. The cocaine solution must be instilled onto untouched corneas.) After instilling equal drops into both eyes, an OSP pupil will not dilate to cocaine, whereas a normal eye will enlarge. A postcocaine anisocoria of 0.5 mm suggests that the odds of an OSP are 77:1; <0.8 mm of anisocoria translates to a 1054:1 chance of OSP; and 1 mm of anisocoria means a 5990:1 chance of OSP.

Paredrine Ophthalmic Solution
Warning! Do not instill Paredrine until 48 hours after instilling cocaine.
- Paredrine ophthalmic solution 1% (hydroxyamphetamine) offers anatomic localization either above or below the level of the mandible (head or chest).
- If the OSP miotic pupil does not dilate to Paredrine, the lesion is "third order," or postganglionic, and above the level of the mandible.
- If the OSP miotic pupil does dilate to Paredrine, the lesion is preganglionic, or "first and second order," and below the level of the mandible.
- Other pupils that do not dilate well to Paredrine include an iris affected by transsynaptic dysgenesis, those of darkly pigmented patients, and dark irides. The diagnostic specificity of Paredrine is 84% for third-order OSP and 97% for first- and second-order OSP. If the post-Paredrine anisocoria is 1 mm, there is an 85% probability for third-order OSP. If there is 2 mm of post-Paredrine anisocoria, there is a 99% probability of OSP.
- Anhidrosis has been employed for anatomic localization of the lesion. If the forehead is hypohidrotic, the lesion is in the head. If the face and cheek are hypohidrotic, the lesion is in the chest. (If the lesion is in the spinal cord, the face and upper half of body become hypohidrotic. If the lesion causing the OSP is in the brainstem, there is anhidrosis over half the face and body.)

Differential diagnosis
Congenital ptosis with physiologic anisocoria.
Dermatochalasis with physiologic anisocoria.
Tonic pupil.
Argyll-Robertson pupil.

Cause
- In adults, 40% of OSP is idiopathic, whereas 8% is neoplastic. Neoplasm is the presenting sign in only 3%.
- 18% of children with neuroblastoma manifest OSP. It is the presenting sign in only 2%. Other causes include benign tumors (e.g., neurofibromas), iatrogenic, idiopathic, and congenital.

Specific causes according to the "three-neuron chain"
Central ("first-order neuron")
Brainstem glioma.
Syringomyelia.
Spinal cord tumor.
Wallenberg's syndrome.
Preganglionic ("second-order neuron")
Cervical trauma.
Cervical arthritis.
Poliomyelitis.
Neural crest tumors.
Pneumothorax.
Lung tumor.
Cervical rib.
Intrathoracic aneurysm.
Neoplasm of thyroid gland or other neck structures.
Postganglionic ("third-order neuron")
Cluster headache.
Nasopharyngeal tumor.
Otitis media.
Internal carotid artery disease (thrombosis, aneurysm, trauma, dissection).
Cavernous sinus syndrome.

Diagnosis continued on p. 248

TREATMENT

Diet and Lifestyle
- No special precautions are necessary.

Pharmacologic Treatment
2.5% Phenylephrine, or apraclonidine (Iopidine) 0.5%, 3 times daily.

Nonpharmacologic Treatment
- No nonpharmacologic treatment is recommended.

Complications
- Heterochromia iridis, straighter hair on side of OSP, or lower brachial plexus palsy (Klumpke's paralysis) all support a congenital cause.
- OSP may be component of telodiencephalic, Foville's, or Wallenberg's syndrome. OSP with a contralateral fourth-nerve paresis suggest a brainstem lesion. Hoarseness and hiccupping in a woman with OSP suggest involvement of the phrenic nerve and recurrent laryngeal nerve from breast cancer at sixth cervical level. OSP with ipsilateral arm pain suggests an apical lung tumor or "Pancoast's syndrome."

Treatment aims
Ptosis repair.

Prognosis
Variable.

Treatment continued on p. 249

247

Oculosympathetic paresis (Horner's syndrome)   (337.9)

DIAGNOSIS—cont'd

Other
- Always review old photographs for long-standing ptosis and anisocoria.
- A computed tomography (CT) scan of the head and neck is indicated.
- Also, in children, obtain 24-hr vanillylmandelic acid levels. ***Every child with a "congenital Horner's" should be screened for a neuroblastoma***.
- Depending on symptoms and signs, may need magnetic resonance imaging (MRI) of brain, neck, upper part of chest, and lung or a mammogram.
- Angiography of carotid artery.

Pearls and Considerations
Facial flushing may be present with preganglionic lesions, whereas ipsilateral orbital pain or migrainelike headache may be present in postganglionic lesions.

Referral Information
Refer for imaging studies to help elucidate organic cause.

TREATMENT—cont'd

- Painful OSP is seen in carotid artery dissection, otitis media, cavernous sinus syndrome, and cluster headache. OSP with an earache suggests carotid artery dissection or otitis media. A neck ache and dysgeusia imply a carotid dissection. OSP that occurs with a headache, red eye, and stuffy nose could be a cluster headache. OSP and shoulder, arm, and chest pain suggest a superior pulmonary sulcus tumor (or Pancoast's syndrome). Hoarseness and hiccuping suggest Vernet's syndrome or phrenic nerve syndrome. Diplopia and an OSP suggest a cavernous sinus syndrome.

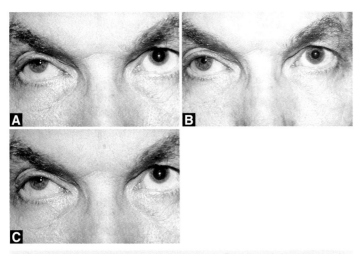

A, This man has Horner's syndrome in his right eye. **B**, Anisocoria is more conspicuous in dark illumination. **C**, Anisocoria 45 minutes after cocaine drop instillation; notice how the normal left pupil has dilated to cocaine, whereas the right pupil is unchanged, creating a greater postcocaine anisocoria.

Key reference

1. Department of Neurology, Mercy Medical Center, Rockville Centre, NY: Stroke following chiropractic manipulation: report of 3 cases and review of the literature, *Cerebrovasc Dis* 13(3):210-213, 2002.

General references

Parmar MS: Horner syndrome, 2006, www.emedicine.com.

Patel S, Ilsen PF: Acquired Horner's syndrome: clinical review, *Optometry* 74(4):245-256, 2003.

Robertson WC, Pettigrew LC: "Congenital" Horner's syndrome and carotid dissection, *J Neuroimaging* 13(4):367-370, 2003.

Walton KA, Buono LM: Horner's syndrome, *Curr Opin Ophthalmol* 14(6):357-363, 2003.

Ophthalmia neonatorum   (771.6)

DIAGNOSIS

Definition
Any conjunctivitis that occurs in the first 4 wk of life.

Synonym
Neonatal conjunctivitis.

Symptom
Irritability.

Signs
Chemical conjunctivitis: watery discharge, injected conjunctivae.

Bacterial conjunctivitis: purulent discharge, injected conjunctivae; corneal ulcer with *Neisseria* gonococcus (from *Neisseria gonorrhoeae*).

Chlamydial conjunctivitis: watery or purulent discharge, injected conjunctivae, pseudomembranes; no follicular conjunctival response.

Herpes simplex conjunctivitis: watery discharge, injected conjunctivae, lid margin vesicles, rare corneal dendrites.

Investigations
Parental sexual history.

Gram stain for all patients:

Neisseria gonococcus: gram-negative intracellular diplococci.

Other bacteria: *Streptococcus* spp., *Staphylococcus* spp., *Escherichia coli*, *Pseudomonas* spp.

Giemsa stain of conjunctiva:

Chlamydia: intracytoplasmic basophilic inclusions (Halberstaedter-Prowazek syndrome).

Herpes simplex: multinucleated giant epithelial cells; Pap stain will exhibit eosinophilic intranuclear inclusions.

Fluorescent and monoclonal antibody studies: *Chlamydia*.

Systemic physical examination:

Chlamydia: pneumonia, rhinitis, nasopharyngitis, tracheitis, otitis media.

Neisseria gonococcus: pneumonia, meningitis, sepsis, septic arthritis.

Herpes simplex: chorioretinitis, encephalitis.

Complications
Chemical conjunctivitis: self-limited, no sequelae.

Bacterial conjunctivitis: *Neisseria* gonococcus is a major concern because it can penetrate intact corneal epithelium; other bacterial keratitis occurs only after epithelial compromise.

Chlamydial conjunctivitis: self-limited, but may result in mild peripheral pannus and scarring; vision is rarely affected.

Herpes simplex conjunctivitis: may lead to corneal scarring and vascularization.

Pearls and Considerations
1. All infants are exposed to infectious organisms in the birth canal. Length of exposure becomes an important factor in development of conjunctivitis as a result of exposure.
2. The most common cause of neonatal conjunctivitis in the United States is *Chlamydia trachomatis*.

Referral Information
Refer to pediatric ophthalmologist and pediatrician for specialty care. In case of *C. trachomatis*, the mother should be referred for *Chlamydia* treatment and testing.

Differential diagnosis
Watery discharge: congenital glaucoma, tear drainage system obstruction, uveitis.
Purulent discharge: tear drainage system obstruction, dacryocystitis.

Cause
Chemical conjunctivitis: from 1% silver nitrate; hyperacute, mild, watery; generally occurs between birth and 3 days; rarely seen as hospitals shifting to erythromycin, tetracycline, and povidone-iodine.
Bacterial conjunctivitis: *Neisseria* gonococcus is very purulent, lids very puffy; generally occurs between 3 and 6 days.
Chlamydial conjunctivitis: generally occurs between 5 and 10 days.
Herpes simplex type II: tends to be unilateral; generally occurs between 7 and 10 days, or later.

Epidemiology
- Beware of simultaneous maternal infection with multiple agents, including lues (syphilis) and human immunodeficiency virus (HIV).
Neisseria gonococcus: 5%-10% of mothers infected at time of birth.
Chlamydia: 5%-10% of mothers infected at time of birth.
Herpes simplex type 2: 1.0%-1.5% of mothers infected at time of birth; type 1 may be seen as well.

Classification
Gonococcal (098.40).

Immunology
- Rapid fluorescent antibody test for *Chlamydia* is useful in diagnosis.

TREATMENT

Diet and Lifestyle

Effective prenatal maternal care and treatment of maternal infection can prevent infection in the newborn.

Pharmacologic Treatment

For Bacterial Conjunctivitis

Follow treatment indicated by culture and Gram stain. For *Neisseria* gonococcus, systemic treatment should be tried in all cases.

Standard dosage	Penicillin G, 50,000 U/kg IM or IV every 12 hr.
Special points	Penicillin-resistant strains are common; follow sensitivities.

- Topical treatment is optional; some prefer erythromycin ointment 4 times daily.

For Chlamydial Conjunctivitis

Standard dosage	Topical 10% sulfa or tetracycline ointment, 4 times daily for 3 wk, *or*
	Erythromycin, 40 mg/kg/day PO for 2-3 wk.

For Herpes Simplex Conjunctivitis

Corneal lesions should be treated with topical vidarabine 9 times daily.

Nonpharmacologic Treatment

For *Neisseria* Gonococcal Infection

Admit patient to hospital isolation unit and lavage secretions hourly from eyes.

Report to public health service; parents may require treatment.

Consider presence of other venereal diseases.

For Chlamydial Conjunctivitis

Patients are usually treated on an outpatient basis unless pneumonia develops between 3 and 13 wk of age.

Report to public health service; parents may require treatment.

Consider presence of other venereal diseases.

For Herpes Simplex Conjunctivitis

Parents may require treatment.

Treatment aims

To preserve clear cornea and quiet eyes.

To prevent additional venereal diseases in parent and child.

Prognosis

- Prognosis is good with early diagnosis and treatment.
- Patients with herpes simplex systemic disease may have devastating neurologic sequelae.

Follow-up and management

As indicated by cause.

- Risk of amblyopia and strabismus if cornea becomes cloudy.

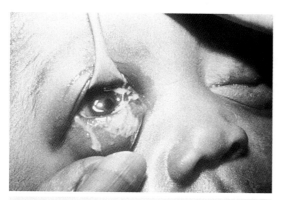

Neisseria conjunctivits.

General references

Dinsmoor MJ: Ophthalmia neonatorum, *Contemp Obstet Gynecol* 37:112-118, 1992.

Prentice MJ, Hitchinson GR, Taylor-Robinson D: A microbiological study of neonatal conjunctivae and conjunctivitis, *Br J Ophthalmol* 61:601-612, 1977.

Rubenstein JB, Jick SL: Disorders of the conjunctiva and limbus. In Yanoff M, Duker JS, editors: *Ophthalmology*, E-dition, St. Louis, 2006, Elsevier.

Sandstrom I, Kallings I, Melen B: Neonatal chlamydial conjunctivitis, *Acta Pediatr Scand* 77:207-212, 1988.

Thygesen: Historical review of oculogenital disease, *Am J Ophthalmol* 71:975-981, 1971.

Optic neuritis   (377.3)

DIAGNOSIS

Definition
Demyelinating inflammation of the optic nerve of unknown etiology.

Synonyms
None; typically abbreviated ON.

Symptoms
Blurred, painful vision: in 92.2% of patients.
Pain on eye movement: before, during, and after visual loss.
Positive visual phenomenon: photopsias on eye movement or auditory induced.
Photophobia.
Depth perception difficulties: Pulfrich stereo phenomenon.
Uhtoff's phenomenon.

Signs
Relative afferent pupillary defect.
Reduced Snellen acuity: the initial median of ON patients is 20/50; ~10% of ON patients have Snellen acuity of 20/20; ~15% have an acuity of finger counting or worse.
Visual field loss: can be diffuse (50%) or local (50%); local defects include altitudinal (29.2%), three-quadrant involvement (14.6%), quadrant (13.2%), hemianopic (11.1%), centrocecal (8.3%), arcuate (6.3%), and other (17.3%); 48% of fellow eyes have an abnormal visual field.
Decreased contrast sensitivity.
Dyschromatopsia.
Reduced brightness sense.
Nerve fiber bundle defects.
Retrobulbar optic neuritis: 65% of patients.
Papillitis: 35% of patients.
Peripapillary hemorrhage: infrequent; 6% of patients.
Multiple sclerosis (MS): associated with anterior uveitis and pars planitis.
Systemic neurologic abnormality.

Investigations
Magnetic resonance imaging (MRI) of brain: to detect high-signal white-matter abnormalities.
MRI of orbit: to rule out orbital lesions.
Lumbar puncture (LP): to detect oligoclonal bands.

Pearls and Considerations
1. In all ON patients, MS must be considered.
2. About a third of ON patients will have papillitis presenting as diffuse edema of the optic nerve head.
3. Loss of vision from ON may be permanent.

Referral Information
Refer to neurologist for imaging and evaluation of possible MS.

Differential diagnosis
Idiopathic: most common.
Ischemic optic neuropathy.
MS (demyelinating disease).
Sarcoid.
Systemic lupus erythematosus.
Wegener's syndrome.
Syphilis.
Sjögren's syndrome.
Dysthyroid optic neuropathy.
Cytomegalovirus.
Leber's mitochondrial optic neuropathy.
Lyme disease.
Cat-scratch disease (Bartonella henselae).
Acute zonal occult outer retinopathy.
Mucocele.

Cause
Forme fruste of MS.
ON demyelination.

Epidemiology
- Female/male ratio is 2:1.
- Whites more affected than blacks.
- Age of onset is 15-40 yr (average, 30 yr).
- Rapid decrease in visual acuity, with maximal visual deficit in ~5 days.
- Incidence is 1-4:100,000 per year.
- Environmental influence against background of genetic susceptibility.

Immunology
An autoimmune inflammatory cascade is believed to mediate myelin destruction in MS.

TREATMENT

Diet and Lifestyle
- No special precautions are necessary.

Pharmacologic Treatment
- High-dose IV corticosteroids followed by a quick oral corticosteroid taper quickens visual recovery but has no effect on final visual outcome. This treatment seems to reduce the risk of developing MS at 2 yr.
- Treatment of ON with oral prednisone more than doubles the risk of a new attack of ON (30%) in either the affected or the fellow eye.
- Treatment with IV methylprednisolone followed by oral prednisone halves the risk of developing a clinical attack of MS at 2 yr in patients with a critical number of white-matter lesions.

Nonpharmacologic Treatment
- No nonpharmacologic treatment is recommended.

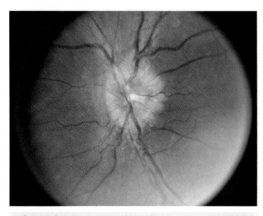

Left eye of a woman age 42 yr who presented with painful visual loss, afferent pupillary defect, dyschromatopsia, and central and arcuate scotoma. Her disc edema is consistent with papillitis. This is distinguished from early papilledema by abnormal optic nerve function.

Prognosis
Visual recovery
- In most ON patients, as per the Optic Neuritis Treatment Trial, visual recovery begins rapidly within 3 wk after the onset of symptoms with or without treatment. Visual recovery seems to plateau at 6 wk but may continue to improve up to 1 yr. At 5 yr, 87% will have an acuity of 20/25 or better, and 94% will have an acuity of 20/40 or better. Visual recovery is less evident in patients with finger-counting vision or worse. These patients have 20/40 acuity or better at 6 mo. Although Snellen acuity may return to normal, many patients have subtle symptomatic visual deficits.
- The probability of experiencing a repeat attack of ON in the same eye or fellow eye is ~20% in 5 yr.

Probability of developing clinically definite multiple sclerosis
- 30% chance of developing clinically definite MS at 5 yr.
- Clinical features of ON associated with a low 5-yr risk of developing clinically definite MS are absence of pain; mild visual loss; and presence of optic disc edema, hemorrhage, or exudate.
- High-signal abnormalities on brain MRI are the strongest predictor of developing MS. At 5 yr the absence of lesions indicates a 16% chance of developing MS (which should not be misinterpreted to mean that MS will not develop). The presence of one or two lesions indicates a 37% risk; three or more lesions, a 51% risk.

General references
Arnold AC: Evolving management of optic neuritis and multiple sclerosis, *Am J Ophthalmol* 139(6):1101-1108, 2005.

Balcer LJ, Galetta SL: Treatment of acute demyelinating optic neuritis, *Semin Ophthalmol* 17(1): 4-10, 2002.

Beck RW, Cleary PA: Optic neuritis treatment trial: one-year follow-up results, *Arch Ophthalmol* 111:773-775, 1993.

Beck RW, Cleary PA, Anderson MM Jr, et al: A randomized, controlled trial of corticosteroids in the treatment of optic neuritis, *N Engl J Med* 326:581-588, 1992.

Beck RW Kupersmith MJ, Cleary PA, Katz B: Fellow eye abnormalities in acute unilateral optic neuritis, *Ophthalmology* 100:691-698, 1993.

Bianchi Marzoli S, Martinelli V: Optic neuritis: differential diagnosis, *Neurol Sci* 22(suppl 2):S52-S54, 2001.

Ergene E: Adult optic neuritis, 2004, www. emedicine.com.

Levin A, Arnold A: *Neuro-ophthalmology*, New York, 2005, Thieme Medical.

Martinelli V, Bianchi Marzoli S: Non-demyelinating optic neuropathy: clinical entities, *Neurol Sci* 22(suppl 2):S55-S59, 2001.

Optic Neuritis Study Group: Visual function 5 year after optic neuritis, *Arch Ophthalmol* 115: 1545-1552, 1997.

Orbital inflammation, acute   (376.0)

DIAGNOSIS

Definition
Acute inflammation of the anterior preseptal and/or posterior orbit.

Synonym
Preseptal cellulitis, orbital cellulitis.

Symptoms
Decreased vision: generally, mildly decreased vision is caused by abnormalities of the tear film secondary to the inflammation; rarely, a rapid loss of vision results from spread of the inflammation to the optic nerve.

Pain and redness: the area of cellulitis tends to be red, warm, and painful (*see* Fig. 1).

Swelling/pressure: the swelling may be so severe as to cause complete closure of the eyelids; also, the swelling often crosses over to involve secondarily the eyelids on the uninvolved side.

Tearing.

Blurred vision: the uninvolved contralateral eye may show blurred vision caused by secondary tearing and eyelid swelling.

Diplopia (double vision): decreased ocular motility results in strabismus and thus double vision.

Signs
Redness of lids.

Chemosis of conjunctiva: may be so severe that the chemotic conjunctiva protrudes through the semiclosed eyelids.

Lid swelling: the patient may present with swelling to such a degree that complete closure of the eyelids occurs.

Exophthalmos (ocular proptosis): inflammation posterior to the septum orbitale (i.e., post-septal extension) may cause exophthalmos, except in children <5 yr of age, in whom exophthalmos does not occur.

Ocular motility problems: the orbital swelling and direct inflammation of the extraocular muscles may limit the mobility of the muscles, resulting in strabismus and diplopia.

Appearance of acute systemic illness.

Investigations
History: especially of sinusitis, orbital trauma, and systemic complaints.

Ocular examination: complete ocular examination (if eyelids are swollen shut completely, local anesthesia may be necessary to examine the eyes adequately), exophthalmometry (measurement of exophthalmos by an exophthalmometer), intraocular pressure, undilated and dilated slit-lamp examinations, and dilated fundus examination.

- A dilated pupil, marked ophthalmoplegia, loss of vision, and afferent pupillary defect are all warning signs of serious orbital cellulitis. Also, phycomycosis (usually *Mucor*) can present as an acute fulminating infection of the sinuses and orbit, generally in an acidotic or immunosuppressed patient.

General examination: general physical examination, white blood count and differential, culture of any ocular purulent material.

Special examination: computed tomography, magnetic resonance imaging, or orbital ultrasound may be indicated, especially if swelling precludes an adequate ocular examination or if an intraocular or orbital foreign body is suspected.

Differential diagnosis
Graves' disease, allergic reaction (angioneurotic edema), pseudotumor of orbit (*see* Orbital inflammation, chronic), Parinaud's oculoglandular syndrome (granulomatous conjunctivitis and ipsilateral enlargement of the preauricular lymph nodes). Wegener's granulomatosis, orbital mucocele, carotid cavernous fistula, orbital neoplasms.

Cause
- Most cases (>60%) arise from infection of contiguous sinuses, especially ethmoiditis and especially in children.
- The most common cause of infectious orbital cellulitis in children is *Haemophilus influenzae*. In adults the most common causes are *Staphylococcus* and *Streptococcus* spp.; can be secondary to trauma, upper respiratory infection, dental abscess, and many other systemic infections.

Epidemiology
- Acute orbital inflammation is rare but extremely important because it is potentially life threatening.

Classification
Preseptal inflammation (orbital cellulitis [376.1]): inflammation contained anterior to the septum orbitale, mainly limited to lids and superficial tissue.

Postseptal extension: inflammation extends posterior to the septum orbitale into orbital tissues.

Associated features
Fever, leukocytosis.
- With posterior spread, signs and symptoms of orbital apex syndrome, cavernous sinus thrombosis, or meningitis may develop.

Pathology
- An acute inflammatory reaction characterized by neutrophils and necrosis is seen.
- Special stains may show a bacterial cause, most often *Staphylococcus aureus* and *Streptococcus* spp.

Diagnosis continued on p. 256

Orbital inflammation, acute   (376.0)

TREATMENT

Diet and Lifestyle
In general, patients who have acute orbital inflammation (most prevalent in children) tend to be acutely ill. Bed rest, warm compresses, and a light diet generally supplement the parenteral antibiotics.

Pharmacologic Treatment
Antibiotic Therapy
- Any purulent material should be cultured.
- Most children need systemic antibiotic therapy. The type of antibiotic used depends on such factors as the Gram-stained appearance of the organism, physician protocol for orbital cellulitis, and results of culture.
- In adults, Gram-stained sections of any purulent material are the best guide to antibiotic therapy. Most physicians start with a broad-spectrum antibiotic while they await the results of culture and sensitivity.
- If cavernous sinus thrombosis is imminent or present, prompt systemic antibiotic therapy can be lifesaving.

Phycomycosis *(Mucor)*
Phycomycosis usually can be recognized easily in hematoxylin-eosin–stained sections by the hyphae, which are large, branching, and contain septa. The fungus tends to invade, causing thrombosis and an immediate threat to both vision and life. Because the acute orbital inflammation may be the initial sign of systemic phycomycosis, proper recognition of this fungal disease can be lifesaving. Immediate IV administration of antifungal agents (generally by an infectious disease expert) is essential. At the same time, prompt attention must be paid to the underlying condition (e.g., diabetes mellitus).

Treatment continued on p. 257

Treatment aims

To preserve vision and ocular function: the key to visual and ocular rehabilitation is prompt therapy; other specialists (e.g., pediatricians, otolaryngologists, oral surgeons, internists) may need to be consulted.

To prevent posterior spread of infection to avoid complications such as orbital apex syndrome, cavernous sinus thrombosis, or meningitis: in the case of posterior spread of the inflammation toward the orbital apex, prompt antibiotic therapy can be lifesaving.

To identify and treat any underlying systemic disease: particularly important in phycomycosis, which often is accompanied by systemic acidosis; the acidosis can be caused by diabetes mellitus, chronic diarrhea, and conditions that cause immunosuppression.

Other treatments

- Any systemic infection (e.g., sinusitis, dental abscess) should be treated accordingly.
- Sinus drainage will have to be performed, generally by an otolaryngologist, in a significant percentage of patients (especially children) who have acute orbital inflammation.

Prognosis

With prompt antibiotic therapy and drainage of any sites where purulent material has formed, the prognosis for visual and ocular rehabilitation is excellent.

Follow-up and management

Close initial follow-up is crucial to determine the effectiveness of therapy and if surgical drainage of any pockets of purulent material is necessary. Also, any systemic problems need to be followed and dealt with appropriately.

DIAGNOSIS—cont'd

Complications
Visual loss, ocular motility problems, orbital apex syndrome.

Cavernous sinus thrombosis: with cavernous sinus involvement, headache, nausea, vomiting, and varying levels of consciousness may occur.

Meningitis: extension of the orbital inflammation posteriorly in the orbit can result in subdural empyema, intracranial abscess, or meningitis.

Pearls and Considerations
Because phycomycosis (Mucor) may present initially in the orbit and because it may be lethal, early recognition by the ophthalmologist may be life saving.

Referral Information
Consider referral to otolaryngologist if spread of infection from adjacent sinuses is suspected.

TREATMENT—cont'd

Nonpharmacologic Treatment

- If sinusitis, otitis, or dental abscess is suspected, consultation with an otolaryngologist or oral surgeon is indicated.
- Any intraorbital purulent material should be drained surgically and cultured. In children, sinus drainage is needed in ~50% of patients. In adults, sinus and abscess drainage is necessary in ~90% of patients.
- Blood cultures are indicated if hematogenous spread is suspected.

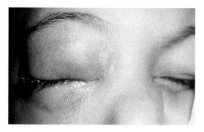

Figure 1   This child has swollen red eyelids (cellulitis) of her right eye caused by acute ethmoiditis.

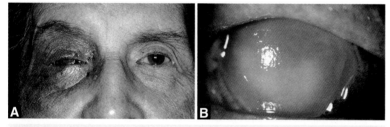

Figure 2   **A,** The red right eye is secondary to panophthalmitis with orbital spread. **B,** On closer observation of the right eye, a hypopyon (pus) is seen behind the cornea in the anterior chamber.

General references

Fairley C, Sullivan TJ, Bartley P, et al: Survival after rhino-orbital-cerebral mucormycosis in an immunocompetent patient, *Ophthalmology* 107(3):555-558, 2000.

Hodges E, Tabbara KF: Orbital cellulitis: review of 23 cases from Saudi Arabia, *Br J Ophthalmol* 73:205-208, 1989.

Klapper SR, Parinely JR, Kaplan SL, et al: Atypical mycobacterial infection of the orbit, *Ophthalmology* 102(10):1536-1541, 1995.

Read RW: Endophthalmitis. In Yanoff M, Duker JS, editors: *Ophthalmology*, E-dition, St Louis, 2006, Elsevier.

Orbital inflammation, chronic   (376.1)

DIAGNOSIS

Definition
An ongoing, low-grade inflammation of the anterior (preseptal) and/or posterior orbit.

Synonyms
None.

Symptoms
Exophthalmos (synonymous with ocular proptosis).

Red, painful eye: if exophthalmos is excessive, exposure keratitis may cause redness and pain in the eye.

Swelling/pressure, tearing, blurred vision, diplopia.

Signs
Exophthalmos: a lesion within the muscle cone causes more exophthalmos than a similar-sized lesion outside the muscle cone: paresis of the extraocular muscles as a result of inflammation (ophthalmoplegia) can cause 2.0 mm of ocular proptosis; in Graves' exophthalmos, extraocular and periorbital muscle involvement by edema, lymphocytic infiltration (mainly CD4+ and CD8+ T cells along with focal accumulations of B, plasma, and mast cells), and mucopolysaccharide deposition are responsible for the exophthalmos.

Chemosis and injection of conjunctiva.

Periorbital and eyelid edema.

Lid lag: especially in Graves' disease.

Ocular motility problems.

Investigations
History: especially of systemic complaints and presence of Graves' disease, sarcoidosis, lymphoma, leukemia, or immunosuppression (e.g., AIDS).

Ocular examination: visual acuity, ocular motility, complete external examination, exophthalmometry (measurement of exophthalmos by an exophthalmometer), intraocular pressure, undilated and dilated slit-lamp examination, dilated fundus examination.

Graves' disease: thyroid function studies can show hypothyroidism, euthyroidism, or hyperthyroidism; can perform computed tomography (CT) or magnetic resonance imaging (MRI) of the orbit, paying particular attention to the extraocular muscles (the best way to diagnose thyroid exophthalmos).

Sarcoidosis: chest radiograph, "blind" conjunctival biopsy, and biopsy of lacrimal gland may be performed to diagnose sarcoidosis.

Infectious agents: the main bacteria that cause chronic orbital inflammation are those that cause tuberculosis (*Mycobacterium tuberculosis*), syphilis (*Treponema pallidum*), and cat-scratch disease (*Bartonella henselae*); the main fungi that cause chronic orbital inflammation are those that cause phycomycosis (*Mucor, Rhizopus*), aspergillosis (*Aspergillus fumigatus*), and sporotrichosis (*Sporotrichum schenckii*); and the main parasites that cause chronic orbital inflammation are those that cause trichinosis (*Trichinella spiralis*), schistosomiasis (*Schistosoma haematobium, S. japonicum*), and cysticercosis (*Cysticercus cellulosae*).

General examination: physical examination, white blood cell count and differential, any other laboratory test as indicated.

Special examination: CT, MRI, orbital ultrasound; these tests are extremely important in diagnosing Graves' disease, orbital mucocele, carotid cavernous fistula, and orbital neoplasms.

Differential diagnosis
Graves' disease, acute orbital inflammation, orbital mucocele, carotid cavernous fistula, orbital neoplasms.

Cause
Granulomatous secondary to bacteria: tuberculosis, syphilis, cat-scratch disease (*Bartonella henselae*).

Granulomatous secondary to fungi: phycomycosis (mucormycosis), sporotrichosis, aspergillosis.

Granulomatous secondary to parasites: trichinosis, schistosomiasis, cysticercosis.

Granulomatous secondary to other entities: sarcoidosis, Wegener's granulomatosis, Crohn's disease, midline lethal granuloma syndrome.

Parinaud's oculoglandular syndrome: granulomatous conjunctivitis and ipsilateral enlargement of preauricular lymph nodes.

Unknown cause: e.g., pseudotumor, benign lymphoepithelial lesion of Godwin.

Epidemiology
- All forms of chronic inflammations of the orbit are rare.
- Although granulomatous infectious orbital inflammation is rare, it is extremely important because it is potentially life threatening, especially phycomycosis (mucormycosis).

Classification
Infectious granulomatous, e.g., phycomycosis (mucormycosis).

Noninfectious granulomatous, e.g., sarcoidosis, Crohn's disease, cat-scratch disease.

Noninfectious nongranulomatous, e.g., pseudotumor.

Associated features
Depend on cause (e.g., sarcoidosis may have multisystem involvement).

Immunology
An immunologic cause has been postulated for several noninfectious entities, but not with certainty.

Diagnosis continued on p. 260

TREATMENT

Diet and Lifestyle

- No special precautions are necessary; however, if the patient is acutely ill (as often occurs with some infectious causes, e.g., phycomycosis), bed rest, warm compresses, and a light diet generally supplement other, more specific treatments.

Pharmacologic Treatment

- If an infectious agent is identified, appropriate therapy should be instituted as soon as possible.
- If exposure keratitis is present, frequent lubrication (even every ½ hour if needed) with either lubricating drops or ointment during the day and ointment at bedtime.

Phycomycosis (Mucormycosis) and Aspergillosis

Both phycomycosis and aspergillosis can present as an acute orbital inflammation (often fulminating) or as a limited chronic form; both can be life threatening. Usually, phycomycosis can be recognized easily in Gram-stained or eosin-hematoxylin–stained sections of purulent material by the hyphae, which are large, branching, and contain septa. The fungus tends to invade early into arterioles, causing thrombosis and therefore posing an immediate threat to both vision and life. Because the acute orbital inflammation may be the initial sign of systemic phycomycosis, proper recognition of this fungal disease can be lifesaving. Similarly, the fungus of aspergillosis can be recognized best (with Grocott or periodic acid–Schiff staining techniques) by its branching, septated hyphae, which are about one fifth the size of *Mucor*. Immediate IV administration of antifungal agents, generally by an infectious disease expert, is essential. At the same time, prompt attention must be paid to the underlying condition (e.g., diabetes mellitus, AIDS, chronic renal disease).

Nonpharmacologic Treatment

- Orbital biopsy may be necessary to establish a diagnosis.
- Often, noninfectious chronic orbital inflammation responds well to corticosteroid or low-dose orbital radiation therapy.

Exposure Keratitis

If conservative therapy (lubricating drops/ointment) is not successful, tarsorrhaphy (lateral or regular) can be performed. With extreme exophthalmos (e.g., advanced thyroid exophthalmopathy), more extreme measures, such as orbital decompression, may be needed.

Treatment aims

To preserve vision and ocular function.

To identify and treat any underlying systemic disease: particularly important in phycomycosis, which often is accompanied by systemic acidosis; the acidosis can result from diabetes mellitus, chronic diarrhea, and conditions that cause immunosuppression; if sarcoidosis presents initially with ocular involvement, the patient must be referred to a primary physician to check for systemic involvement and future monitoring.

Other treatments

- Any systemic infection or noninfectious condition (e.g., tuberculosis, AIDS, phycomycosis, sarcoidosis) should be treated accordingly.

Prognosis

- With prompt, appropriate therapy, the prognosis for visual and ocular rehabilitation is excellent in most of the conditions.
- The key to visual and ocular rehabilitation is prompt therapy. Other specialists (e.g., pediatricians, otolaryngologists, oral surgeons, internists) may need to be consulted.

Follow-up and management

- Close initial follow-up is essential to monitor the effectiveness of therapy.
- Long-term follow-up is necessary to recognize any early recurrence. Also, any systemic problems need to be followed up and dealt with appropriately.

Treatment continued on p. 261

Orbital inflammation, chronic   (376.1)

DIAGNOSIS—cont'd

Complications
Exposure keratitis, visual loss, uveitis, intraocular involvement.
Strabismus and diplopia (double vision).
Systemic involvement and even death (e.g., from phycomycosis).

Pearls and Considerations
Topic too broad to make specific recommendations.

Referral Information
Refer to appropriate subspecialist based on suspected etiology of inflammation (e.g., endocrinologist for Graves' disease).

TREATMENT—cont'd

Suspected Sarcoidosis

If chest radiograph is not helpful, a "blind" conjunctival biopsy can be performed; "blind" refers to not seeing any nodule within the conjunctiva in the inferior cul-de-sac. Under topical anesthesia, the conjunctiva in the inferior cul-de-sac is tented up, and a strip of conjunctiva approximately 8 × 3 mm is removed with a scissors. Suturing is usually not needed.

If a conjunctival nodule (granuloma) is detected clinically, this should be included in the biopsy. It is extremely important to communicate with the pathologist that a strip of four to six sections should be placed on one glass slide and repeated at three different levels. This procedure yields 12-18 sections in which to search for the subconjunctival noncaseating granuloma characteristic of sarcoidosis.

General references

Bartalena L, Marocci C, Bogazzi F, et al: Relation between therapy for hyperthyroidism and the course of Graves' ophthalmology, *N Engl J Med* 338(2):73-78, 1998.

Carta A, D'Adda T, Carrara F, et al: Ultrastructural analysis of external muscle in chronic progressive external ophthalmoplegia, *Arch Ophthalmol* 118(10):1141-1145, 2000.

Fairley C, Sullivan TJ, Bartley P, et al: Survival after rhino-orbital-cerebral mucormycosis in an immunocompetent patient, *Ophthalmology* 107(3):555-558, 2000.

Tsubota K, Fujita H, Tsuzaka K, et al: Mikulicz's disease and Sjögren's syndrome, *Invest Ophthalmol Vis Sci* 41(7):1666-1673, 2000.

Pars planitis (363.21)

DIAGNOSIS

Definition
Intraocular inflammation, primarily of the anterior vitreous.

Synonym
Intermediate uveitis (IU).

Symptoms
Floaters.
Decreased vision.
Photophobia.

Signs
Mild anterior-chamber inflammation.
Cells in the anterior vitreous.
Cellular aggregations in the vitreous "snowballs."
"Snowbanking": white exudative material over the inferior ora serrata [1,2].
Peripheral retinal vascular sheathing.
Cystoid macular edema.
Posterior subcapsular cataract.
Secondary glaucoma.
Peripheral retinal neovascularization.
Vitreous hemorrhage.
Peripapillary edema.

Investigations
History and appropriate laboratory studies: to rule out Lyme disease, sarcoidosis, toxoplasmosis, tuberculosis, syphilis, multiple sclerosis.
Complete ocular examination including peripheral depression: to view the inferior ora serrata.
Fluorescein angiography: to rule out diffuse vascular leakage.
Optical coherence tomography: to rule out cystoid macular edema.

Complications
Cystoid macular edema.
Peripheral neovascularization.
Cataract.
Vitreous hemorrhage.
Secondary glaucoma.
Epiretinal membranes.
Traction or rhegmatogenous detachment.

Pearls and Considerations
1. Pars planitis tends to follow a prolonged course of exacerbations and remissions.
2. Children tend to have worse visual outcomes with IU than adults.

Referral Information
Refer to retinal specialist for vitrectomy or intravitreal steroids as appropriate.

Differential diagnosis
Tumors (e.g., reticulum cell sarcoma, malignant melanoma, leukemia, retinoblastoma).
Retinitis pigmentosa.
Rhegmatogenous retinal detachment.
Asteroid hyalosis.
Amyloidosis.
Intraocular foreign body.
Endophthalmitis.

Cause
- Pars planitis is a chronic inflammatory disorder of unknown cause.

Epidemiology
Usually found in patients age 14-40 yr.
Bilateral in 80% of patients.
May remain active for many years.

Pathology
Peripheral lymphocytic cuffing of venules.
Loose fibrovascular membrane.

TREATMENT

Diet and Lifestyle
- No special precautions are necessary.

Pharmacologic Treatment
- Steroid therapy is used in patients with cystoid macular edema. Treatment usually consists of intravitreal injection of steroid and often needs to be repeated.
- Cytotoxic agents are reserved for intractable cases.
- Oral therapy may be necessary if the vitreous infiltrate causes decreased vision.

Nonpharmacologic Treatment
Cryoablation: of the pars plana membrane or in severe cases.

Peripheral laser or cryoablation: to neovascularization.

Vitrectomy: for dense vitreous infiltrates with or without traction that cause significant visual loss.

Treatment aims
To prevent secondary complications (e.g., chronic cystoid macular edema, vitreous hemorrhage).

Prognosis
- Clinical course is usually self-limited with gradual improvement of vision.
- Cases can smolder with intermittent acute exacerbation, limiting the visual end result because of chronic cystoid macular edema.

Follow-up and management
- Patients are followed every few months, depending on the severity of disease, response to treatment, and rate of recurrence.

Key references
1. Welsh RB, Maumenee AE, Wahler HE: Peripheral posterior segment inflammation, vitreous opacities and edema of the posterior pole: pars planitis, *Arch Ophthalmol* 64: 540-549, 1960.
2. Henderly DE, Haymond RS, Rao NA, Smith RE: The significance of the pars plana exudate in pars planitis, *Am J Ophthalmol* 103:669-671, 1987.

General references
Read RW, Zamir E, Rao NA: Nongranulomatous inflammation: uveitis, endophthalmitis, panophthalmitis and sequelae. In Tasman W et al, editors: *Duane's clinical ophthalmology* (CD-ROM), Baltimore, 2004, Lippincott Williams & Wilkins.
Smith RE: Pars planitis. In Ryan SJ, editor: *Retina*, vol 2, St Louis, 1989, Mosby, pp 637-645.

Phacoanaphylactic endophthalmitis   (360.19)

DIAGNOSIS

Definition
Inflammation of the ocular tissues secondary to rupture of the crystalline lens.

Synonyms
Phacoimmune endophthalmitis.

Symptoms
- Phacoanaphylactic endophthalmitis always follows a penetrating ocular injury in which the lens is ruptured; characterized by a zonal granulomatous inflammatory reaction centered around the ruptured lens (*see* Figs. 1 and 2), with symptoms of:

Photophobia.
Ocular irritation or pain.
Blurred vision.

Signs
Red eye secondary to ciliary injection.
Evidence of previous penetrating ocular injury.
Mutton-fat keratic precipitates.
Corneal edema secondary to glaucoma.

Investigations
History: penetrating ocular injury.
Visual acuity test.
Complete ocular examination: including undilated and dilated slit-lamp examination.
Dilated fundus examination.

Complications
Decreased visual acuity.
Glaucoma.
Cataract.
Macular edema.
Retinal detachment.
Phthisis bulbi: the end stage of ocular disease—a shrunken, functionless eye.

Cause
The disease occurs under special conditions that involve an abrogation of tolerance to lens proteins that are organ specific but not species specific. Lens proteins, if exposed to the systemic circulation, normally are recognized as "self." If they were not, phacoanaphylactic endophthalmitis would occur regularly (instead of rarely) after disruption of the lens capsule.

Pearls and Considerations
As with other forms of endophthalmitis, this is a true medical emergency.

Referral Information
Refer immediately for surgical removal of remaining pieces of the lens.

Differential diagnosis
Anterior iridocyclitis.
Phacolytic glaucoma.
Sympathetic uveitis.
Vogt-Koyanagi-Harada syndrome.

Epidemiology
- Phacoanaphylactic endophthalmitis only occurs when the lens capsule is traumatically ruptured and only rarely.

Immunology
Phacoanaphylactic endophthalmitis, an autoimmune condition, may result from the breakdown or reversal of central tolerance at the T-cell level. Small amounts of circulating lens protein normally maintain T-cell tolerance, but it may be altered as a result of trauma, possibly through the adjuvant effects of wound contamination, bacterial products, or both. After the abrogation of tolerance to lens protein, antilens antibodies are produced and reach the lens remnants in the eye, where an antibody-antigen reaction takes place (phacoanaphylactic endophthalmitis).

Pathology
A zonal granulomatous inflammation surrounds lens remnants. Activated neutrophils surround and seem to dissolve or "eat away" lens material, probably releasing proteolytic enzymes, arachidonic acid metabolites, and oxygen-derived free radicals. Epithelioid cells and occasional (sometimes in abundance) multinucleated inflammatory giant cells are seen beyond the neutrophils. Lymphocytes, plasma cells, fibroblasts, and blood vessels (i.e., granulation tissue) surround the epithelioid cells. Usually the iris is encased in the inflammatory reaction and inseparable from it. The uveal tract generally shows a reactive, chronic nongranulomatous inflammatory reaction.

TREATMENT

Diet and Lifestyle
- No special precautions are necessary.

Pharmacologic Treatment
- Phacoanaphylactic endophthalmitis basically is a surgical disease. However, the usual precautions (e.g., topical antiglaucoma drops for accompanying glaucoma, topical corticosteroids to reduce inflammation) are recommended before surgery.

Nonpharmacologic Treatment
Surgery: removing the remaining lens remnants may relieve the situation.

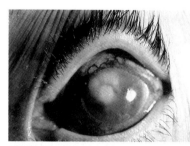

Figure 1 This patient had an extracapsular cataract extraction. Endophthalmitis developed postoperatively, and the eye was enucleated.

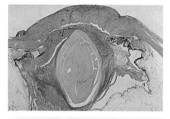

Figure 2 The lens remnant, mainly nucleus, shows a zonal type of granulomatous reaction, consisting of surrounding epithelioid cells and giant cells surrounded by lymphocytes and plasma cells, which in turn are surrounded by granulation tissue. The lens capsule is ruptured posteriorly.

Treatment aims
To preserve vision.

Other treatments
- Treatment of any glaucoma and inflammation usually is necessary. Corticosteroid and antiglaucoma drops usually suffice.

Prognosis
- The prognosis for vision is guarded.
- Often the inflammation is so violent that useful vision is destroyed before the inflammation can be resolved.

Follow-up and management
- Long-term follow-up is indicated, especially if permanent glaucoma results.

General references
Inomata H, Yoshikawa H, Rao NA: Phacoanaphylaxis in Behçet's disease: a clinicopathologic and immunohistochemical study, *Ophthalmology* 110(10):1942-1945, 2003.
Marak GE: Phacoanaphylactic endophthalmitis [major review], *Surv Ophthalmol* 36(5):325-339, 1992.

Phakomatoses

DIAGNOSIS

Definition
A group of different diseases characterized by multiple tumors (benign or malignant) developing in different organs of the body.

Synonyms
None; see terms used for specific tumors.

Symptoms
- Phakomatoses are a heredofamilial group of congenital tumors that have disseminated, benign (usually) hamartomas (tumors of tissue normally found in an area) in common.

Neurofibromatosis
Facial deformities (i.e., cosmetic problems), **multiple skin tumors, ocular proptosis (exophthalmos), blurred vision.**

Sturge-Weber Syndrome
Facial blemish (i.e., cosmetic problems secondary to "port-wine stain"), **blurred vision:** *see* Fig. 1.

Von Hippel's Disease
Blurred vision: *see* Fig. 2.

Tuberous Sclerosis
Facial blemish (i.e., cosmetic problems secondary to adenoma sebaceum), **mental impairment, blurred vision.**

Signs
Neurofibromatosis (237.71)
Café au lait spots, cutaneous neurofibromas, thickening of conjunctival and corneal nerves, Lisch iris nodules (characteristic of neurofibromatosis type 1 and present in ~90% of patients by age 6 yr: *see* Fig. 3), **intraocular uveal and neural retinal hamartomas, orbital plexiform neurofibromas and neurilemomas** (orbital neurofibroma often presents with typical S-shaped deformity of upper lid), **optic nerve glioma** (~25% of patients who have optic nerve gliomas have neurofibromatosis, almost exclusively in type 1), **glaucoma** (especially when upper eyelid involved).

Sturge-Weber Syndrome (Meningocutaneous Angiomatosis) (759.7)
Choroidal cavernous hemangioma (tends to involve choroid diffusely and blend into surrounding normal choroid), **facial nevus flammeus or port-wine stain** (usually along distribution of trigeminal nerve), **glaucoma** (~30% of patients; especially when upper eyelid involved).

Von Hippel's Disease (Angiomatosis Retinae) (759.6)
Neural retinal capillary hemangioma (similar to cerebellar capillary hemangioma), **neural retinal exudates** (even when capillary hemangioma located in peripheral retina, exudates can appear in macula and cause blurred vision; in a child, any unexplained macular exudation may indicate von Hippel's disease or Coats' disease), **glaucoma** (usually angle-closure glaucoma secondary to iris neovascularization and peripheral anterior synechiae associated with long-standing retinal detachment).

Tuberous Sclerosis (Bourneville's Disease) (759.5)
Facial cutaneous adenoma sebaceum, glial hamartomas (giant drusen) of optic disc (these can be misdiagnosed as optic disc edema; however, the history and other clues, e.g., adenoma sebaceum and retinal glial hamartomas, should make the diagnosis obvious), **glial (astrocytic) hamartomas of neural retina** (~53% of patients).

Differential diagnosis
- Retinal hemangiomas, astrocytic hamartomas, choroidal hemangiomas, orbital neurofibromatoses and neurilemomas, and giant drusen of the optic disc all can occur primarily without phakomatoses.
- Neuromas, café au lait spots, and prominent corneal nerves—all similar to findings in neurofibromatosis—may also be seen in multiple endocrine neoplasia, which is caused by an abnormality of chromosomes 11q13 and 10q11.2.

Cause
Neurofibromatosis type 1: irregular autosomal dominant; chromosome 17 (band 17q11.2).

Neurofibromatosis type 2: irregular autosomal dominant; chromosome 22 (band 22q12).

Sturge-Weber syndrome: irregular autosomal dominant.

Von Hippel's disease: congenital; autosomal dominant with incomplete penetrance; short arm of chromosome 3.

Tuberous sclerosis: irregular autosomal dominant; long arm of chromosome 39.

Epidemiology
Neurofibromatosis type 1: prevalence 1:3000-4000.

Neurofibromatosis type 2: prevalence 1:50,000.

Sturge-Weber syndrome: very rare.

Von Hippel's disease: prevalence 1:40,000.

Tuberous sclerosis: incidence 0.56:100,000 person-years; prevalence 10.60:100,000.

Pathology
Neurofibromatosis type 1: depends on type of tumor (e.g., neurofibroma, optic nerve glioma).

Neurofibromatosis type 2: depends on type of tumor (e.g., eighth-nerve tumor [neurilemoma], meningioma).

Sturge-Weber syndrome: choroidal cavernous hemangioma.

Von Hippel's disease: retinal capillary hemangioma.

Diagnosis continued on p. 268

TREATMENT

Diet and Lifestyle
- If blindness is anticipated, the family should be informed of the many interventions available to blind patients.
- Central nervous system lesions in von Hippel's disease, Sturge-Weber syndrome, and tuberous sclerosis may require considerable modification of lifestyle.

Pharmacologic Treatment
- No pharmacologic treatment for phakomatoses is available; however, the secondary effects (e.g., glaucoma) can be treated.

Nonpharmacologic Treatment
- The phakomatoses should be treated surgically as indicated.
- Generally, the optic nerve glioma found in neurofibromatosis should be treated conservatively. Because the tumor is essentially a benign hamartoma, the indications for removal depend on factors other than the tumor (e.g., exophthalmos may cause exposure keratitis). Deciding whether to remove only the orbital optic nerve glioma or both the globe and the glioma is based on clinical data.
- An orbital neurofibroma may cause severe ocular proptosis and exposure keratitis, and removal of the neurofibroma may be warranted.
- Choroidal hemangiomas in Sturge-Weber syndrome tend to leak fluid, resulting in a secondary serous neural retinal detachment. This can be treated by laser photocoagulation, usually in a scatter form over the tumor.
- In von Hippel's disease, if exudation has decreased vision, cryotherapy of the peripheral retinal lesion or laser photocoagulation of the lesion's feeder vessels may cause partial or complete resolution of the exudate.
- Usually, no specific therapy is needed in tuberous sclerosis.

Treatment aims
To preserve vision.

Cosmetic aims
- The facial adenoma sebaceum in tuberous sclerosis (port-wine stain) and the facial deformities of neurofibromatosis can be extremely upsetting to patients. Cosmetic surgery often can change their outlook on life.

Other treatments
- Other treatments are aimed at the multiple systemic abnormalities associated with the phakomatoses.
- The eye care physician can provide guidance to patients and their families regarding expectations and additional help.

Prognosis
- Prognosis for vision and for life depends on the type of tumor that develops.

Follow-up and management
- Long-term follow-up is essential because different tumors can develop at various ages; also, benign tumors may become malignant.

Treatment continued on p. 269

DIAGNOSIS—cont'd

Investigations

History (including family history), **complete external examination, visual acuity testing, refraction, intraocular pressure, undilated and dilated slit-lamp examination, dilated fundus examination.**

Pearls and Considerations

Varied and specific to the type of underlying disorder; topic too broad.

Referral Information

Refer to primary care physician and/or plastic surgeon for intervention as appropriate based on the specific condition.

TREATMENT—cont'd

Complications

- Neurofibromatosis, Sturge-Weber syndrome, and von Hippel's disease all can be associated with glaucoma, retinal exudation and detachment, and eventually blindness.
- Neurofibromatosis of the orbit can cause exophthalmos, which can become marked and result in exposure keratitis.
- Neurofibromatosis of the optic nerve can cause optic nerve glioma and subsequent blindness.
- The neural retinal lesions of tuberous sclerosis disease generally remain stationary.

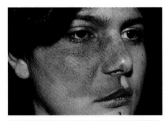

Figure 1 Sturge-Weber syndrome. Port-wine stain is present along the distribution of the trigeminal nerve.

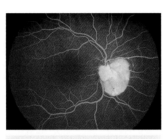

Figure 2 Angiomatosis retinae (von Hippel's disease). Fluorescein angiography shows a retinal capillary hemangioma of the optic nerve. *(Courtesy GE Lang.)*

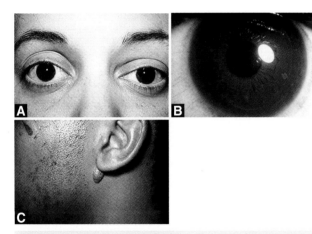

Figure 3 Neurofibromatosis. **A,** Orbital plexiform neurofibroma has caused proptosis of the right eye. **B,** Iris shows multiple spiderlike melanocytic nevi (Lisch nodules), characteristic of neurofibromatosis. **C,** Nodule under ear is a neurofibroma.

General references

Akiyama H, Tanaka T, Itakura H, et al: Inhibition of ocular angiogenesis by an adenovirus carrying the human von Hippel–Lindau tumor-suppressor gene in vivo, *Invest Ophthalmol Vis Sci* 45(5): 1289-1296, 2004.

Amirikia A, Scott IU, Murray TG: Bilateral diffuse choroidal hemangiomas with unilateral facial nevus flammeus in Sturge-Weber syndrome, *Am J Ophthalmol* 130(3):362-364, 2000.

Gutmann DH, Aylsworth A, Carey JC, et al: The diagnostic evaluation and multidisciplinary management of neurofibromatosis 1 and neurofibromatosis 2, *JAMA* 278(1):51-57, 1997.

Palena PV, Augsberger JJ: Phakomatoses. In Tasman W et al, editors: *Duane's clinical ophthalmology* (CD-ROM), Philadelphia, 2004, Lippincott Williams & Wilkins.

Shields JA, Eagle RC Jr, Shields CL, et al: Aggressive retinal astrocytomas in 4 patients with tuberous sclerosis complex, *Arch Ophthalmol* 123(6):856-863, 2005.

Pseudoexfoliation of the lens   (366.11)

DIAGNOSIS

Definition
Accumulation of white flakes at the pupillary margin and on the anterior surface of the lens.

Synonyms
None; often abbreviated PEX.

Symptoms
- Patients are usually asymptomatic, and PEX is discovered on routine examination. *See also* Glaucoma, pseudoexfoliative (365.52).

Signs
- PEX is bilateral in slightly >50% of cases. In following a patient for years, the clinician may note PEX in one eye. This usually prompts a careful examination of the other eye, which generally is normal. Continued examination of the uninvolved eye can result in normal findings until suddenly, years later, the second eye becomes involved.

PEX material (PEXM): dandruff-like material on the pupillary margin of the undilated pupil; usually the earliest sign (*see* Fig. 1).
- After dilation the anterior surface of lens shows a characteristic thin, homogeneous, white deposit centrally located and surrounded by a relatively clear zone, which in turn is surrounded by a more peripheral, coarse, granular "hoarfrost" material that extends to the equator. In aphakic and pseudophakic eyes, PEXM may appear years after cataract surgery on the pupillary border, anterior and posterior surfaces of the lens implant, anterior hyaloid surface, and vitreous framework. (*See* Figs. 2 and 3.)

Corneal endothelial abnormalities: may include powdery PEXM on the internal corneal surface and within its cytoplasm (seen as intraendothelial inclusions).

"Leathery" and poorly dilating iris: PEXM collects on the posterior surface of the iris and acts as a strut. Also, atrophy of the iris dilator muscle fibers occurs, causing difficulty in dilating.

Subtle iridodonesis and phacodonesis: seen in many patients; caused by an instability of the zonules supporting the lens.

Spontaneous subluxation and dislocation of the lens: rare.

Glaucoma: will develop in ~8% of patients, and an additional 12% will be glaucoma suspects (ocular hypertension); the cumulative probability for PEX eyes to develop abnormally high intraocular pressure is ~5% in 5 yr and 15% in 10 yr; the cause of the glaucoma is not known; both mechanical (PEXM "clogging" the trabecular meshwork) and genetic theories have been proposed.

Findings similar to those of pigment dispersion syndrome: the iris pigment epithelium undergoes degeneration, liberating melanin pigment. This pigment can deposit on the posterior surface of the cornea (pseudo-Krukenberg spindle) in the anterior-chamber angle and within the trabecular meshwork, mimicking the pigment dispersion syndrome; an early sign is a pigmented linear deposit lying on the corneal side of Schwalbe's line, called Sampaolesi's line.

Investigations
Visual acuity testing.
Refraction.
Intraocular pressure.
Undilated and dilated slit-lamp examination.
Gonioscopy.
Dilated fundus examination.

Differential diagnosis
Pigment dispersion syndrome.
Inflammatory deposits on lens surface.

Cause
- The cause is unknown.

Epidemiology
- PEX of the lens has a worldwide distribution but seems to be most common in Scandinavian people (especially those living in Norway and Finland) and is rare in African people.
- PEX probably is inherited (possibly autosomal dominant) with incomplete penetrance.
- PEX tends to involve an older population, mainly ages 60-80 yr.

Classification
- Generally, PEX of the lens is classified as unilateral or bilateral, with or without elevated intraocular pressure.

Associated features
- PEXM has been found histologically in the following structures:
Ocular: iris, ciliary body, posterior ciliary vessels, palpebral and bulbar conjunctiva, eyelid, orbital tissue.
Nonocular: skin, lung, heart, liver, gallbladder, kidney, cerebral meninges.
- The significance of the systemic findings is not known.

Pathology
- PEXM appears eosinophilic in routine histology and is found prominently on the anterior surface of the lens, the posterior surface of the iris, and the internal surface of the ciliary body. The material stains positively with periodic acid–Schiff; it probably is a type of basement membrane.

Diagnosis continued on p. 272

TREATMENT

Diet and Lifestyle

- No special precautions are necessary.

Pharmacologic Treatment

- Pharmacologic treatment has no effect on PEX unless glaucoma develops.

Nonpharmacologic Treatment

- Unless a cataract develops, no treatment is necessary for the lens. Any associated glaucoma should be treated appropriately.

Cataract Surgery in PEX Eyes

- Complications occur more frequently in patients with PEX syndrome. The instability of the zonules supporting the lens often leads to a subtle iridodonesis and phacodonesis in many patients and, rarely, spontaneous lens subluxation (lens in posterior chamber but not in its normal location) and dislocation (lens not in posterior chamber but in vitreous or anterior chamber).

Treatment aims
To control any associated glaucoma.

Other treatments

- Because of the increased risk associated with cataract surgery in PEX patients, appropriate care must be taken if a cataract develops.
- Informed consent is extremely important, especially considering the increased risk of cataract surgery in PEX patients (*see* Nonpharmacologic treatment). Also, the patient must be informed that careful postoperative follow-up (including long-term follow-up) is essential because of the increased risk of developing glaucoma.

Prognosis

- If no other vision-threatening ocular conditions are present, cataract extraction and IOL implantation result in >90% visual improvement to an acuity of $\geq 20/40$.

Follow-up and management

- The cumulative probability of PEX eyes developing abnormally high intraocular pressure (IOP) is ~5% in 5 yr and ~15% in 10 yr. Long-term follow-up is therefore mandatory.
- Patients with PEX of the lens should be considered glaucoma suspects and followed up yearly if IOP is normal. If IOP is elevated, appropriate testing (e.g., visual fields, optic nerve photos) should be performed and follow-up visits tailored to the individual patient.

Treatment continued on p. 273

Pseudoexfoliation of the lens   (366.11)

DIAGNOSIS—cont'd

Complications
Secondary open-angle glaucoma.
Increased chance of complications during cataract surgery.

Pearls and Considerations
1. Can lead to pseudoexfoliative glaucoma, the most common secondary open-angle glaucoma worldwide.
2. True exfoliation syndrome only occurs with heat or infrared changes in the anterior lens capsule.

Referral Information
Refer to glaucoma specialist for argon laser or selective laser trabeculoplasty.

TREATMENT—cont'd

- The instability of the cataractous PEX lens during surgery can lead to capsular tears and vitreous loss. Some advocate nuclear-expression extracapsular cataract (ECC) surgery, and others recommend phacoemulsification ECC surgery; level of comfort and experience should guide the surgeon's choice of procedure.
- Another question is whether to put the intraocular lens (IOL) implant into the "lens bag" or on top of the bag into the ciliary sulcus. Initially, many surgeons thought that it was safer to put the IOL into the sulcus. Then the pendulum swung strongly to in-the-bag insertions. However, many surgeons now prefer in-the-sulcus insertions because of the recent findings of subluxated and dislocated IOLs years after in-the-bag insertions.

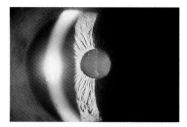

Figure 1 The earliest indication of PEX of the lens in the undilated pupil is the presence of dandruff-like material on the pupillary edge of the iris and on the anterior surface of the lens in the region of the pupillary margin.

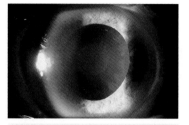

Figure 2 Partial dilation shows a plaque of PEX on the surface of the central lens and the beginning (from 12-6 o'clock positions) of the peripheral rim of PEX material.

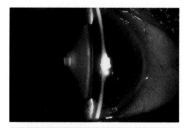

Figure 3 The slit beam passes through the central plaque.

General references

Bleich S, Roedl J, von Ahsen N, et al: Elevated homocysteine levels in aqueous humor of patients with pseudoexfoliation glaucoma, *Am J Ophthalmol* 138(1):162-164, 2004.

Pons ME, Eliassi-Rad B: Glaucoma, pseudoexfoliation, 2006, www.emedicine.com.

Puska P: Unilateral exfoliation syndrome: conversion to bilateral exfoliation and to glaucoma: a prospective 10-year follow-up study, *J Glaucoma* 11(6):517-524, 2002.

Puska P, Tarkkanen A: Exfoliation syndrome as a risk factor for cataract development: five-year follow-up of lens opacities in exfoliation syndrome, *J Cataract Refract Surg* 27(12): 1992-1998, 2001.

Pseudotumor cerebri (benign intracranial hypertension)   (348.2)

DIAGNOSIS

Definition
Papilledema associated with idiopathic intracranial hypertension.

Synonyms
Benign intracranial hypertension.

Symptoms
- 5%-10% of patients are asymptomatic, and papilledema is detected on routine eye examination.

Headache: 90% of patients.

Transient visual obscuration: 54% of patients.

Diplopia: 36% of patients.

Painful neck stiffness: 31% of patients.

Pulsatile tinnitus (usually on right side): 27% of patients.

Signs
- Normal visual acuity; no afferent pupillary defect unless chronic atrophic papilledema.

Papilledema: can be acute, chronic, or chronic atrophic.

Visual field loss: includes arcuate nerve fiber bundle loss, enlarged blind spot, constricted visual fields, inferior nasal field depression, decreased color vision (by Ishihara color plates), and cecocentral and central scotomas.

Modified Dandy's Diagnostic Criteria [1]
1. Patient is awake and alert.
2. Signs and symptoms of increased intracranial pressure (ICP).
3. Absence of localized neurologic signs except for sixth-nerve palsy.
4. Opening pressure of cerebrospinal fluid (CSF) on lumbar puncture (LP) is >200 mm H_2O and is of normal composition.
5. Normal ventricles and normal study on computed tomography (CT) and magnetic resonance imaging (MRI).
   - Relative afferent pupillary defects may occur if there is asymmetric visual field loss or chronic atrophic papilledema in one eye.

Investigations
To avoid brainstem herniation, **CT** of head before LP to rule out intracranial lesion.

Threshold visual fields, Goldmann visual field, contrast sensitivity, CT or MRI, magnetic resonance arteriography and venography, LP (cell count, glucose, protein, opening-pressure cytology, VDRL), **erythrocyte sedimentation rate, complete blood count, rapid plasma reagin test, fluorescent treponemal antibody absorption test, calcium (Ca^{++}), phosphorus, thyroxine, blood urea nitrogen, electrolytes.**

Complications
Progressive loss of vision, secondary vein occlusion from papilledema.

Factors that may influence visual loss: hypertension, older age, myopia, anemia, chronic disc edema of >4 diopters, optochoroidal shunts, subretinal hemorrhage.

Disc infarction, choroidal folds, vein occlusion.

Pearls and Considerations
Associated optic atrophy may lead to permanent vision loss and is the only permanent morbidity associated with idiopathic intracranial hypertension.

Referral Information
Refer to neurologist or neuro-ophthalmologist for complete workup and imaging; consider referral to nutritionist for assistance with weight reduction therapy.

Differential diagnosis
Lateral sinus or superior sagittal sinus thrombosis.
Combination of anomalous discs, obesity, and migraine.
Papilledema from an intracranial mass.
Bilateral perioptic neuritis.
Spinal cord tumor.

Cause
Idiopathic.
- Decreased rate of CSF absorption, increased rate of CSF formation, increased venous ICP, and increased brain interstitial fluid (edema).
- Secondary causes: vitamin A, tetracycline, nalidixic acid, anabolic steroids, lithium.

Epidemiology
- Incidence is 13:100,000 in women ages 20-40 yr who are 10% above their ideal body weight. Incidence increases to 19:100,000 if they are 20% above their ideal body weight.
- There is no racial predilection.
- 92% of patients are women.
- In children the gender ratio is equal, and obesity is not as important. The child may become irritable, apathetic, and somnolent instead of suffering headache. Children have a higher prevalence of sixth-nerve palsy than adults. They may develop a third- or fourth-nerve palsy and a unilateral lower-motor-neuron facial palsy or skew deviation. Dandy's criteria do not apply to children (see Signs).
- In men, pseudotumor cerebri may be a different disease. Dural arteriovenous malformations may be causative.
- Although familial pseudotumor cerebri has many causes, no genetic linkage studies have been done.

Pathology
Unknown.

TREATMENT

Diet and Lifestyle
Weight loss: the one proven treatment for pseudotumor cerebri.
Behavior modification.

Pharmacologic Treatment
Standard dosage   Carbonic anhydrase inhibitor: acetazolamide (Diamox), 250-1000 mg in 1-4 divided doses, or 500-mg sustained-release capsules twice daily.
Furosemide, 20-80 mg, maximum 600 mg/day.
Digoxin, 0.25 mg/day.

- There is no role for long-term use of steroids in pseudotumor cerebri.

Nonpharmacologic Treatment
Optic nerve fenestration.
Serial LPs.
Lumboperitoneal shunt.
Subtemporal decompression.
Gastric reduction surgery.

Associated Features [1]
Association Criteria
1. Associated feature satisfies the Dandy criteria (*see* Signs).
2. Underlying condition should be proved to increase ICP.
3. Treatment of the association should improve it.
4. Properly controlled studies should show an association.

Proven associations (meet all 4 criteria for association): obesity.

Likely associations (meet 3 criteria but lacks case-control studies): chlordecone (Kepone), hypervitaminosis A.

Probable associations (meet 2 criteria): steroid withdrawal in children, hypothyroid children receiving replacement therapy, ketoprofen and indomethacin in Bartter's syndrome, hypoparathyroidism, Addison's disease, uremia, iron deficiency anemia, tetracycline, nalidixic acid, danazol, lithium, amiodarone, phenytoin, nitrofurantoin, ciprofloxacin, nitroglycerin.

Possible associations (meet 1 criterion): menstrual irregularity, oral contraceptive use, Cushing's syndrome, vitamin A deficiency, minor head trauma, Behçet's syndrome.

Unlikely (no criteria met): hyperthyroidism, steroid ingestion, immunization.

Unsupported: pregnancy, menarche.

Treatment aims
To prevent or reverse vision loss.

Prognosis
- Severe, permanent visual impairment occurs in 25% of patients in months to years.
- 80% improve visual function in 8 mo with treatment.
- Recurrence rate is 10%-40%.

Follow-up and management
- Patients should have serial visual function evaluation.
- Monitor visual function with visual fields, color vision, contrast sensitivity, Snellen acuity, and optic disc photos.

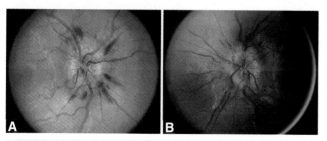

Acute papilledema in a woman (height 5 ft, 2 in; weight 300 lb) who had an opening pressure of 450 mm H_2O. Note elevation of optic disc with flame-shaped hemorrhages.

Key reference
1. Wall M, George D: Idiopathic intracranial hypertension (pseudotumor cerebri): a prospective study of 50 patients, *Brain* 114:155-180, 1991.

General references
Friedman DI: Papilledema and pseudotumor cerebri, *Ophthalmol Clin North Am* 14(1): 129-147, 2001.
Goodwin J: Pseudotumor cerebri, 2006, www.emedicine.com.
Mathews MK, Sergott RC, Savino PJ: Pseudotumor cerebri, *Curr Opin Ophthalmol* 14(6):364-370, 2003.
Movsas TZ, Liu GT, Galetta SL, et al: Current neuro-ophthalmic therapies, *Neurol Clin* 19(1):145-172, 2001.

DIAGNOSIS

Definition
Refractive disorder: condition in which light entering the eye does not focus at the retina.
Accommodation disorder: weakness or abnormality in the near-focusing system.

Synonyms
None; associated terms and conditions: myopia, nearsightedness, hyperopia, farsightedness, presbyopia, astigmatism, accommodative insufficiency, convergence insufficiency, accommodative spasm.

Symptoms
Decreased visual acuity at distance and/or near-fixation.
Visual discomfort (asthenopia).

Signs
Squinting.
Holding objects closely to or far away from the eyes.

Investigations
Refraction: to ascertain the patient's refractive error.
- Consideration of the patient's lifestyle and visual needs.

Complications
Progressive myopia: associated with uncorrected astigmatism in young children.
Amblyopia: associated with uncorrected anisometropia (differing refractive errors in the two eyes) in the following circumstances (D, diopters):
Hyperopia >1.75 D difference.
Myopia >2.50 D difference.
Astigmatism >1.50 D difference.
- Children who have high hyperopia (>4.00 D) are at increased risk for developing accommodative esotropia. Those who have hyperopia >6.00 D may have bilaterally decreased distance visual acuity for months after appropriate glasses prescription. Some term this "bilateral amblyopia," but it may represent bilateral dishabituation.

Associated Features
- Myopia may be caused by increased axial length (normal adult globe length 23.5 mm), increased curvature of the cornea *(keratoconus)* or lens *(spherophakia),* or movement of the lens toward the cornea.
- Hyperopia may be caused by decreased axial length *(microphthalmos),* decreased curvature of the cornea *(cornea plana)* or lens, or backward movement of the lens away from the cornea.
- Astigmatism is caused by deformity of the cornea or lens. Usually, the cornea is more curved in one meridian than another. *Lenticular* astigmatism occurs if the lens is tilted or subluxed. *Irregular* astigmatism is caused by irregular deformity of the cornea; it cannot be corrected with spectacles and requires contact lens correction.

Pathology
- The optic disc in myopia is oblique; the temporal edge is flattened and the nasal edge elevated. The retinal pigment epithelium and Bruch's membrane do not extend to the temporal disc edge; the choroid extends farther. The exposed sclera is viewed through transparent retina as a white crescent.
- Patients with extremely high myopia are at risk for retinal breaks and detachments, breaks in Bruch's membrane with macular hemorrhage, and vitreous degeneration.
- Patients with high hyperopia are at risk for angle-closure glaucoma.

Pearls and Considerations
Topic too broad for specific recommendations.

Referral Information
None.

Differential diagnosis
Decreased visual acuity from any pathologic ocular condition.
High hyperopia: seen in nanophthalmos, in which the eye is small but has no other gross abnormalities.
Macular hypoplasia and thickened sclera: the latter predisposes to choroidal effusion and retinal or choroidal detachment.

Cause
- Cause is often unknown, but refractive errors tend to run in families.
- Myopia with onset in school years has been attributed to prolonged near work.
- All refractive errors represent mismatch between axial length of the eye and power of refractive surfaces (primarily the cornea and lens).
- Patients who have myopia focus light from the horizon (when accommodation is relaxed) in front of the retina; patients who have hyperopia focus light behind the retina.
- Patients who have astigmatism focus a point of light on the horizon into a complex form that can be in front of, behind, or straddling the retina.
- Occasionally, patients with normal axial length and refractive surface power have a refractive error caused by movement of the lens-iris diaphragm. Myopia occurs if the lens moves forward; hyperopia occurs if the lens moves backward.

Epidemiology
- Some populations (Asiatic) have higher incidences of myopia than others (Aboriginal Australians).
- In Western Europe the chance of a child developing myopia is 48% if both parents are myopic, 24% if one is myopic, and 8% if neither parent is myopic.
- Many young children have bilateral symmetric astigmatism that resolves by 3 yr of age.
- Typically, young children have modest hyperopia, which decreases slowly throughout adolescence; some become myopic at that time. A much smaller group is myopic in young childhood, and myopia continues to increases as the child grows.

TREATMENT

Diet and Lifestyle
- The influence of diet and lifestyle on the development of refractive errors is unproved; some claim nutrition plays a role in the development of myopia and would prescribe nutritional supplements.
- Prolonged near work in the young child has been speculated to cause increased accommodative tone and increased axial length.

Pharmacologic Treatment
- Atropinization of young children with progressive myopia to prevent prolonged accommodation has been studied, but the results are equivocal; some children become more myopic, others do not.

Nonpharmacologic Treatment
Glasses and contact lenses: the traditional means of refractive correction; bifocal glasses have been prescribed to myopic patients to prevent accommodation at near-fixation and presumably prevent the development of axial enlargement.

Refractive surgery (radial keratotomy, photorefractive keratotomy): can be performed for suitable adults who require improved visual acuity without the use of glasses or contact lenses; patient selection is critical because this surgery involves cutting a normal cornea and is occasionally associated with corneal infection or perforation.

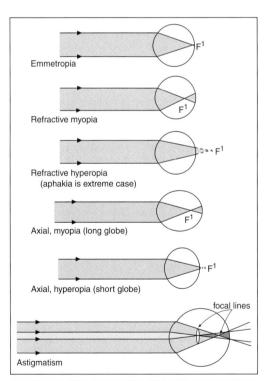

Patients with emmetropia focus light precisely on the retina; those with myopia focus light in front of the retina; and those with hyperopia focus light behind the retina. Patients with astigmatism do not focus light precisely to a point but rather to a complicated three-dimensional figure in space called a *conoid*.

Treatment aims
To improve visual acuity and decrease ocular discomfort.
- Patients with unequal refractive errors *(anisometropia)* may require special lenses to provide the two eyes with equal image sizes. *Aniseikonia* (unequal image sizes) may prevent comfortable single binocular vision.

Other treatments
- Children in some Eastern countries perform daily eye-massage exercises in school to prevent myopia development.

Prognosis
- Children generally accept a new prescription without difficulty; caution should be exercised before changing the prescription of an older person.

Follow-up and management
- Children who have refractive errors are generally examined yearly; adults are examined every 2 yr.

General references
Goss DA: Attempts to reduce the rate of increase of myopia in young people: a critical literature review, *Am J Optom Physiol Opt* 59:828-841, 1982.

McBrien N, Moghaddam HO, Reeder AP: Atropine reduces experimental myopia and eye enlargement via a nonaccommodative mechanism, *Invest Ophthalmol Vis Sci* 34:205-215, 1993.

O'Leary DJ, Millodot M: Eyelid closure causes myopia in humans, *Experientia* 35:1478-1479, 1979.

Wallman J, Turkel J, Trachtman J: Extreme myopia produced by modest changes in early visual experience, *Science* 201:1249-1251, 1978.

Retinal artery occlusion (362.31)

DIAGNOSIS

Definition
Blockage of an artery supplying the retina (can be the central artery or an arterial branch).

Synonyms
None; common abbreviations include BRAO (branch retinal artery occlusion) and CRAO (central retinal artery occlusion).

Symptoms
Acute, severe, painless loss of vision.

Signs
BRAO (*see* Fig. 1)
- May see one or more emboli in a branch arteriole.

Cotton-wool spots.
Arteriolar narrowing.
Retinal whitening: in distribution of the blocked arteriole.

CRAO (*see* Fig. 2)
Retinal whitening.
Cherry-red spot in the fovea.
Narrowing or segmentation of retinal arterioles.
Optic nerve pallor: can be seen in the late stages.

Investigations
BRAO

Fluorescein angiography: will help map out the area of retinal involvement.
Noninvasive carotid artery blood flow studies.
Echocardiography.

CRAO

Fluorescein angiography: demonstrates delayed, or even complete lack of, retinal arterial filling.
Echoretinography (ERG): shows a reduction in the B-wave amplitude.
Systemic workup: carotid artery noninvasive testing, echocardiography, erythrocyte sedimentation rate if temporal arteritis suspected; further studies should be considered if sickle cell disease, intravenous drug use, or hyperviscosity syndromes are suspected.

Complications
BRAO

Neovascularization of the retina: from ischemia.

CRAO

Neovascularization of the retina, iris, or angle.
Neovascular glaucoma.

Pearls and Considerations
1. CRAO is a true ocular emergency requiring immediate intervention.
2. Afferent pupillary defect will be present in CRAO.
3. Less than 10% of eyes with CRAO will eventually develop rubeosis iridis in the affected eye.
4. >90% of BRAO events involve the temporal vessels.
5. Patients with CRAO have a high 5-yr mortality rate because of cardiovascular disease and stroke.
6. If no cholesterol plaque is seen and the patient is in the appropriate age group, a sedimentation rate needs to be done to rule out temporal arteritis.

Referral Information
Refer to a retinal specialist for further evaluation and treatment immediately.

Differential diagnosis
BRAO
Transient retinal ischemia.
Tansient visual disturbance.
Commotio retinae secondary to trauma.
Arteriolar vasospasm.
CRAO
Ophthalmic artery occlusion.

Cause
BRAO
Embolization of a branch retinal arteriole from atherosclerotic plaque in the carotid artery or a calcific heart valve: most common cause.
Atrial myxoma in younger patients.
Talc emboli associated with IV drug use.
Intranasal cocaine causing arteriolar spasm.
Fat emboli after long-bone fractures.
CRAO
Thrombosis or embolic blockage to the central retinal artery; the most common source of emboli comes from the carotid arteries.

Epidemiology
BRAO
Most patients will resume a vision of 20/40 or better, although the paracentral scotoma can be visually disabling in some patients.
Most patients will have a permanent visual field defect in the area of retinal distribution supplied by that arteriole.
CRAO
90% of patients will have vision less than finger-counting range.
Up to 25% of patients will describe a preceding episode of transient visual loss.
5-yr mortality results from myocardial infarction in ~40% of patients.

Pathology
BRAO
Similar to that seen with CRAO, although the area of retinal necrosis confined to the inner layers of the retina is small; the outer layers are well preserved; late in the healing phase, the inner layer of the retina becomes acellular.
CRAO
Initially, ishemic necrosis seen, followed by acellular scarring of the inner retinal layers.

TREATMENT

Diet and Lifestyle
- Diet that promotes cardiovascular health, including decreased fat and salt intake, is indicated.

Pharmacologic Treatment
- An aspirin a day may help prevent future episodes of BRAO and is recommended for CRAO patients with a negative workup who are in the atherosclerotic age range.
- In selected patients (e.g., monocular patients presenting within 180 minutes), the risks and benefits need to be discussed thoroughly before considering administration of intravenous tissue plasminogen activator. This may lead to reperfusion and restoration of vision in some patients.

Nonpharmacologic Treatment
For BRAO
- If there is evidence of retinal neovascularization, sector laser photocoagulation in the distribution of the ischemia is recommended.

For CRAO
- Prompt evaluation within 180 min of the occlusion of the central retinal artery is optimal before irreparable damage to the retina occurs.
- If the patient is seen within this time frame, a paracentesis should be performed in an attempt to lower the intraocular pressure.
- Digital ocular massage may be able to dislodge the clot and improve vision; although rarely successful it should be attempted, since there are minimal side effects to the maneuver, the most common being bradycardia from the oculo-cardiac reflex.

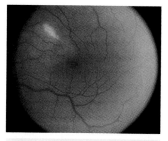

Figure 1 Supratemporal branch occlusion (BRAO) with intraretinal whitening in the superior macula and a prominent cotton-wool spot.

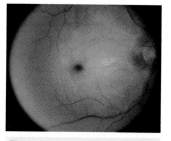

Figure 2 Central occlusion (CRAO) with diffuse whitening of the posterior pole, cherry-red spot in the fovea, and telangiectasia of the optic nerve vessels.

Treatment aims
BRAO

Prompt workup to rule out any treatable causes that would decrease future morbidity.

CRAO

To lower intraocular pressure and vasodilate the arterioles to dislodge the emboli into a smaller branch arteriole.

Other treatments
CRAO

Panretinal photocoagulation should be instituted for evidence of iris, angle, or retinal neovascularization and for associated secondary glaucoma.

Prognosis
BRAO
- Most patients see an improvement in vision as the retinal edema resolves.
- Patients will have a relative scotoma in the distribution of the occlusion that may be permanent.

CRAO
- Prognosis for normal vision is poor; however, central vision may be spared if a patent cilioretinal artery is present.
- If suspected, temporal arteritis must be ruled out in an attempt to preserve vision in the fellow eye.

Follow-up and management
BRAO
- Patients should be followed closely for the first 6 mo to look for signs of neovascularization.

CRAO
- Patients should be followed every 4 wk to look for signs of neovascular glaucoma, which has been reported in up to 10% of patients.

General references
Brown GC, Magargal LE: Central retinal artery obstruction and visual acuity, *Ophthalmology* 89:14-19, 1982.

Brown GC, Magargal LE, Simeone FA, et al: Arterial obstruction and ocular neovascularization, *Ophthalmology* 89:139-146, 1982.

Heyreh SS, Kolder HE, Weingeist TA: Central retinal artery occlusion and retinal tolerance time, *Ophthalmology* 87:75-78, 1980.

Sharma S, Brown GC: Retinal artery obstruction. In *Retina*, ed 4, E-dition, St Louis, 2006, Elsevier.

Retinal degeneration, peripheral cystoid   (362.62)

DIAGNOSIS

Definition
Cystlike spaces associated with focal thinning of the peripheral retina.

Synonyms
None.

Symptoms
• Patients are asymptomatic.

Signs
Small, stippled areas of the inner retinal surface just posterior to the ora serrata: often aligned with the dentate processes; more frequently found inferotemporally and supratemporally.

Investigations
Visual acuity testing.
Slit-lamp biomicroscopic examination.
Dilated fundus examination.

Complications
• The cystoid spaces may coalesce into retinoschisis cavities that over time may cause peripheral visual loss.

Pearls and Considerations
Often detected with careful inspection of retina on routine examination.

Referral Information
No referral necessary.

Differential diagnosis
• Lattice degeneration.
• Bullous retinoschisis.

Cause
Peripheral degeneration.

Epidemiology
• Most adults will have evidence of typical cystoid degeneration by age 20 or older. Over time the cysts may coalesce to form typical retinoschisis.
• 18% of adults will have reticular cystoid degeneration, 41% of whom will have bilateral involvement. This can develop into reticular retinoschisis over time.

Classification
• Classification is based on pathologic findings:
Typical cystoid degeneration.
Reticular cystoid degeneration: often found posterior to areas of typical cystoid degeneration; more common inferotemporally.

Pathology
Reticular cystoid degeneration: cysts are found in the nerve fiber layer.
Typical cystoid degeneration: cysts are found between the outer plexiform layer and the inner nuclear layer.

TREATMENT

Diet and Lifestyle
- No special precautions are necessary.

Pharmacologic Treatment
- No pharmacologic treatment is recommended.

Nonpharmacologic Treatment
- No nonpharmacologic treatment is recommended.

Treatment aims
None.

Prognosis
Excellent.

Follow-up and management
Follow up with annual dilated eye examinations.

General references
Byer NE: Cystic retinal tuft and miscellaneous peripheral retinal findings. In Albert DM, Jakobiec FA, editors: *Principles and practice of ophthalmology*, vol 2, Philadelphia, 1994, Saunders, pp 1067-1068.

DIAGNOSIS

Definition

Separation of the sensory retina from the retinal pigment epithelium (RPE).

Rhegmatogenous retinal detachment: a retinal detachment caused by one or more full-thickness breaks in the retina.

Nonrhegmatogenous tractional retinal detachment: a retinal detachment caused by mechanical force from vitreoretinal adhesions.

Nonrhegmatogenous serous retinal detachment: a retinal detachment that results from an accumulation of subretinal fluid.

Synonyms

None; often abbreviated RD.

Symptoms

Rhegmatogenous RD

Flashes; floaters.

Veil- or curtain-like loss of vision: starting in the peripheral visual field and progressing toward the center.

Nonrhegmatogenous RD (Serous and Tractional)

Progressive loss of vision, floaters, pain.

Signs

Rhegmatogenous RD

Decreased central and peripheral vision, pigment in the anterior vitreous, detached retina with or without identifiable breaks in the retina.

Nonrhegmatogenous Serous RD

- Serous detachment of the retina is secondary to fluid building up in the subretinal space without evidence of a retinal break. These detachments take on a typical bullous, convex appearance and have a characteristic "shifting of fluid" when the patient changes from an erect to a supine position.

Nonrhegmatogenous Tractional RD

- Tractional detachment is caused by vitreoretinal fibroproliferative membranes that form on the surface of the retina; with contraction, the retinal surface takes on a concave appearance. These RDs occasionally advance to the ora serrata.

Investigations

Rhegmatogenous RD

Careful history: ask if the patient is nearsighted; if history of trauma or history of recent eye surgery or laser, check visual acuity and visual fields by confrontation.

Slit-lamp evaluation: of the anterior vitreous looking for pigment dispersion.

Dilated fundus examination: with peripheral depression to look for retinal breaks.

Examination of the posterior vitreous: look for a vitreous detachment.

Nonrhegmatogenous Serous RD

Slit-lamp and indirect ophthalmoscopic examination: of peripheral retina to rule out a break; a contact lens may improve peripheral view; scleral depression should be performed to view adequately the retinal–ora serrata junction.

- Serous detachment lacks corrugated appearance and pigmented demarcation line.

Differential diagnosis

Rhegmatogenous RD

Exudative retinal detachment, choroidal hemorrhage, choroidal tumor.

Nonrhegmatogenous RD

Rhegmatogenous RD.

Cause

Rhegmatogenous RD

- Retinal breaks cause fluid from the vitreous to seep under the surface of the retina, elevating the retina off the RPE. Pigment cells are released from the RPE through the break and then layer on the retinal surface.
- Approximately 10% of patients with a symptomatic posterior vitreous detachment will have a retinal tear. If there is an associated vitreous hemorrhage, the incidence increases to 70% [1,2].
- RD after trauma is usually secondary to retinal dialysis. The most common sites of retinal dialysis are inferotemporal or supranasal. Also, irregular radially oriented retinal tears are seen in relation to trauma.

Nonrhegmatogenous tractional RD

Proliferative diabetic retinopathy, sickle cell retinopathy, hypertensive retinopathy, retinopathy of prematurity, familial exudative vitreoretinopathy.

Nonrhegmatogenous serous RD

Choroidal tumors, Harada's disease, posterior scleritis, idiopathic central serous retinopathy, idiopathic uveal effusion syndrome, nanophthalmos, malignant hypertension/toxemia of pregnancy, optic nerve pit, morning glory syndrome, coloboma of the optic nerve or retina.

Epidemiology

Rhegmatogenous RD

- 30% of rhegmatogenous RDs are secondary to lattice degeneration, although a very small proportion of patients with lattice degeneration develop detached retinas [3].

Pathology

Rhegmatogenous RD

Fluid in the subretinal space with a full-thickness break in the retina.

Diagnosis continued on p. 284

TREATMENT

Diet and Lifestyle
Rhegmatogenous RD

- Safety glasses should be worn by individuals with high-risk characteristics (e.g., high myopia, increased axial length, large patches of lattice).
- Avoid contact sports if the individual has high-risk characteristics.

Nonpharmacologic Treatment
For Rhegmatogenous RD

Laser: to wall off the detached area if it is peripheral and if only a small area is detached.

Pneumatic retinopexy with cryotherapy: if the break is above the 4 and 8 o'clock positions.

Scleral buckle and cryotherapy: with or without drainage of subretinal fluid.

Vitrectomy, laser, gas or silicone-oil tamponade: most commonly done in pseudophakic patients.

For Nonrhegmatogenous RD (Serous and Tractional)

Pars plana vitrectomy with membrane delamination: indicated for tractional RDs that threaten the fovea.

Treatment aims
Rhegmatogenous RD

To prevent extension of the RD into the macular region.

To reattach the retina.

Nonrhegmatogenous RD

To preserve vision.

Prognosis
Rhegmatogenous RD

- The prognosis depends on the involvement of the macula, size of the break, and duration of the detachment. If the macula is off, the longer the retina is detached, the more permanent the damage to the retina. Larger breaks are more difficult to repair due to the formation of proliferative vitreoretinopathy.

Nonrhegmatogenous RD

- The overall prognosis depends on the underlying condition causing the detachment.

Follow-up and management
Rhegmatogenous RD

Careful education for patients with high-risk characteristics.

Yearly dilated eye examination for patients with lattice degeneration.

Nonrhegmatogenous RD

Varies for each cause.

Treatment continued on p. 285

DIAGNOSIS—cont'd

Complications
Rhegmatogenous RD

Decreased intraocular pressure (IOP): common; IOP can be elevated rarely.

Cataract formation.

Proliferative vitreoretinopathy: contraction and folding of the retina secondary to membrane formation on the retinal surface.

Peripheral neovascularization, permanent visual loss, inflammation in the vitreous, iris neovascularization.

Nonrhegmatogenous Serous RD

Permanent visual loss: from disruption of the RPE layer.

Nonrhegmatogenous Tractional RD

Retinal break: from advancing vitreoretinal traction; creates a combined tractional-rhegmatogenous RD.

Visual loss: will occur if the traction advances to involve the macula.

Pearls and Considerations

1. All patients with predisposing peripheral degenerations (e.g., lattice degeneration) should be advised of the signs and symptoms of RD.
2. Three factors must be present for a rhegmatogenous RD to occur:
   a. Liquefaction of the vitreous (factors that contribute to liquefaction include cataract extraction, trauma, high myopia, and intraocular inflammation).
   b. Tractional force.
   c. Presence of a retinal break.
3. Rhegmatogenous RD has a familial component; siblings of an RD patient are three times more likely to experience a rhegmatogenous RD.

Referral Information
Immediate referral to a retinal specialist for surgical repair is indicated.

TREATMENT—cont'd

Other Treatments
For Rhegmatogenous RD

Laser prophylaxis to symptomatic retinal breaks (breaks associated with flashes and floaters).

Laser prophylaxis to areas of lattice degeneration, atrophic holes, or asymptomatic horseshoe-shaped tears in the fellow eye, in patients with a history of RD (remains controversial).

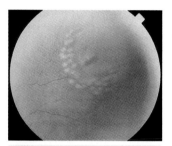

Figure 1 Peripheral horseshoe-shaped retinal break with surrounding laser photocoagulation.

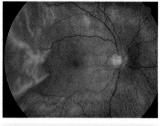

Figure 2 Rhematogenous RD with elevation and corrugation of the retina temporal to the fovea.

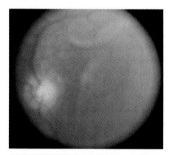

Figure 3 Serous RD in patient with recurrent Harada's disease involving the macula.

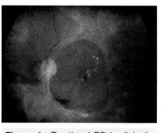

Figure 4 Tractional RD in diabetic patient. Note the concave appearance of the retinal elevation caused by contraction of fibrovascular tissue emanating from the optic nerve and arcade vessels.

Key references
1. Bouldry EE: Risk of retinal tears in patients with vitreous floaters, *Am Ophthalmol* 96:783-787, 1983.
2. Tasman WS: Posterior vitreous detachment and peripheral retinal breaks, *Trans Am Acad Ophthalmol Otolaryngol* 72:217-224, 1968.
3. Benson WE, Morse PH: The prognosis of retina detachment due to lattice degeneration, *Ann Ophthalmol* 10:1197-1200, 1978.

General references
Oh KT, Hartnett MT, Landers MB: Pathogenetic mechanisms of retinal detachment. In *Retina*, ed 4, E-dition, St Louis, 2006, Elsevier.
Young LHY, D'Amico DJ: Retinal detachments. In Albert DM, Jakobiec FA, editors: *Principles and practice of ophthalmology*, vol 2, Philadelphia, 1994, Saunders, pp 1084-1092.

DIAGNOSIS

Definition
A family of inherited degenerative disorders of the retinal structure.

Synonyms
See diseases below.

Symptoms
Best's Disease (Vitelliform Macular Dystrophy, 362.76)
Blurry vision.
Metamorphopsia.
Decreased vision.

Stargardt's Disease (Fundus Flavimaculatus, 362.75)
Gradual decrease in central vision: by teenage years.
Decreased color vision: red-green dyschromatopsia.

Signs
Best's Disease
Based on the stage of the disease: *see* Classification.

Stargardt's Disease
Decreased vision: in the 20/100 range.
Absolute central scotoma.
Acquired red-green dyschromatopsia.
Yellow-white irregular flecks: at level of retinal pigment epithelium (RPE).
Beaten-metal or bull's-eye appearance of the macula.

Investigations
Best's Disease
Careful family history.
Electro-oculogram: abnormal ratio of <1.5 (normal >1.8).
Full electroretinograms (ERGs): normal.
Fluorescein angiography: shows areas of blockage by the vitelliform lesion.

Stargardt's Disease
Dark adaptation is normal.
Fluorescein angiography: shows a classic silent choroid with window-defect changes caused by alteration of RPE.
Full ERGs: normal.

Complications
Best's Disease
Secondary choroidal neovascularization.

Stargardt's Disease
Decreased vision to legal blindness: by the 20s.
Secondary choroidal neovascularization.

Pearls and Considerations
Topic too broad for specific recommendations.

Referral Information
Refer for genetic counseling as appropriate.

Differential diagnosis
Stargardt's disease
Toxic maculopathy.
Cone-rod degeneration.

Cause
Best's disease
Autosomal dominance seen in individuals of European, Hispanic, and African ancestry.
Stargardt's disease
Autosomal recessive inheritance with variable penetrance.

Epidemiology
Stargardt's disease
- 80% of patients will have >20/40 vision.
- Only 4% of patients will have <20/200 vision.

Classification
Best's disease
Stage 1. Previtelliform: normal fundus appearance with normal vision.
Stage 2. Vitelliform: occurs in early childhood; patients are asymptomatic, and disease often goes undetected; a yellow lesion 0.5-2.0 disc diameters in size is often seen in the macula under the RPE, resembling yolk of an egg.
Stage 3. Pseudohypopyon: usually occurs in teenage years; the lipofuscin breaks through the RPE and settles inferiorly in the subretinal space.
Stage 4. "Scrambled egg": yellow deposits scattered throughout the posterior pole; varying amounts of RPE atrophy and hypertrophy.
- A variant of Best's disease occurs at an older age. Multiple vitelliform lesions throughout the posterior pole can be seen.

Pathology
Best's disease
Excessive lipofuscin-like material in the RPE cells throughout the posterior pole, particularly in the fovea [1].
Stargardt's disease
Accumulation of a lipofuscin material at the apical level of the RPE cells [2].

TREATMENT

Diet and Lifestyle
- No special precautions are necessary.

Pharmacologic Treatment
- No pharmacologic treatment is recommended.

Nonpharmacologic Treatment
- Patients with either disease should receive genetic counseling.

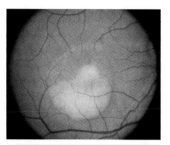

Figure 1 Stage 3 Best's disease. Note the layered pseudohypopyon. The lipofuscin has broken through the RPE and settled inferiorly in the subretinal space.

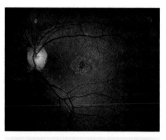

Figure 2 Stargardt's disease. Note the yellow-white irregular flecks at the level of the RPE and the beaten-metal appearance of the macula.

Treatment aims
None.

Prognosis
Best's disease
Good, with vision in the 20/40-20/60 range.
Stargardt's disease
Legal blindness.

Follow-up and management
Best's disease
- Educate the patient on the signs of secondary choroidal neovascularization.
- Annual eye examinations.
- Because it is a dominant inheritance pattern, all family members should be examined.

Stargardt's disease
- Education on the symptoms of secondary choroidal neovascularization.

Key references
1. Frangieh GT, Green WR, Fine SL: A histopathologic study of Best's vitelliform dystrophy, *Arch Ophthalmol* 100:1115-1121, 1982.
2. Eagle RC, Lucier AC, Bernadino VB Jr, et al: Retinal pigment epithelial abnormalities in fundus flavimaculatus: a light and electron microscope study, *Ophthalmology* 87:1189-1200, 1980.

General reference
Deutman AF, Hoyng CB, van-Lith Verhoeven JJC: Macular dystrophies. In *Retina*, ed 4, E-dition, St Louis, 2006, Elsevier.

DIAGNOSIS

Definition
Obstruction of a vein draining the retina (can be the central vein or a branch retinal vein).

Synonyms
None; common abbreviations are CRVO (central retinal vein occlusion) and BRVO (branch retinal vein occlusion).

Symptoms
BRVO

Decreased vision.

Floaters: indicates vitreous hemorrhage.

CRVO

Loss of vision, decreased vision: related to degree of obstruction, ischemia.

Eye pain: if associated elevation in intraocular pressure (IOP).

Floaters: indicates a vitreous hemorrhage.

Signs
BRVO

Intraretinal hemorrhages: distributed in one quadrant of the retina.

Cotton-wool spots.

Retinal edema.

Intraretinal lipid.

Vitreous hemorrhage.

Neovascularization: of the disc or elsewhere.

CRVO

Intraretinal hemorrhages: in all four quadrants.

Cotton-wool spots.

Lipid exudates.

Retinal edema.

Vitreous hemorrhage.

Neovascularization: of the retina, iris, or angle.

Elevated IOP.

- Collateral vessels on the optic nerve head imply a resolved occlusion.

Investigations
BRVO

Fluorescein angiography: to assess retinal capillary perfusion and ischemia, retinal leakage, and extent of occlusion.

Optical coherence tomography: to assess degree of macular edema and response to treatment.

CRVO

IOP: to rule out glaucoma.

Gonioscopy: to rule out angle neovascularization.

Fluorescein angiography: used to determine if there is retinal ischemia, edema, or neovascularization.

Optical coherence tomography: to gauge level of macular edema and response to treatment.

Systemic blood pressure.

Laboratory studies: complete blood count with differential, rapid plasma reagin, antinuclear antibodies, anticardiolipin antibodies, serum protein electrophoresis.

Electroretinogram: depressed B/A-wave amplitude indicates retinal ischemia. This test is rarely ordered, because fluorescein can usually be done to detect ischemia.

Differential diagnosis
Trauma, vasculitis, severe anemia, ocular ischemic syndrome.

Cause
Hypertension, chronic open-angle glaucoma, atherosclerosis, history of cardiovascular disease, oral contraceptives, chronic elevated systemic hypertension, glaucoma, diabetes mellitus, syphilis, antiphospholipid antibody syndrome, blood dyscrasias, collagen vascular diseases.

Epidemiology
BRVO

- Two thirds involve the supratemporal retinal vein; occurs at the crossing of the artery and vein that share a common adventitial sheath.
- 50% have associated decreased vision secondary to macular edema.
- Occurs in the fifth and sixth decades of life.

CRVO

- Peak incidence in those >60 yr of age; more common in men.
- 30% are ischemic.
- 60% with >10 disc areas of ischemia will develop neovascular glaucoma within 90 days.
- 70% are nonischemic; may convert to ischemic within first 3-6 mo.

Classification
Ischemic versus nonischemic BRVO/CVRO.

- In patients with ischemic BRVO, if >5 disc diameters of capillary nonperfusion on fluorescein angiography, they are at risk of developing neovascularization of the retina [1].
- Ischemic CRVOs have extensive hemorrhage in all four quadrants of the retina, more cotton-wool spots, marked macular edema, and a presenting vision of <20/200. Fluorescein angiography usually shows 10 disc areas of capillary nonperfusion.
- Nonischemic CRVOs have mild disc edema, mild dilation of retinal veins, and intraretinal hemorrhages in all four quadrants of the retina. Macular edema may develop gradually. Presenting visual acuity implies prognosis.

Pathology
BRVO: contraction of the sheath, increased rigidity of the crossing artery, atherosclerosis, and thrombotic occlusion of the corresponding vein [2].

CRVO: occlusion of the central retinal vein occurs behind the lamina cribrosa in the substance of the optic nerve or where the vein enters the subarachnoid space; can see blood throughout all layers of the retina.

Diagnosis continued on p. 290

TREATMENT

Diet and Lifestyle

- No precautions are necessary.

Pharmacologic Treatment
For BRVO

- Lower IOP if elevated.
- Discontinue oral contraceptives if applicable.
- Intravitreal Kenalog (triamcinolone) or Avastin (bevacizumab) for macular edema.

For CRVO

- Intravitreal triamcinolone or bevacizumab for macular edema. Bevacizumab can also be used to decrease the neovascular drive if vessels still growing after panretinal layer.
- Lower IOP if there is evidence of glaucoma.

Standard dosage   Nonselective β-blocker (timolol, metipranolol, or levobunolol), 1 drop twice daily.

Selective β-blocker (betaxolol 0.5%), 1 drop twice daily.

Topical carbonic anhydrase inhibitor, 1 drop 3 times daily.

Oral carbonic anhydrase inhibitor (acetazolamide), 250 mg 4 times daily or 500 mg twice daily.

- If there is evidence of iris neovascularization, administer atropine sulfate 1%. One drop twice daily is recommended to maintain long-term pupillary dilation.

Treatment aims

To maintain IOP within the normal range.

To resolve intraretinal hemorrhage and macular edema.

Prognosis

BRVO: often depends on presenting visual acuity; better in patients without macular ischemia.

CRVO: often depends on visual acuity, level of ischemia.

Follow-up and management
BRVO

- Every 4-6 wk to look for evidence of edema or neovascularization.

CRVO

- Every 4 wk for at least 6 mo; gonioscopy at all visits to look for evidence of angle neovascularization.
- Fundus photographs to document changes and allow future comparison.
- Fluorescein angiography for patients suspected of ischemic CRVO or if evidence of macular edema; often this needs to be repeated within the first 6 mo if clinical signs of progression.

Treatment continued on p. 291

DIAGNOSIS—cont'd

Complications
BRVO

Vitreous hemorrhage, neovascularization of the disc and elsewhere, retinal macular edema.

CRVO

Retinal macular edema, optic nerve and retinal neovascularization, neovascular glaucoma.

Vitreous hemorrhage: from optic nerve or peripheral retinal neovascularization.

Pearls and Considerations
1. The earlier CRVO is treated, the lower the risk of developing ocular neovascularization.
2. BRVO almost always occurs at arteriovenous crossings.

Referral Information
Refer to a retinal specialist for laser photocoagulation as indicated.

TREATMENT—cont'd

Nonpharmacologic Treatment
For BRVO

Grid laser photocoagulation: for macular edema and vision >20/40 without evidence of macular ischemia [3].

Sector panretinal photocoagulation: for ischemic BRVO for evidence of retinal or optic nerve neovascularization.

For CRVO

- Panretinal photocoagulation for ischemic CRVOs is recommended when there is evidence of iris or angle neovascularization with or without elevated IOP [4]. It is also recommended when severe ischemia as documented by fluorescein angiography is present.
- Focal grid laser therapy for macular edema has not shown significant benefit in the older population [5].

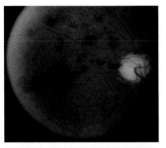

Figure 1 BRVO involving the supratemporal vein. The intraretinal blot hemorrhages extend into the macula and respect the horizontal midline.

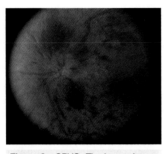

Figure 2 CRVO. The hemorrhages involve all four quadrants of the posterior pole and dilated venous system.

Key references
1. Branch Retinal Vein Occlusion Study Group: Argon laser scatter photocoagulation for prevention of neovascularization and vitreous hemorrhage in branch retinal vein occlusion, *Arch Ophthalmol* 104:34-41, 1986.
2. Yanoff M. Fine BS, editors: Neural (sensory) retina. In *Ocular pathology*, ed 4, Barcelona, Spain, 1996, Mosby, p 491.
3. Branch Retinal Vein Occlusion Study Group: Argon laser photocoagulation for macular edema and branch vein occlusion, *Am J Ophthalmol* 98:271-282, 1984.
4. Central Retinal Vein Occlusion Study Group: A randomized clinical trial of early panretinal photocoagulation for ischemic central retinal vein occlusion, *Ophthalmology* 102:1434-1443, 1995.
5. Central Retinal Vein Occlusion Study Group: Evaluation of grid pattern photocoagulation for macular edema in central retinal vein occlusion, *Ophthalmology* 102:1425-1433, 1995.

General references
Phillips S, Fekrat S, Finkelstein D: Branch retinal vein occlusion. In *Retina*, ed 4, E-dition, St Louis, 2006, Elsevier.
Mruthyunjaya P, Fekrat S: Central retinal vein occlusion. In *Retina*, ed 4, E-dition, St Louis, 2006, Elsevier.

Retinitis pigmentosa   (362.74)

DIAGNOSIS

Definition
A group of disorders characterized by progressive retinal dysfunction, cell loss, and atrophy of the retinal tissue.

Synonym
"Night blindness"; commonly abbreviated RP.

Symptoms
Decreased night vision (nyctalopia).
Decreased color vision.
Loss of peripheral vision.
Blurry vision.

Signs
Pigment clumping or "bone spicule formation" in the peripheral retina: *see* figure.
Areas of retinal pigment atrophy.
Arteriolar attenuation.
Optic nerve "waxy" pallor.
Pigmented cells in the vitreous.
Stellate pattern to posterior lens capsule opacification.
Cystoid macular edema.
Epimacular membrane.

Investigations
Careful family history: to detect any history of blindness.
Careful drug history: to rule out pseudo-RP as a possible cause.
Full-color examination.
Goldmann visual field analysis: to look for constriction and ring scotomas.
Electroretinography: results usually abnormal to nonrecordable.
- Rule in or out possible systemic associations:
   Phytanic acid level: rule out Refsum disease.
   Cardiology consult: to rule out heart block.
   Peripheral blood smear: to look for acanthocytosis.
Genetic counseling and workup.
- Examine family members for possible subclinical levels of disease.

Complications
Decreased vision.
Cataracts.
Cystoid macular edema.
Drusen in the optic nerve head.

Classification
Hereditary RP: autosomal dominant most common; autosomal recessive; X-linked most severe.
Kearns-Sayre syndrome.
Usher's syndrome.
Refsum disease.
Vitamin A deficiency.
Congenital stationary night blindness.

Differential diagnosis
Toxic retinopathy secondary to pheno-thiazines, congenital rubella, syphilis, resolution of previous retinal detachment (serous or rhegmatogenous), vitamin A deficiency, choroideremia, end-stage Stargardt's disease, gyrate atrophy, congenital stationary night blindness, diffuse unilateral neuroretinitis.

Cause
Hereditary or spontaneous RP
Autosomal dominant: late onset, less severe.
Autosomal recessive: variable onset and severity.
X-linked recessive: least frequent, most severe, earliest onset.
RP associated with systemic disease
Refsum disease: elevated phytanic acid levels.
Bassen-Kornsweig syndrome: deficiency in lipoproteins and malabsorption of vitamins A, D, E, and K.
Kearns-Sayre syndrome: progressive chronic progressive external ophthalmoplegia limitation of ocular motility, ptosis, and heart block before 20 yr of age.
Usher's syndrome: hearing loss.
β-Lipoproteinemia: acanthocytosis of red blood cells.

Epidemiology
- RP affects 1:5000 individuals worldwide.
- 44% are isolated.
- 16% autosomal dominant.
- 31% autosomal recessive.
- 9% X-linked recessive [1].

Associated features
See Cause section.

Pathology
Photoreceptor loss.
RPE hyperplasia into the retina and surrounds retinal vessels.
Arteriolar thickening and hyalinization of vessel walls.
Diffuse or sectorial atrophy with late gliosis in the optic nerve.

Diagnosis continued on p. 294

TREATMENT

Diet and Lifestyle
Genetic counseling.
Low-vision training and aids for activities of daily living.
Vocational rehabilitation.
Protective eyewear with ultraviolet-absorbing lenses.

Pharmacologic Treatment
- Treat underlying cause if associated with a systemic syndrome.
- Supplement vitamins E and C and carotene.

Treatment aims
To monitor vision.
To detect secondary side effects early.

Prognosis
Guarded, because of gradual progression of visual field loss and development of macular edema.

Follow-up and management
- Patients should have a baseline visual field examination and electroretinography performed annually; visual field examination should be performed annually until visual field is stable.

Treatment continued on p. 295

DIAGNOSIS—cont'd

Pearls and Considerations

1. The term "retinitis" is misleading because it implies inflammation, which is not part of the pathologic process of RP.
2. Night problems typically present within the first or second decade of life.
3. Night blindness is not diagnostic of RP; it can occur with other retinal disorders as well.
4. Color vision in RP usually remains good until vision is worse than 20/40.
5. Bone spicule formation results from the migration of pigment after retinal pigment epithelium (RPE) cells disintegrate.

Referral Information

Refer for genetic counseling or advanced diagnostic techniques as appropriate.

TREATMENT—cont'd

Nonpharmacologic Treatment
- No nonpharmacologic treatment is recommended.

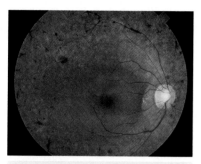

Typical appearance of a patient with retinitis pigmentosa with bone spicule formation and retinal attenuation.

Key reference

1. Kalloniatis M, Fletcher EL: Retinitis pigmentosa: understanding the clinical presentation, mechanisms and treatment options, *Clin Exp Optom* 87(2):65-80, 2004.

General references

Wang DY, Chan WM, Tam PO, et al: Gene mutations in retinitis pigmentosa and their clinical implications, *Clin Chim Acta* 351(1-2):5-16, 2005.

Weleber RG, Gregory-Evans K: Retinitis pigmentosa and allied disorders. In *Retina*, ed 4, E-dition, St Louis, 2006, Elsevier.

Weleber RG, Kurz DE, Trzupek KM: Treatment of retinal and choroidal degenerations and dystrophies: current status and prospects for gene-based therapy, *Ophthalmol Clin North Am* 16(4):583-593, 2003.

Retinopathy of prematurity   (362.21)

DIAGNOSIS

Definition
A vasoproliferative disorder affecting extremely premature infants.

Synonyms
None; often abbreviated as ROP.

Symptoms
Cicatricial ROP: decreased visual acuity resulting from myopia, astigmatism, retinal detachment, and distortion of fovea.

Glaucoma and cataract: tearing, photophobia.

Signs
Strabismus.

Leukokoria: from retinal detachment.

Corneal clouding: from glaucoma.

Pseudoexotropia: from temporal foveal displacement.

Investigations
Periodic retinal examinations: in infants at risk for ROP, i.e., infants born before 36 wk of gestation and weighing <2500 g at birth.

- Infants receiving supplemental oxygen or requiring multiple transfusions are also at increased risk.

Complications
Total or partial retinal detachment: as infant, child, or adult.

Strabismus.

Refractive errors.

Anisometropic or strabismic amblyopia.

Glaucoma.

Cataract.

Corneal clouding.

Band keratopathy.

Phthisis bulbi.

Associated Features
Active Disease

Stage 1: demarcation line between avascular and vascular retina.

Stage 2: ridge between avascular and vascular retina, becomes elevated and thickened.

Stage 3: neovascular tissue arising from ridge (*see* figure).

Stage 4: partial retinal detachment.

Stage 5: total retinal detachment.

Stages and Zones Used to Determine Need for Treatment

Zone I: area in posterior pole corresponding to a circle that encloses the disc and has a radius of twice the distance from the disc to the macula.

Zone II: area between Zone I and a circle that is centered on the optic disc and that is tangential to the nasal ora serrata.

Zone III: area that includes the remaining temporal crescent of retina. This area is the last to be vascularized.

Differential diagnosis
Familial exudative vitreoretinopathy: autosomal dominant; no history of prematurity or O_2 supplementation; irides rarely engorged.

Incontinentia pigmenti: skin lesions early in life; X-linked dominant; lethal in males; avascular peripheral retinas, but retinal neovascularization and iris engorgement are rare.

Maternal cocaine ingestion: rarely associated with peripheral retinal neovascularization in infant.

Cause
- Prematurity is major cause. Smallest, sickest infants tend to have worst ROP, which is stimulated by removal from enriched O_2 source. No level of inspired O_2 is totally safe but is required by infants to prevent severe neurologic disease.
- ROP is associated with hypercarbia, multiple exchange transfusions, presence of intraventricular hemorrhage, respiratory distress syndrome, and sepsis.
- Racial and familial tendencies may exist. Severe, vision-threatening ROP occurs more frequently in white infants of low birth weight than in black infants.

Epidemiology
- In 1989, a fetus with weight of 700 g at 25 wk of gestation had 50% chance of survival. In 1979, ROP blinded ~550 babies.

Incidence of ROP by birth weight

<1000 g: 80%.

1001-1250 g: 60%.

1251-1500 g: 20%.

>1501 g: 8%.

Severity in infants >1501 g (+ disease is iris engorgement, retinal vascular tortuosity, and engorgement in infants with active ROP):

No ROP: 50%.

<Stage 2+ ROP (ridge + disease): 36%.

>Stage 2+ ROP: 12%.

Pathology
Acute ROP: true shunt at retinal ridge with obliteration of capillaries around arterioles and venules; neovascular tufting from ridge to vitreous and lens; with regression, neovascular buds develop from mesenchyme of ridge.

Progressive, severe, active ROP: neovascular tissue develops from posterior border of the ridge.

Diagnosis continued on p. 298

TREATMENT

Prevention of Prematurity
- Compulsive, universal prenatal care should prevent some cases of prematurity.

Pharmacologic Treatment
- Vitamin E (α-tocopherol) at physiologic doses has been shown to decrease the incidence and severity of cicatricial ROP in infants with active ROP, but is less potent in the smallest premature infants. At higher doses, its use is associated with increased risk of necrotizing enterocolitis and *Escherichia coli* sepsis.
- Calf-lung surfactant treatment for acute respiratory distress syndrome in uncontrolled studies shows promise in decreasing the incidence and severity of active and cicatricial ROP.

Nonpharmacologic Treatment
Laser or Cryotherapy
- Laser is the preferred method of treatment because of the ease of use and lack of external trauma, although cryotherapy can be used if laser is unavailable. The recommendation of the Early Treatment for Retinopathy of Prematurity group is that earlier treatment ("prethreshold") has better outcomes than traditional timing of treatment ("threshold"). Retinal ablative therapy is recommended for:
1. ROP any stage in Zone I with plus disease (dilation of posterior pole retinal vessels).
2. Zone I Stage 3 ROP without plus distance.
3. Zone II Stages 2 or 3 ROP with plus disease.

Treatment aims
To resolve retinal neovascularization.
To foster progression of vascular development to ora serrata.
To ensure absence of strabismus, glaucoma, corneal decompensation, and posterior-pole vascular distortion and traction.
Hyperopic, equal refractive error in each eye.

Other treatments
As appropriate for complications.

Prognosis
- 3.5 yr after cryogenic therapy for threshold ROP, letter acuity, grating acuity, and posterior-pole status were improved in treated versus untreated eyes.
- Treated eyes still had a 26% chance of unfavorable posterior-pole structural status, and patients who had active ROP in the posterior retina had poor outcomes even with cryogenic treatment.
- Few eyes undergoing retinal detachment repair with vitrectomy will have better than hand-motions vision.

Follow-up and management
- Premature infants at risk for ROP who have incomplete retinal vascular development should be examined every other week until vascular development is complete to the ora serrata.
- Infants who have active ROP should be examined weekly (or more frequently) until the ROP regresses or they reach a threshold for treatment with cryogenic or diode laser (stage 3+ disease with ≥6 hr of retinal neovascularization).
- Many surgeons are treating posterior ROP at the first sign of "plus disease."
- Sequelae of ROP (e.g., amblyopia, glaucoma, strabismus, retinal traction) are managed as usual.

Treatment continued on p. 299

DIAGNOSIS—cont'd

Pearls and Considerations

1. Most severe cases can lead to irreversible, total blindness.
2. Oxygen is no longer thought to be a causative agent of ROP; newborns need to receive adequate oxygenation to grow into healthy infants able to leave the neonatal intensive care unit.

Referral Information

Refer to appropriate subspecialist for management of lingering complications (e.g., amblyopia).

TREATMENT—cont'd

Nonpharmacologic Treatment

- Cryogenic or diode laser treatment to avascular retina in infants with prethreshold ROP has been shown to decrease incidence and severity of severe, blinding cicatricial ROP.
- Ten years after treatment, eyes treated with laser had mean best-corrected visual acuity of 20/66, and eyes treated with cryotherapy had best-corrected visual acuity of 20/182, reflecting less retinal dragging in laser-treated eyes.
- Retinal detachment repair is anatomically successful in ~50%, but reattached retina rarely functions, and the visual outcome is usually very poor (hand motions or light perception).

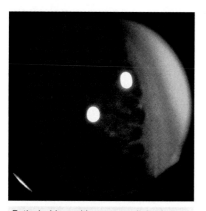

Retinal ridge with neovascularization on posterior border (stage 3 active ROP).

General references

Chan CC, Roberge FG, Whitcup SM, et al: 32 cases of sympathetic ophthalmia, *Arch Ophthalmol* 113:597, 1995.

Cryotherapy for Retinopathy of Prematurity Cooperative Group: 3½ year outcome: structure and function, *Arch Ophthalmol* 111: 339-350, 1993.

Early Treatment for Retinopathy of Prematurity Cooperative Group: Revised indications for the treatment of retinopathy of prematurity: results of the early treatment for retinopathy of prematurity randomized trial, *Arch Ophthalmol* 121:1684-1694, 2003.

Higgins RD: Retinopathy of prematurity, 2006, www.emedicine.com.

Ng EY, Connolly B, McNamara A, et al: A comparison of laser photocoagulation with cryotherapy for threshold retinopathy of prematurity at 10 years, *Ophthalmology* 109:928-935, 2002.

Palmer EA et al: Retinopathy of prematurity. In *Retina*, ed 4, E-dition, St Louis, 2006, Elsevier.

Shindo Y, Ohno S, Usi M, et al: Immunogenetic study of sympathetic ophthalmia, *Tissue Antigens* 49:111, 1997.

Rubeosis iridis (364.42) and neovascular glaucoma (365.63)

DIAGNOSIS

Definition
Rubeosis iridis: neovascularization of the iris.

Neovascular glaucoma (NVG): increase in intraocular pressure (IOP) secondary to blockage of aqueous outflow by neovascularization in the anterior-chamber angle.

Synonyms
None.

Symptoms
Pain: a prominent feature in acute NVG; in early cases before the development of full-blown inflammatory NVG, patients may be relatively pain free.

Loss of vision: marked loss of vision is also prominent early in the course of NVG.

Signs
Hyperemia: marked conjunctival and episcleral vessel engorgement is common.

Greatly elevated IOP.

Corneal edema: epithelial and sometimes stromal edema are seen in response to the rapid increase in IOP.

Inflammation: usually a marked inflammatory response with anterior-chamber flare and cells.

Anterior-chamber hemorrhage: red blood cells in the anterior chamber are often present; occasionally a spontaneous layered hyphema will occur.

Neovascularization of the iris and angle: abnormal new blood vessels are seen on the surface of the iris stroma and in the angle crossing the scleral spur and growing on the trabecular meshwork (*see* figure); these vessels impart a red color to the iris and angle, thus the term *rubeosis iridis;* early in the course of the disease, fine tufts of vessels are barely visible in the peripupillary area; later, fine vessels are seen in the angle; as the disease advances, the entire iris and angle are involved; the vessels may become quite large.

Ectropion uveae: often seen in NVG (*see* figure).

Gonioscopic findings: the angle may be open early in the course of disease; more typically, a nonpupillary block angle closure results from extensive peripheral anterior synechiae.

Investigations
Retinal evaluation: NVG is usually a manifestation of retinal vascular disease; occasionally it may be seen associated with intraocular neoplasms; careful examination of the posterior pole and peripheral retina is indicated; if the fundus cannot be seen, B-scan ultrasonography should be performed.

Carotid evaluation: some cases of NVG are seen in association with carotid occlusive disease; if a retinal cause is not apparent, noninvasive carotid flow and ultrasound studies are indicated.

Complications
Intraocular hemorrhage: anterior-chamber hemorrhage from the fragile rubeotic vessels is common; vitreous hemorrhages are also seen.

Pearls and Considerations
1. Retinal ischemia is the most important factor leading to the development of NVG.
2. Generally, NVG is poorly responsive to treatment, and preserving vision is difficult.

Referral Information
1. Refer to glaucoma specialist for immediate and aggressive care.
2. Refer to retinal specialist as needed for treatment of underlying cause.

Differential diagnosis
- The differential diagnosis includes other acute inflammatory glaucomas:
Acute angle-closure glaucoma.
Uveitic glaucoma.
Acute traumatic glaucoma and hyphema.
- Neovascularization of the anterior segment resembling rubeosis may also be seen in Fuchs' heterochromic iridocyclitis and pseudoexfoliation syndrome.

Cause
Rubeosis is thought to result from the production of an intraocular angiogenic factor by ischemic retina. This factor provokes the growth of a fibrovascular membrane over the surface of the iris and trabecular meshwork. As the membrane contracts, it pulls the peripheral iris into the angle, causing peripheral anterior synechiae and progressive closure of the angle. As the ocular ischemia progresses, the pressure increases, and the abnormal blood vessels leak more; an inflammatory response occurs, leading to the complete clinical picture.

Classification
Rubeosis with NVG is seen in a variety of disease conditions that produce retinal ischemia. The most common causes are central retinal vein occlusion, proliferative diabetic retinopathy, carotid occlusive disease, and ocular ischemic syndrome.

Associated features
- In susceptible eyes the risk of NVG is increased after intraocular surgery, especially cataract surgery and pars plana vitrectomy.

Pathology
- Proliferation of vascular endothelial cells and smooth muscle fibroblasts over the surface of the iris produces the fibrovascular membrane characteristic of rubeosis iridis.

TREATMENT

Diet and Lifestyle

Diabetic control: proliferative diabetic retinopathy is a common cause of NVG; the risk of developing this complication is significantly reduced if the diabetes is well controlled with diet and medication.

Control of hypertension, cholesterol: other causes of NVG are often related to hypertension and arteriosclerosis; careful attention to dietary intake of fat and salt, as well as control of any existing hypertension, may reduce the risk of developing ocular vascular disease.

Pharmacologic Treatment
For Intraocular Pressure

During the acute phase, hyperosmotics and aqueous suppressants are useful to lower IOP, reduce pain, and reduce corneal edema to allow better visualization of the anterior segment and retina. After more definitive nonpharmacologic treatments, long-term treatment for glaucoma may be needed, as with any chronic glaucoma. Miotics should be avoided in NVG because of their effect on vascular permeability.

For Inflammation

Topical steroids and atropine are very useful for treating the associated inflammation and pain.

Analgesics

Patients with severe pain may require systemic analgesics.

Nonpharmacologic Treatment
Panretinal Photocoagulation

Ischemic retina must be treated with panretinal photocoagulation to eliminate the angiogenic stimulus. Treatment should be initiated immediately and should be sufficiently extensive to destroy all ischemic retina. More than one session may be needed. If the retina cannot be seen, panretinal cryotherapy should be performed.

Filtering Surgery

Once the panretinal photocoagulation has been completed, filtering surgery is indicated if the IOP cannot be controlled medically. The failure rate with filtration is extremely high, and the use of antifibrotics (e.g., mitomycin-C or 5-fluorouracil) is usually indicated. In severe or recalcitrant cases, use of an aqueous tube-shunt device or cyclophotocoagulation may be useful. The results of treatment for NVG are generally among the worst for any common glaucoma.

Treatment aims
To adequately treat ischemic retina.
To control pain and inflammation.
To control IOP and preserve visual function.

Prognosis
The prognosis for patients with NVG is poor. Patients are often unresponsive to treatment. Complications of treatment (e.g., hypotony) are common. Vision rarely returns to normal and is often greatly reduced despite treatment. Early recognition and adequate treatment of retinal ischemic disease before the development of rubeosis is the best way to prevent NVG and preserve visual function.

Follow-up and management
• Because the underlying cause of NVG often is a systemic problem that affects both eyes, careful evaluation and prophylactic treatment of the fellow eye are important.

Neovascular glaucoma showing neovascularization of the surface of the iris (rubeosis) and ectropion uveae at the pupil.

General references
Eid T, Katz LJ, Spaeth GL, Augsberger JJ: Tube-shunt surgery versus neodymium:YAG cyclophotocoagulation in the management of neovascular glaucoma, *Ophthalmology* 104: 1692-1700, 1997.
Khan YA, Ahmed IIK: Glaucoma, neovascular, 2006, www.emedicine.com.
McGrath DJ, Ferguson JG, Sanborn GE: Neovascular glaucoma. In *Focal points clinical modules for ophthalmologists,* vol 15, no 7, San Francisco, 1997, American Academy of Ophthalmology.
Shields MB: Glaucomas associated with disorders of the retina, vitreous, and choroid. In *Textbook of glaucoma,* ed 4, Baltimore, 1998, Lippincott Williams & Wilkins, pp 269-286.
Tsai JC, Feuer WJ, Parrish RK II, Grajewski AL: 5-Fluorouracil filtering surgery and neovascular glaucoma: long-term follow-up of the original pilot study, *Ophthalmology* 102:887-893, 1995.
Wand M: Neovascular glaucoma: new approaches to inhibition of angiogenesis, *J Glaucoma* 3:178-181, 1994.

Seventh-nerve palsy (facial)   (351.0)

DIAGNOSIS

Definition
Loss of function of the seventh cranial (facial) nerve.

Synonyms
Bell's palsy.

Symptoms
Unable to hold food or liquid in mouth while eating.
Corner of mouth droops.
Weak platysma: makes shaving difficult.
Ipsilateral hyperacusis.
Aguesia: decreased taste to anterior two thirds of tongue.
Aching pain around jaw or behind ear.

Signs
Muscles of facial expression are paretic on side of lesion.
Eyebrow droops.
Palpebral fissure widens.
Eyelid does not close.
Punctum turns outward.
Forehead and nasolabial folds are lost.
Ala nasi is immobile on respiration.

Investigations
Complete blood count.
Erythrocyte sedimentation rate.
Two-hour postprandial blood sugar.
Rapid plasma reagin.
Fluorescent treponemal antibody absorption test.
Angiotensin-converting enzyme.
Lyme titer.
Neuroimaging: if palsy not isolated.

Complications
Filamentary keratitis.
Aberrant regeneration of seventh nerve.

Pearls and Considerations
1. The seventh cranial nerve carries parasympathetic fibers to the nose, palate, and lacrimal glands, as well as motor nerves to the facial muscles.
2. A diabetic patient's risk of Bell's palsy is up to 29% higher than that of the nondiabetic population.

Referral Information
Refer to appropriate subspecialist, depending on the suspected underlying etiology of paralysis.

Differential diagnosis
Cerebellopontine angle tumor.
Geniculate ganglionitis (Ramsay-Hunt syndrome).

Cause
Common
Idiopathic (Bell's palsy).
Rare
Herpes simplex virus (HSV).
Varicella-zoster virus (VZV).
Cytomegalovirus (CMV).
Epstein-Barr virus (EBV).
Rubella.
Lyme disease.
Syphilis.
Human immunodeficiency virus (HIV).
Sarcoid.
Leprosy.

Epidemiology
- 20:100,000 population per year.
- 45.1:100,000 pregnant women per year.

Classification
Upper-motor-neuron seventh-nerve palsy: weakness of only the lower two thirds of the face contralateral to a supranuclear lesion.
Lower-motor-neuron seventh-nerve palsy: all muscle actions of facial expression are lost on the side of the lesion.

Pathology
Edema of the seventh nerve in the fallopian canal.
Infection.
Compression.

TREATMENT

Diet and Lifestyle
- No special precautions are necessary.

Pharmacologic Treatment
Standard dosage   Prednisone, 60 mg for 5 days tapered within 14 days.

Special points   Administer during the first 48 hr; treatment is controversial.

Nonpharmacologic Treatment
Artificial tears.

Tape eyelids closed.

Moist chamber patches.

Tarsorrhaphy.

Treatment aims

To protect the cornea.

Other treatments

Facial massage.

Electrical stimulation.

Prognosis
- Facial-nerve conduction studies 3-5 days after onset can indicate prognosis.
- Complete loss of conduction indicates wallerian degeneration and poor prognosis.
- Normal latencies and amplitudes at 5 days suggest excellent prognosis for recovery.

General references

Adour KK, Wingerd J: Idiopathic facial paralysis (Bell's palsy): factors affecting severity and outcome in 446 patients, *Neurology* 24: 1112-1116, 1974.

Esslen E: *The acute facial palsies*, New York, 1977, Springer-Verlag.

Monnell K, Zachariah SB: Bell palsy, 2005, www.emedicine.com.

Morgan M, Nathurami D: Facial palsy and infection: the unfolding story, *Clin Infect Dis* 14:263-271, 1992.

Sixth-nerve palsy (abducens)   (378.54)

DIAGNOSIS

Definition
Loss of function of the sixth cranial (abducens) nerve.

Synonyms
None.

Symptoms
Horizonal diplopia: greater at distance.
- Some patients experience pain; others do not.

Signs
Head turn.
Crossed eyes.

Investigations
Complete blood count.
Erythrocyte sedimentation rate.
Two-hour postprandial blood sugar.
Rapid plasma reagin.
Fluorescent treponemal antibody absorption test.
Lyme titer.
Magnetic resonance imaging of brain and orbits.
- Look for signs that distinguish a sixth-nerve palsy from mimicking conditions:
  Greater abduction of the paretic eye with ductions than with versions.
  Slowed abducting saccades of the paretic eye.
  Negative forced ductions.
  Diminished abducting optokinetic nystagmus of the paretic eye.
  Anti-acetylcholine antibody test, Tensilon (edrophonium) test to rule out myasthenia gravis.
  Thyroid function test.
  Forced-duction test to rule out Graves' disease.
  Lumbar puncture; increased intracranial pressure can cause nonlocalizing sixth-nerve palsy.

Pearls and Considerations
See table.

Referral Information
None.

Differential diagnosis
Duane retraction syndrome type I.
Spasm of the near reflex.
Graves' orbitopathy.
Myasthenia gravis.
Loss of horizontal fusional reserves.

Cause
Adults
Neoplasm.
Trauma.
Aneurysm.
Ischemic-vasculopathic.
Children
Neoplasm.
Trauma.
Febrile illness.
By age group
- 1-15 yr: viral; febrile illnesses; postimmunization; Gradenigo syndrome; pontine glioma.
- 15-35 yr: demyelinating.
- 35-50 yr: nasopharyngeal carcinoma; meningioma.
- ≥55 yr: ischemic vascular; giant cell arteritis.

Classification
- Sixth-nerve palsy can be acute or chronic.
- Chronic sixth-nerve palsy is one that persists for ≥6 mo and is usually a harbinger of serious intracranial disease.

Associated features
See table.

Anatomic localization of a "complicated" sixth-nerve palsy: the checklist examination

What to look for	Anatomic location	Cause
Sixth-nerve paresis plus contralateral hemiplegia (Raymond syndrome)	Pons	Infarction, demyelination, tumor, trauma
Sixth- and seventh-nerve paresis plus contralateral hemiplegia (Millard-Gubler syndrome)	Ventral pons	Infarction, demyelination, tumor, trauma
Gaze palsy, seventh- and eighth-nerve paresis, facial analgesia, and Horner's sign (Foville syndrome)	Dorsal pons	Infarction, demyelination, tumor, trauma
Bilateral sixth-nerve paresis	Clivus; subarachnoid space	Tumor (nonlocalizing)
Papilledema	Subarachnoid space	Nonlocalizing
Sixth-nerve paresis plus pain and decreased hearing (Gradenigo syndrome)	Petrous apex	Infection, thrombosis, compression, fracture
Sixth-nerve paresis plus decreased tearing and hearing, and Horner's sign	Cavernous sinus	Tumor, thrombosis, fistula, infection, trauma, aneurysm
Sixth-nerve paresis plus third- and fourth-nerve paresis, V1, Horner's sign, and proptosis	Cavernous sinus	Tumor, thrombosis, fistula, infection, trauma, aneurysm
Sixth-nerve paresis plus second-nerve paresis and proptosis	Orbital apex/superior orbital fissure	Tumor

TREATMENT

Diet and Lifestyle
- No special precautions are necessary.

Pharmacologic Treatment
Oculinum injection.

Nonpharmacologic Treatment
Segment patch on glasses for distance.
Base-out prism for distance.
Surgical intervention: based on whether the patient can abduct beyond midline, can reach midline, or cannot achieve primary position.

Treatment aims
To restore and maintain single, simultaneous, binocular vision in primary position at distance and near.

Prognosis
- Vasculopathic sixth-nerve palsies should resolve in 3 mo.
- Patients with traumatic sixth-nerve palsies may take up to 1 yr to recover.

Follow-up and management
- Monitor patients every few weeks for secondary contracture during recovery period. Once the medial rectus muscle begins to contract, it is unlikely to relax.

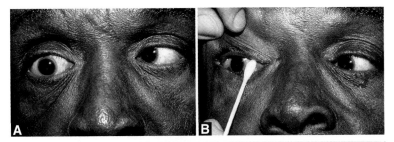

A, This man demonstrates a right abduction deficit in his attempt to look to the right. **B,** Modified forced duction easily moves the right eye into abduction. He has a "negative" forced-duction test consistent with a right sixth-nerve palsy.

General references
Bellusci C: Paralytic strabismus, *Curr Opin Ophthalmol* 12(5):368-372, 2001.
Rucker JC, Tomsak RL: Binocular diplopia: a practical approach, *Neurologist* 11(2):98-110, 2005.

Skin tumor, benign   (216.1)

DIAGNOSIS

Definition
Noncancerous growth or mass on the lid.

Synonyms
None.

Symptoms
Growth or mass on lid.
Generally painless.

Signs
Seborrheic keratosis (702.19): waxy, sharply demarcated; appears stuck to surface.
Papilloma (skin tags): appear as skin-colored filiform lesions (*see* Fig. 1).
Warts (078.1): firm growth with a papillomatous surface.
Inclusion cyst (374.84): single whitish nodule filled with keratin.
Xanthelasma (374.51): yellowish raised plaques (*see* Fig. 2).
Molluscum (078.0): skin-colored, dome-shaped lesion with umbilicated center (*see* Fig. 3).
Actinic keratosis (702.0): small erythematous lesions with overlying scales.

Investigations
History: duration of lesion, growth of lesion, previous type or similar lesions.
Biopsy: suspected lesion to rule malignancy.
• Investigate similar lesions elsewhere on body.

Complications
• Some of the benign lesions (e.g., actinic keratosis) may have a premalignant potential and therefore should be excised.

Pearls and Considerations
Varied, and dependent on type of lesion.

Referral Information
Refer for biopsy and excision.

Differential diagnosis
• Other benign lesions include:
  Verruca.
  Keratosis.
  Nevus.
  Sebaceous adenoma.
  Syringoma.
  Hydrocystoma.
  Hemangioma.
  Lymphangioma.
  Xanthelasma.
  Chalazion.
  Sarcoid.
  Pyogenic granuloma.
  Neurofibroma.

Cause
Warts: associated with human papillomavirus (HPV).
Xanthelasma: in one third of people, associated with lipid abnormalities.
Molluscum: poxvirus.

Pathology
Seborrheic keratosis: papillomatous lesion above the skin surface that contains basaloid-type cells and keratin cysts.
Papilloma: fingerlike projection of hyperkeratosis with a fibrovascular core.
Inclusion cysts: cysts lined with squamous epithelium and keratin filling the lumen of the cyst.
Xanthelasma: dermal thickening with fat-filled macrophages.
Molluscum: key feature is intracytoplasmic molluscum bodies that appear eosinophilic in the deep layers and become basophilic in the superficial layers before breaking through and shedding into the tears.
Actinic keratosis: lesion above the skin surface that demonstrates hyperkeratosis and thickening.

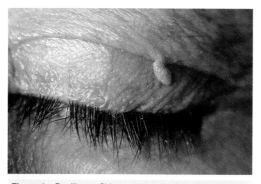

Figure 1 Papilloma. Skin tag protrudes from the left upper lid. Histologically, this was a squamous cell papilloma.

TREATMENT

Diet and Lifestyle
- No special precautions are necessary.

Pharmacologic Treatment
- No pharmacologic treatment is recommended.

Nonpharmacologic Treatment
- Most treatments are associated with biopsy of the lesion (incisional/excisional) to establish the diagnosis and remove the lesion.

Treatment aims
To remove lesion.

Other treatments
- Fulguration has been used for some benign lesions, but definitive diagnosis is not possible because of inability to obtain a specimen for microscopic examination.

Prognosis
- Excision of lesions results in cure, with no significant risk of associated disease entities.

Follow-up and management
As needed to ensure healing of incisional area and to verify suspected pathology so as not to overlook an occult malignant lesion.

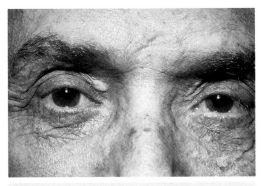

Figure 2   Xanthelasma. Yellow placoid lid lesion is present superior nasally in each eye (larger in the right upper lid).

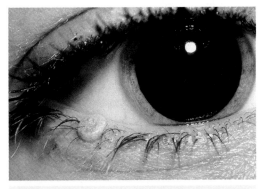

Figure 3   Molluscum. Raised lesion with an umbilicated center is present temporally at the right lower lid margin. The lesion contains packets of molluscum bodies that are characteristic.

General references
Fraunfelder F, Roy F, editors: *Current ocular therapy*, Philadelphia, 2000, Saunders.
Hornblass A et al: *Oculoplastic, orbital, and reconstructive surgery*, vol 2, Baltimore, 1990, Lippincott Williams & Wilkins.
Older J, editor: Benign tumors and related conditions. In *Eyelid tumors: clinical diagnosis and surgical treatment*, New York, 1987, Raven Press, pp 27-45.
Tasman W, Jaeger E, editors: *Duane's clinical ophthalmology*, vol 4, Philadelphia, 2006, Lippincott- Raven.
Yanoff M, Fine B: *Ocular pathology: a color atlas*, Philadelphia, 2002, Lippincott.

Skin tumor, malignant   (173.1)

DIAGNOSIS

Definition
Cancerous mass or growth on the lid.

Synonyms
None.

Symptoms
- Because of the slow growth and lack of associated symptoms, patients may allow the lesion to grow to a fair size before seeking a medical opinion.

Basal Cell Carcinoma

Slow-growing, painless lesion that may ulcerate, bleed, or crust: *see* Fig. 1.

Squamous Cell Carcinoma

Painless, enlarging mass: *see* Fig. 2.

Sebaceous Gland Carcinoma

Simulates a benign lesion (especially a chalazion), but may present as chronic lid irritation or blepharoconjunctivitis; loss of lashes over lesion is common.

Signs
Basal Cell Carcinoma

Starts as discrete nodule (usually on lower lid, inner canthus), with the central area eventually becoming ulcerated.

Squamous Cell Carcinoma

Discrete, flat, slightly erythematous lesion: with overlying vessels and scaling; frequently, loss of eyelashes.

Sebaceous Gland Carcinoma

Predilection for upper lid; lesion shows minimal ulceration; possible manifestations of unilateral conjunctivitis, blepharoconjunctivitis, lid thickening; may simulate a chalazion.

Investigations
Basal Cell Carcinoma

- If spread is suspected, consider computed tomography scan to rule out spread to globe, bone, or sinuses.

Squamous Cell and Sebaceous Gland Carcinoma

- Biopsy lesion to ensure the diagnosis; evaluate regional lymph nodes to rule out distant spread (<0.5%).

Complications
Basal Cell Carcinoma

Locally infiltrative; rarely metastasizes.

Squamous Cell Carcinoma

Small percentage shows distant metastasis.

Pearls and Considerations
Varied, and dependent on the type of lesion.

Referral Information
Refer to oculoplastics specialist or dermatologist for biopsy and treatment.

Differential diagnosis
Various benign or malignant tumors of the lid.

Cause
Basal cell carcinoma
Most often seen in patients age 60-80 yr.
- ~5%-15% of lesions occur in patients age 20-40 yr.
- Although never proved, there is circumstantial evidence of increased occurrence from prolonged sun exposure.

Squamous cell carcinoma
One tenth to four tenths (0.1-0.4) as common as basal cell lesions; associated increased incidence with prolonged sun exposure.

Sebaceous gland carcinoma
Approximately the same frequency as squamous cell carcinoma; cause unknown.

Epidemiology
Basal cell carcinoma
Most common malignancy of eyelid; accounts for 90% of all carcinomas.

Squamous cell carcinoma
Rare eyelid malignancy; accounts for about 7%; occurs more in fair-skinned and elderly individuals; thought to be sun related.

Sebaceous gland carcinoma
Rare malignancy; increased female predominance, with a mortality rate of ~22%.

Classification
Basal cell carcinoma types
Nodular, ulcerative, syringoid, adenoid, basosquamous, multicentric, recurrent, morpheaform, sclerosing.

Pathology
Basal cell carcinoma
May take on several appearances: solid masses of uniform cells with basophilic nuclei, peripheral palisading of basal cells, or strands or cords of cells that appear in an "Indian file" pattern.

Squamous cell carcinoma
Deep dermal findings of keratin-producing, squamous neoplastic cells.

Sebaceous gland carcinoma
Numerous cells resembling sebaceous elements with mitotic figures; the cells may stain positively for fat.

TREATMENT

Diet and Lifestyle

Because malignant skin tumors are most often seen on the most sun-exposed surfaces, it is believed that ultraviolet light may be a predisposing factor. Therefore, avoidance of intense sun exposure is recommended for patients with documented lesions.

Pharmacologic Treatment

Squamous Cell Carcinoma

- If distant metastases are present, chemotherapy may be warranted.

Nonpharmacologic Treatment

Basal Cell Carcinoma

Irradiation: generally not used at present; effective only in early stages.

Excision: excision by frozen section, Mohs' technique, or wide excision, with various types of reconstruction to ensure that clear margins are obtained.

Cryotherapy: freeze/thaw technique with use of thermocouple to ensure freezing to −25° C is effective for small lesions (<1 cm).

Squamous Cell Carcinoma

Wide excision of lesion by techniques such as Mohs' and frozen section; if there is periorbital involvement, exenteration is the treatment of choice.

Sebaceous Gland Carcinoma

Wide excision of tumor, with lymph node evaluation and possible radical neck dissection.

Treatment aims
To remove the malignant lesion to prevent local or systemic spread.

Other treatments
- For lesions that are nonresectable (particularly sebaceous cell carcinomas), orbital radiation may be warranted.

Prognosis
- With wide excision and no evidence of metastasis, surgery results in a cure for the malignancies. However, sebaceous lesions have a high incidence of recurrence (~33%) and metastasis (~23%).

Follow-up and management
- Once a malignancy is found, ongoing monitoring for additional malignancies or metastatic sites is warranted. There is a marked increase in head-and-neck basal cell lesions found in patients with previous eyelid malignancies.

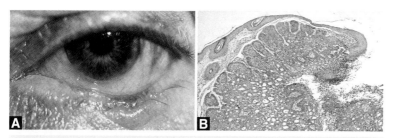

Figure 1 Basal cell carcinoma. **A,** Middle outer portion of the left lower lid contains an indurated, ulcerated, nontender lesion. **B,** Histologically, basal cell carcinoma arises from the overlying surface epithelium and invades the dermis. Characteristically, the nests of basal cells demonstrate peripheral palisading.

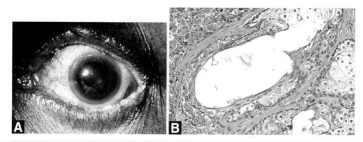

Figure 2 Sebaceous gland carcinoma. **A,** Eyelids are diffusely thickened, indurated, and show some loss of eyelashes. Sebaceous carcinoma can present as a lesion simulating a chalazion or, as shown here, can masquerade as a chronic lid inflammation. **B,** Histologically, the malignant sebaceous cells (*left* and *upper left*) can be seen arising from relatively normal sebaceous cells on the right.

General references
Fraunfelder F, Roy F, editors: *Current ocular therapy,* Philadelphia, 2000, Saunders.
Hornblass A et al: *Oculoplastic, orbital, and reconstructive surgery,* vol 2, Baltimore, 1990, Williams & Wilkins.
Older J, editor: *Eyelid tumors: clinical diagnosis and surgical treatment,* New York, 1987, Raven Press.
Tasman W, Jaeger E, editors: *Duane's clinical ophthalmology,* vol 4, Philadelphia, 2006, Lippincott-Raven.
Yanoff M, Fine B: *Ocular pathology: a color atlas,* Philadelphia, 2002, Lippincott.

Third-nerve palsy (oculomotor), partial   (378.51) and complete   (378.52)

DIAGNOSIS

Definition
Loss of function of the third cranial (oculomotor) nerve.

Synonyms
None.

Symptoms
Ptosis.

Vertical and horizontal diplopia.

Pain: present almost always with aneurysmal third-nerve palsy and pituitary apoplexy; variable with diabetic third-nerve palsy.

- *Acute onset* suggests ischemic vascular disease and aneurysm.
- *Progressive* implies compressive lesion.

Signs
Ophthalmoparetic eye.

Eye unable to elevate, depress, or adduct.

Ptosis: subtle to profound.

Pupil may be spared or involved:

- In adults, a painful, pupil-involving third-nerve paresis means an aneurysm at the junction of the internal carotid and posterior communicating arteries.
- A pupil-sparing third-nerve paresis can only be cited in a complete third-nerve palsy; usually vasculopathic in adults ≤50 yr of age.
- A relative pupil-sparing third-nerve paresis means that the pupil is minimally reactive to light in the setting of a complete third-nerve palsy. Some physicians interpret this as being "pupil involving," whereas others interpret it as "pupil sparing."

Vitreous hemorrhage (Terson's syndrome): suggests an intracranial bleed from an aneurysm.

Signs of aberrant regeneration.

Visual loss: in pituitary apoplexy.

Pilocarpine 1% constricts pupil, unlike pupils dilated with other pharmacologic agents.

Investigations
- Immediately hospitalize patients with painful, pupil-involving third-nerve paresis.

Computed tomography and arteriography.

Magnetic resonance imaging and arteriography.

Lumbar puncture.

Two-hour postprandial blood sugar.

Erythrocyte sedimentation rate.

Rapid plasma reagin.

Complications
Subarachnoid bleed.

Coma.

Death.

Pearls and Considerations
1. In a true isolated oculomotor palsy, the presumed location of the lesion is in the subarachnoid space.
2. Compression of the third nerve by an aneurysm at the junction of the internal carotid and posterior communicating arteries is considered a true neuro-ophthalmologic emergency. This is a life-threatening condition.

Referral Information
Refer to neuro-ophthalmologist as appropriate.

Differential diagnosis
Myasthenia gravis.
Graves' orbitopathy.
Inflammatory orbital pseudotumor.
Internuclear ophthalmoplegia.
Ocular skew torsion.

Cause
Adults
Aneurysm, tumor, infarction, idiopathic, trauma, infection (e.g., syphilis).
Children
Congenital, trauma, inflammation, neoplasm, aneurysm and ischemia (rare).

Associated features
Weber's syndrome
Third-nerve palsy.
Contralateral hemiparesis.
Benedikt's syndrome
Third-nerve palsy.
Contralateral hemiparesis.
Contralateral involuntary movements or tremor.
- Lesion affects the third-nerve fascicle, cerebral peduncle, substantia nigra, and red nucleus.
Claude's syndrome
Third-nerve palsy.
Contralateral ataxia.
Asynergy.
Dysdiadochokinesia.
- Fourth-nerve palsy and sensory loss may be included. Lesion affects the third-nerve fascicle, red nucleus, superior cerebellar peduncle, and sometimes the fourth nerve, medial lemniscus, and medial longitudinal fasciculus.
Nothnagel's syndrome
Bilateral, asymmetric third-nerve palsies.
Gait ataxia.
Nystagmus.
- Lesion affects both third-nerve fascicles and the superior and inferior colliculi.
Cavernous sinus syndrome
Oculosympathetic paresis.
Sensory loss in V1, V2, sixth nerve, and fourth nerve; proptosis up to 4 mm.
- The involvement of the optic nerve constitutes a superior orbital fissure/orbital apex syndrome.

TREATMENT

Diet and Lifestyle
- No special precautions are necessary.

Pharmacologic Treatment
- No pharmacologic treatment is recommended.

Nonpharmacologic Treatment
- No nonpharmacologic treatment is recommended.

Prognosis
- A vasculopathic third-nerve paresis resolves in 3 mo, although a compressive etiology may persist.
- A compressive/inflammatory third-nerve paresis may develop signs of aberrant regeneration, including:

Pseudo-Graefe sign (eyelid fails to follow the eye downward).

Eyelid synkinesia (eyelid elevates in adduction and drops in abduction).

Light-gaze dissociation pupil (pupil fails to respond to light but constricts to adduction, elevation, or depression).

Limitation of elevation and depression of the eye with occasional retraction of the globe on attempted vertical movement.

Adduction of the involved eye on attempted elevation or depression.

Monocular vertical optokinetic nystagmus.

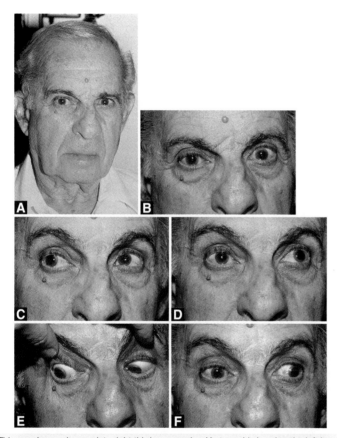

A, This man has an incomplete right third-nerve palsy. He turns his head to the left because of decreased innervation to the right medial rectus muscle. **B,** The left eyelid is retracted to compensate for his partial right ptosis, and a small left hypertropia is measurable in primary gaze. **C** and **D,** The left hypertropia is more pronounced in upgaze because of paretic right superior rectus and right inferior oblique muscle. **E,** In downgaze the left hypertropia reverses to a right "hypertropia" because of a paretic right inferior rectus muscle. **F,** The right exotropia increases in left gaze because of weak right medial rectus muscle.

General references

Johnston JL: Parasellar syndromes, *Curr Neurol Neurosci Rep* 2(5):423-431, 2002.

Miller NR, Lee AG: Adult-onset acquired oculomotor nerve paresis with cyclic spasms: relationship to ocular neuromyotonia, *Am J Ophthalmol* 137(1):70-76, 2004.

Moster ML: Paresis of isolated multiple cranial nerves and painful ophthalmoplegia. In Yanoff M, Duker JS, editors: *Ophthalmology*, E-dition, St Louis, 2006, Elsevier.

Tonic pupil   (379.46)

DIAGNOSIS

Definition
An enlarged, nonreactive pupil.

Synonym
Adie's tonic pupil.

Symptoms
Anisocoria.

"Funny looking" pupil.

Mid-dilated to small pupil.

The larger pupil in bright illumination: the same pupil is sometimes the smaller one in dim illumination.

Light-near dissociation pupil.

Blurred vision: from accommodative paresis.

Difficulty reading.

Photophobia.

"Brow ache": from ciliary spasm with near work.

Signs
Sector sphincter paralysis.

Stromal spread.

Stromal streaming.

Ectropion uvea.

Vermiform pupil movements.

Investigations
- Low-dose pilocarpine 0.125% yields constriction of pupils with cholinergic denervation sensitivity. Normal pupils do not constrict to such low concentration of pilocarpine.
- Check microhemagglutination assay–*Treponema pallidum* (MHA-TP) and rapid plasma reagin to rule out syphilis.
- May need brain magnetic resonance imaging.

Pearls and Considerations
1. Typically, the affected pupil is larger than pupil in fellow eye.
2. Vermiform movements of the iris are often visible at the slit lamp.
3. The tonic pupil will typically react to 0.1% pilocarpine, whereas the normal pupil will not.

Referral Information
None.

Differential diagnosis
Posterior synechia.
Traumatic iridoplegia.
Aberrant regeneration of the third nerve.
Tectal pupils (dorsal midbrain syndrome).
Argyll-Robertson pupils.

Cause
Damage to the ciliary ganglion.

Epidemiology
Idiopathic tonic pupil
Female/male ratio is 2.6:1.
Age of onset is 20-40 yr.
90% of patients present unilaterally.
Involvement of the fellow eye is common.

Classification
Local tonic pupil
Varicella.
Retrobulbar injection.
Orbital tumor.
Orbital surgery.
Neuropathic tonic pupil (bilateral)
Diabetes.
Syphilis.
Sarcoid.
Idiopathic (Adie's tonic pupil)

Associated features
Accommodative paresis, tonicity, and induced astigmatism at near gaze.
Idiopathic tonic pupil
Decreased corneal sensation.
Diminished deep tendon reflexes.

TREATMENT

Diet and Lifestyle
- No special precautions are necessary.

Pharmacologic Treatment
Cycloplegia: for the tonic pupil with a tonicity cramp; prescribe reading glasses to match the near point between the two eyes.

Nonpharmacologic Treatment
Patch.
Cosmetic contact lens.

Treatment aims
To normalize appearance of pupil.
To synchronize near points between the two eyes with reading lenses.
To relieve cramping with tropine medication.

Prognosis
- Mid-dilated pupil tends to become more miotic over time.
- Direct light reflex remains impaired.
- Fellow eye will become involved at a rate of 4%/yr, so at the end of 20 yr, 50% of patients will have bilateral involvement.

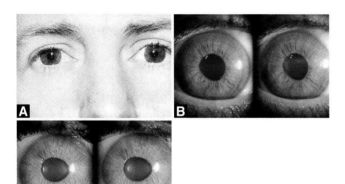

A, This woman has bilateral Adie's tonic pupils. **B,** Stereophotograph of the right eye in which a segmental paralysis of the pupillary sphincter from the 6 o'clock to the 9 o'clock positions is associated with a spreading of the iris stroma. **C,** Stereophotograph of the left eye in which the pupil assumes a polygonal appearance with segmental paresis from the 3 o'clock to the 6 o'clock positions.

General references
Foroozan R, Buono LM, Savino PJ, Sergott RC: Tonic pupils from giant cell arteritis, *Br J Ophthalmol* 87(4):510-512, 2003.
Kawasaki A: Physiology, assessment, and disorders of the pupil, *Curr Opin Ophthalmol* 10(6):394-400, 1999.
Wilhelm H: Neuro-ophthalmology of pupillary function: practical guidelines, *J Neurol* 245(9): 573-583, 1998.

DIAGNOSIS

Definition
Drug toxicity of the posterior segment.

Synonyms
None.

Symptoms
Chloroquine and Hydroxychloroquine
Often asymptomatic; **photophobia, nyctalopia, photopsias**.

Phenothiazines
Blurry vision, decreased night vision, brown color to vision.

Methanol
White, blurry vision.

Signs
Chloroquine and Hydroxychloroquine
Corneal whorls, poliosis, irregular macular pigmentation, loss of foveal reflex, classic bull's-eye maculopathy: *see* figure.
Peripheral pigmentation: gives pseudoretinitis pigmentosa appearance; **bone spicule formation, arteriolar attenuation, optic nerve pallor**.

Phenothiazines
Granularity to postequatorial fundus: found early, although early on fundus may be normal.
Transient edema of optic nerve and retina.
Large patches of increased pigmentation: may give appearance of bone spiculization.
Large areas of depigmentation and atrophy.

Methanol
Nystagmus, poorly reactive dilated pupils.
Edema of optic nerve and retina: retinal edema spreads out along major arcades.
Central or cecocentral scotomas.

Investigations
Chloroquine and Hydroxychloroquine
Amsler grid: screening to look for central and paracentral scotomas.
Goldmann perimetry: small paracentral scotomas sparing fixation superiorly.
Electroretinography: abnormal in advanced retinopathy.
Electro-oculogram: reduced with more retinopathy.
Fluorescein angiography: highlights the pigmentation changes (*see* figure).

Phenothiazines
Careful history: to determine the use of antipsychotic medication.
Slit-lamp and dilated fundus examination.
Fluorescein angiography: demonstrates window-defect changes in pigment layer.
• Reduction in the photopic and scotopic electroretinogram.
Abnormal dark adaptation.

Methanol
Careful history: to determine if the patient had been drinking solvents or homemade liquors; although the usual method of poisoning is through ingestion, patients may also develop toxicity from vapors or skin contact.

Pearls and Considerations
An open line of communication with the patient's prescribing physician is key to effective management of toxic retinopathies.

Referral Information
Refer/co-manage these cases with the prescribing physician.

Differential diagnosis
Chloroquine and hydroxychloroquine
Retinitis and pseudo–retinitis pigmentosa.
Phenothiazines
Retinitis pigmentosa, syphilis, rubella.
Methanol
Increased intracranial pressure, causing papilledema.

Cause
Chloroquine and hydroxychloroquine
Have an affinity for pigmented structures in the eye; half-lives also increase as the dosage increases.
Phenothiazines
The mechanism of injury is unknown.
Methanol
Ingestion or exposure to methanol.

Epidemiology
• Toxic retinopathy affects ~10% of unmonitored patients receiving chloroquine and 3%-4% of patients taking hydroxychloroquine. Incidence increases with both dose and duration.

Classification
• Chloroquine and hydroxychloroquine are members of quinolone drug family.

Associated features
Chloroquine and hydroxychloroquine
Hydroxychloroquine used to treat rheumatoid arthritis, systemic lupus erythematosus; chloroquine used to treat malaria.
Methanol
Metabolic acidosis, depressed level of consciousness, respiratory distress, coma, death.

Pathology
Chloroquine and hydroxychloroquine
• Outer segments of the retina degenerate, often sparing the fovea.
• Pigment migrates to the retina.
• Ganglion cells develop membranous cytoplasmic bodies within 1 wk of treatment.
Methanol
• It is believed that the damage is caused by axoplasmic stasis, and that permanent damage is caused by secondary swelling of the optic nerve and retina [1,2].

TREATMENT

Diet and Lifestyle
- No special precautions are necessary.

Pharmacologic Treatment
Chloroquine and Hydroxychloroquine
- Discontinue the drug when symptoms begin.

Phenothiazines
- Discontinue the drug when symptoms of decreased vision begin will allow reversal of the symptoms.
Standard dosage   Thioridazine, 300 mg/day (maximum 800 mg/day).

Methanol
- Intravenous ethanol acts as a competitive inhibitor of the metabolism of methanol.

Nonpharmacologic Treatment
Chloroquine, Hydroxychloroquine, and Phenothiazines
- No nonpharmacologic treatment is recommended.

Methanol
Respiratory support.
Treatment of the metabolic acidosis.
Dialysis.

Complications
Chloroquine and Hydroxychloroquine
- Most severe toxic retinal findings are due to chloroquine. Hydroxychloroquine infrequently causes a maculopathy.
- If found early, functional and fundus changes should return to normal with discontinuation of the chloroquine or hydroxychloroquine. If not, irreversible visual damage can occur.

Phenothiazines
- The risk of retinopathy is dose related. Even if the medication is discontinued, the pigmentary changes can continue.

Methanol
Severe visual loss: can occur from ingesting as little as 1 oz of methanol; the more severe the retinal findings, the more severe the eye damage.

Treatment aims
Chloroquine and hydroxychloroquine
To discontinue use once maculopathy has started.
Phenothiazines
To discontinue the use of the phenothiazine once symptoms start.
To titrate the dosage of the medication to stay within the guidelines.

Prognosis
Chloroquine and hydroxychloroquine
Good, if doses are monitored and patients are followed carefully.
Phenothiazines
Good, if caught early.
Methanol
- Usually, vision should improve within 6 days; if not, improvement is unlikely.

Follow-up and management
Chloroquine and hydroxychloroquine
Amsler grid: for patient home monitoring; look for central scotomas or paracentral scotomas.
Macular visual field: annually during the first 3 yr, when most of the toxicity generally develops [3].
Color vision monitoring.
Phenothiazines
- All patients on this type of medication should have a baseline eye examination and should be followed periodically if symptoms begin.
Methanol
- Optic atrophy and excavation usually occurs after 1-2 mo.

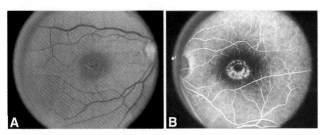

Retinopathy caused by chloroquine and hydroxychloroquine. **A,** Color photograph of the right eye of a patient with increasing pigmentation in the macula. **B,** Fluorescein angiogram of the same patient's left eye showing window-defect hyperfluorescence corresponding to the area of pigment alteration.

Key references
1. Hayrah MS, Hayreh SS, Baumbach GL, et al: Methyl alcohol poisoning. III. Ocular toxicity, *Arch Ophthalmol* 95:1851-1859, 1977.
2. Baumbach GL, Cancilla PA, Martin-Amat G, et al: Methyl alcohol poisoning. IV. Alterations in morphological findings of the retina and optic nerve, *Arch Ophthalmol* 95:1859-1865, 1977.
3. Fishman GA: Retinal toxicity with the use of chloroquine or hydroxychloroquine. In Heckenlively JR, Aden GB, editors: *Principles and practice of electrophysiology of vision*, St Louis, 1991, Mosby, pp 594-599.

DIAGNOSIS

Definition
A malignant lesion occurring in the uveal tract.

Synonyms
None.

Symptoms
- Patients can be asymptomatic.

Blurry or decreased vision: from extension of tumor into fovea, fluid in fovea, or tumor contact with lens.

Photopsias, visual field defects, dark spot on iris.

Signs
Elevated pigmented lesion of iris, ciliary body, or choroid.

Iris melanomas: usually arise from an existing iris nevus; will have an elevated nodular area; prominent vessels may be present in the lesion; pigmentation may vary; *see* Fig. 1.

Ciliary body and choroidal tumors: often takes on characteristic collar-button appearance when the tumor breaks through Bruch's membrane; pigmentation may vary; may have associated orange lipofuscin pigment on the surface; often associated with serous retinal detachment when tumor exceeds 4 mm in height; although most tumors are pigmented, ~20% are amelanotic; anterior tumors extending to involve ciliary body will have prominent episcleral vessels; *see* Figs. 2 and 3.

Investigations
Clinical history: not useful when trying to differentiate choroidal melanoma from other simulating lesions, except for metastasis.

Gonioscopy: for iris and ciliary body lesions, to look for pigment dispersion in the angle and to determine if lesion is arising from iris or extending anteriorly from ciliary body.

Dilated fundus examination: usually makes the diagnosis in >95% of cases of ciliary body and choroidal malignant melanoma.

Fluorescein angiography: may have a characteristic "double circulation" in choroidal malignant melanoma; scleral transillumination is usually blocked by the ciliary body and choroidal tumor.

Ultrasonography: of ciliary body and choroidal melanoma; *B mode:* acoustically silent zone within the tumor, choroidal excavation, orbital shadowing; *A mode:* medium-to-low internal reflectivity. Ultrasound is the most useful diagnostic tool to determine response to treatment.

Computed tomography (CT), magnetic resonance imaging (MRI): not always necessary. Expensive to perform; increased uptake of the tumor on T1-weighted MR images for larger tumors [1]. Most useful to determine extraocular extension of tumor.

Fine-needle biopsy: useful when diagnosis is difficult and chance of metastatic disease exists, although interpretation of the tissue is difficult.

Differential diagnosis
Choroidal nevus: usually asymptomatic; flat or <1.5 mm in thickness; sharply defined borders; drusen on surface; fluorescein angiography shows early hypofluorescence; serous detachment and secondary hemorrhage are rare (*see* Fig. 4).

Choroidal melanocytoma: often jet black in appearance, does not enlarge, and usually develops around the optic disc (*see* Fig. 5).

Subretinal hemorrhage: secondary to age-related macular degeneration, macroaneurysm, or choroidal hemorrhage.

Metastatic disease: usually more than one lesion in the choroid; these tumors are usually less pigmented, are more likely found in the posterior pole, and often involve the macula; serous retinal detachment is also possible (*see* Fig. 6).

Choroidal osteoma: cream-colored, calcified macular or peripapillary lesion; relatively flat; more common in women; bilateral in 10%-20%; calcification can be documented by ultrasound or CT scan (*see* Fig. 7).

Choroidal hemangioma.

Retinal pigment epithelial tumors.

Congenital hypertrophy of the pigment epithelium (CHRPE).

Cause
Controversial; some believe primary ocular melanoma arises from a preexisting nevus; others believe they develop de novo.

Epidemiology
- Iris melanomas are rare. Late metastasis is possible, occurring 20-30 yr after diagnosis despite excision of the original ocular lesion.
- Ciliary body melanomas have the highest rate of metastasis and are thought to develop because of the anterior location and relatively high blood flow rate through the ciliary body.
- Choroidal melanoma has a 50% mortality rate after enucleation at 10-15 yr, with a peak incidence at 3 yr.

Pathology
- Melanomas can be spindle A, spindle B, epithelioid, or mixed tumors. Epithelioid and mixed cell tumors carry a worse prognosis.

Diagnosis continued on p. 318

TREATMENT

Diet and Lifestyle
- No special precautions are necessary.

Pharmacologic Treatment
- If metastatic disease, then may need to refer for systemic chemotherapy. Extremely poor prognosis if becomes metastatic.

Nonpharmacologic Treatment
For Iris Melanoma
- Most pigmented iris lesions are benign, so observation is recommended. If there is documented evidence of growth, local excision through an iridectomy or iridocyclectomy should be performed.

For Ciliary Body and Choroidal Melanoma

Enucleation: least common treatment modality; Collaborative Ocular Melanoma Study showed that enucleation and plaque radiation therapy were equally effective for the prevention of metastatic disease.

Radiation therapy: two methods are in use:
- *Brachytherapy:* a plaque containing radioactive seeds is applied directly to episcleral surface of eye directly exterior to the tumor; common isotopes used are ^{60}Co, ^{106}Ru, and ^{125}I; plaque remains in place to deliver 80-100 Gy to the tumor apex.
- *Charged particle (proton or helium) beam radiotherapy:* tumor base is located, and tantalum buttons are surgically sewn to the sclera; radiation is administered while monitoring position of the eye and tumor by fluoroscopy.

Treatment continued on p. 319

Treatment aims
To decrease the risk of tumor growth and metastasis while trying to maintain vision in the eye.

Prognosis
- Cell type is important for determining prognosis in all types of uveal melanoma.
- Iris melanomas are rare and have a better prognosis, but metastasis can occur 20-30 yr after excision of the tumor.
- For choroidal melanoma, three important factors that imply a worse prognosis are anterior location of tumor margin, cellular pleomorphism, and presence of extrascleral extension.

Follow-up and management
- Fundus photographs and ultrasound measurements should be taken of all lesions. This allows the physician to study the tumor margins carefully on subsequent visits.
- Follow-up management largely depends on the site, location, and associated features of the tumor, which is beyond the scope of this book. Most patients with uveal melanoma are followed by retina specialists or ocular oncologists, who have a better understanding of these lesions.

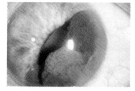

Figure 1 Iris melanoma showing the elevated amelanotic nodule with a pigmented base. Note the prominent vasculature.

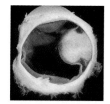

Figure 3 Gross specimen of a choroidal melanoma showing the mushroom-shape configuration.

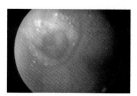

Figure 2 Choroidal melanoma with elevated pigmented lesion and surface pigmentation. Yellow dots in the vitreous represent asteroid hyalosis.

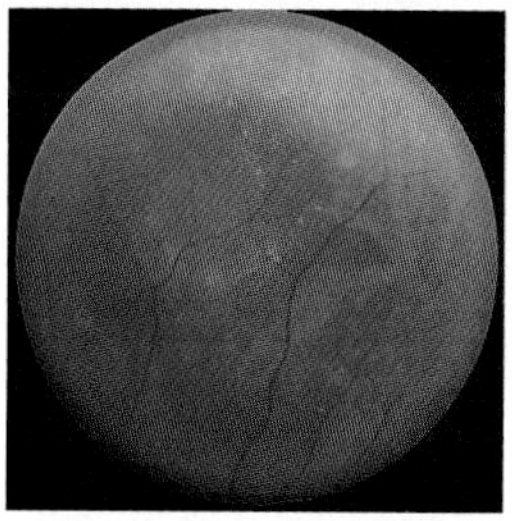

Figure 4 Choroidal nevus. Note the feathery borders, flat appearance, and drusen on the surface.

Uveal malignant melanoma, primary   (190.6)

DIAGNOSIS—cont'd

Complications

Intraocular

Glaucoma, decreased vision, loss of vision, cataract, pain and discomfort, serous retinal detachment, hemorrhage into the anterior chamber and vitreous.

Systemic

Metastasis: usually occurs in the liver and then in the lungs, bone, and skin.

Death.

Pearls and Considerations

1. Uveal tract melanoma is the most common ocular tumor in adults.
2. Can metastasize through the bloodstream to other parts of the body, especially the liver.
3. Patients with increasing astigmatic refractive changes need to have a thorough peripheral retinal examination to rule out a ciliary body melanoma as the cause of the astigmatism.

Referral Information

Refer to ocular oncologist as appropriate.

TREATMENT—cont'd

Laser photocoagulation: reserved for tumors <3 mm in thickness and 7 mm in largest basal dimension. Used infrequently. Has mostly been replaced by transpupillary thermal therapy (TTT).

Surgical resection: reserved for anterior choroidal and ciliary body tumors; tedious and complicated surgery. Done infrequently.

Observation: a suspicious nevus may be observed to document growth before instituting therapy. Not all nevi that grow are melanomas.

Transpupillary thermal therapy (TTT): commonly used for small- to medium-sized tumors. Uses infrared laser light with a large spot size to induce hyperthermia; results in regression of tumor and is done in the office.

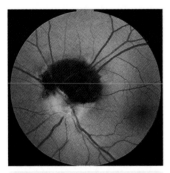

Figure 5 Melanocytoma. Note the jet-black color with feathery borders.

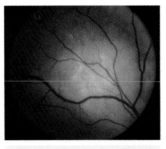

Figure 6 Choroidal metastasis with creamy-yellow choroidal infiltrate located superior to the optic nerve in a patient with metastatic nasopharyngeal carcinoma.

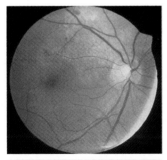

Figure 7 Choroidal osteoma with areas of retinal pigment epithelium atrophy located supratemporally to the optic nerve.

Key reference

1. Augsburger JJ: Intraocular neoplasms. In Podos SM, Yanoff M, editors: *Textbook of ophthalmology*, vol 2, pp 11.1-11.19, 1992.

General references

Augsberger JJ, Damato BE, Bornfeld N: Uveal melanoma. In Yanoff M, Duker JS, editors: *Ophthalmology*, E-dition, St Louis, 2006, Elsevier.

Mukai S, Gragoudas ES: Diagnosis of choroidal melanoma. In Albert DM, Jakobiec FA, editors: *Principles and practice of ophthalmology*, Philadelphia, 1994, Saunders, pp 3209-3217.

Sahel JA, Marcus DM, Albert DM: Nevus and melanocytoma. In Albert DM. Jakobiec FA, editors: *Principles and practice of ophthalmology*, Philadelphia, 1994, Saunders, pp 3244-3251.

DIAGNOSIS

Definition
Inflammation of the uveal tract after a penetrating ocular injury.

Synonym
Sympathetic ophthalmia.

Symptoms
- Sympathetic uveitis always follows a penetrating ocular injury to one eye (the "exciting" eye) and is characterized by a bilateral granulomatous uveal inflammatory reaction with the following symptoms:

Photophobia in the noninjured ("sympathizing") eye: *see* Fig. 1.

Ocular irritation or pain.

Blurred vision in the noninjured (sympathizing) eye.

Trouble with near vision (difficulty with accommodation).

Signs
Red eye secondary to ciliary injection.

Evidence of previous ocular injury: in rare cases the injury occurred years before the onset of uveitis, and the patient does not remember.

Bilateral mutton-fat keratic precipitates: *see* Fig. 2.

Bilateral uveitis: the presentation of sympathetic uveitis has a wide spectrum, from an anterior uveitis or focal choroiditis to a severe panuveitis; Dalen-Fuchs nodules are tiny areas of focal choroidal inflammation most often seen in the midperiphery but also in the posterior pole. (*See* Fig. 3.)

Papillitis (inflammation of optic nerve head).

Exudative retinal detachment.

Investigations
History: a penetrating ocular injury, usually with uveal prolapse; generally after a 2-wk "safe period"; most cases (80%) occur 3 wk to 3 mo after the injury, and both eyes are affected; rarely, sympathetic uveitis can occur years after a penetrating ocular injury.

Visual acuity test.

Refraction.

Complete external examination.

Intraocular pressure.

Undilated and dilated slit-lamp examination.

Dilated fundus examination.

Fluorescein angiography: can be helpful; characteristically, multiple tiny areas of fluorescein hyperfluorescence that spread with time (leakage) are noted.

Differential diagnosis
Vogt-Koyanagi-Harada syndrome.
Bilateral phacoanaphylactic endophthalmitis.
Multifocal choroiditis.
Other causes of bilateral uveitis.

Cause
- Cause appears to be a delayed type of hypersensitivity reaction of the uvea to antigens localized on the retinal pigment epithelium or uveal melanocytes.

Epidemiology
- Sympathetic uveitis occurs after intraocular surgical trauma (<0.007%) and penetrating nonsurgical ocular trauma (>0.200%).
- The incidence is higher in men than women because more men sustain penetrating ocular injuries than women.
- Two peaks of frequency occur:
  Children <10 yr: most likely because of the increased occurrence of nonsurgical penetrating ocular injuries in this age group.
  Adults >60 yr: most likely because of the increased occurrence of intraocular surgery in this age group.

Associated features
- Cutaneous and neurologic findings, similar to those found in Vogt-Koyanagi-Harada syndrome (alopecia, poliosis, vitiligo, dysacousia, tinnitus, vertigo, cerebrospinal fluid pleocytosis), rarely accompany sympathetic uveitis.

Immunology
- Lymphocytic choroidal infiltrate is composed almost exclusively of T lymphocytes.

Pathology
- Histologic hallmarks of choroidal inflammatory infiltrate include bilateral granulomatous (epithelioid cells) uveal reaction, sparing of the choriocapillaris, epithelioid cells containing phagocytosed uveal pigment, and Dalen-Fuchs nodules (epithelioid cells between retinal pigment epithelium and Bruch's membrane).

Diagnosis continued on p. 322

TREATMENT

Diet and Lifestyle
- No special precautions are necessary.

Pharmacologic Treatment
- Intensive topical and systemic corticosteroids should be started as soon as possible.

Standard dosage   Prednisone, 1.0-1.5 mg/kg daily.

Special points   After control of the inflammation, taper the systemic corticosteroid and institute alternate-day therapy until the inflammation has cleared. After the inflammation has cleared, treatment should be continued for 3-6 mo with alternate-day therapy in the range of 10-20 mg of oral prednisone.

In patients who are intolerant or do not respond to corticosteroids, periocular or immunosuppressive therapy (e.g., cyclosporine, methotrexate, chlorambucil, or azathioprine) along with reduced dosage of oral corticosteroid therapy may be indicated.

Treatment aims
To preserve vision in both eyes.
- Even though sympathetic uveitis is rare, it can be (and often is) a blinding disease. Therefore, aggressive, rapid therapy is necessary if any chance exists of preserving visual function.

Other treatments
- Therapy aimed at T-cell subsets is being investigated. Most investigations of alternate therapy focus on patients who do not respond (or only partially respond) to high-dose corticosteroid therapy.

Prognosis
- Approximately 60% of patients will retain visual acuity of ≥20/60; however, ~33% will have visual acuity of <20/200.

Follow-up and management
- Long-term follow-up is indicated to treat the entity and to protect against recurrence. Relapses occur in >50% of patients and may not occur for a few years after seemingly successful therapy.

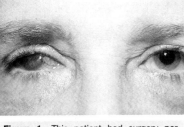

Figure 1 This patient had surgery performed on his right eye. A few months later the right eye became inflamed, and photophobia developed in the left eye. The blind right eye was enucleated, and sympathetic uveitis was found.

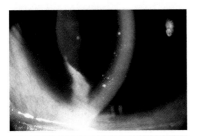

Figure 2 Large mutton-fat keratic precipitates are seen on the posterior surface of the cornea.

Treatment continued on p. 323

DIAGNOSIS—cont'd

Complications

Decreased visual acuity: worst case is bilateral blindness; approximately one third of patients are left with a visual acuity of <20/200 (legal blindness); the exciting (injured) eye may have better vision than the sympathizing eye.

Band keratopathy.

Hypotony.

Glaucoma.

Cataract.

Chorioretinal scarring: after the inflammation resolves, chorioretinal scarring occurs and may be severe in the peripheral retina and macula in approximately one third of patients; chorioretinal scarring in the region of the macula may be responsible for central visual loss in some patients.

Macular edema.

Retinal detachment.

Phthisis bulbi: the end stage of ocular disease—a shrunken, functionless eye.

Pearls and Considerations

1. If pain in nontraumatized eye is out of proportion to ocular findings, need to consider early sympathetic ophthalmia as the cause.
2. Sympathetic ophthalmia is a bilateral disease, so both eyes will have evidence of uveitis.

Referral Information

Needs immediate referral to ophthalmologist for aggressive immunosuppressive therapy.

TREATMENT—cont'd

Nonpharmacologic Treatment
Enucleation

- Enucleation of the injured eye before the second eye becomes involved protects against the development of sympathetic uveitis.
- Prophylactic corticosteroids do not prevent sympathetic uveitis.
- In general, after a penetrating ocular injury with uveal prolapse, if no potential for useful vision exists, the injured eye should be enucleated within 2 wk of injury. Enucleation of an injured eye that has a potential for navigational (i.e., "getting around") visual function is not justified, because the injured eye may ultimately turn out to have a better visual acuity than the sympathizing eye.
- Because of the 2-wk safe period, every effort should be made to salvage the injured eye as soon as possible after the injury. The surgery often consists of immediate repair of the laceration of the ocular coats, often accompanied (at the same time or shortly thereafter) by vitreous surgery, which includes evacuation of any hemorrhage in the vitreous compartment and repair of any retinal tears or detachment.

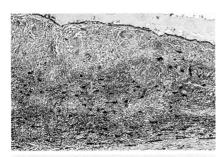

Figure 3 Histologically, sympathetic uveitis is characterized by a diffuse granulomatous inflammation. The pale area represents epithelioid cells, and the dark areas consist mainly of lymphocytes. Sparing of the choriocapillaris is seen.

General references

Albert DM, Diaz-Rohena R: A historical review of sympathetic ophthalmia and its epidemiology, *Surv Ophthalmol* 34(1):1-14, 1989.

Damico FM, Kiss S, Young LH: Sympathetic ophthalmia, *Semin Ophthal* 20(3):191-7, 2005.

Vitreous detachment, posterior (379.21)

DIAGNOSIS

Definition
Separation of the vitreous gel from the retina.

Synonyms
None; usually abbreviated PVD.

Symptoms
Flashing lights.
Floaters.

Signs
Free-floating ring of formed vitreous in front of optic nerve: also known as a *Weiss ring*.

Investigations
History.
Slit-lamp and dilated eye examination.
360-degree scleral depression: should be performed to rule out retinal tears.

Complications
Vitreous hemorrhage.
Retinal tears.
Retinal detachment.

Pearls and Considerations
Vitreous detachment is a normal degenerative process in the aging eye, and most people will develop it in time. The vast majority of patients require no treatment.

Referral Information
Needs to be referred to an ophthalmologist within 24 hr of onset of symptoms to rule out associated pathologies such as retinal tear or retinal detachment.

Differential diagnosis
Ocular migraine can cause swirling or "zigzag" flashing lights.
Vitritis can cause floaters.

Cause
- Age-related vitreous changes lead to synchysis and vacuolization of the vitreous.

Epidemiology
- 37% of myopic patients have had a PVD at an earlier age.
- The prevalence of PVD formation increases with age and greater axial length [1].
- Approximately 10% of patients with a symptomatic PVD will have a retinal tear [2].

Pathology
Vacuolization and synchysis of the vitreous.

TREATMENT

Diet and Lifestyle
- No special precautions are necessary.

Pharmacologic Treatment
- No pharmacologic treatment is recommended.

Nonpharmacologic Treatment
- No nonpharmacologic treatment is recommended.

Treatment aims
To reassure the patient.
To teach the signs and symptoms of a retinal detachment to the patient.

Prognosis
Good.

Follow-up and management
- Symptomatic patients with acute PVD associated with flashes and floaters should be seen at 1 wk, then at 1 mo. If the dilated eye examination with scleral depression is normal, an annual follow-up examination is appropriate.

Key references
1. Yonemoto J, Noda Y, Mashara N, Ohno S: Age of onset of posterior vitreous detachment, *Curr Opin Ophthalmol* 7:73-79, 1996.
2. Tasman WS: Posterior vitreous detachment and peripheral retinal breaks, *Trans Am Acad Ophthalmol Otolaryngol* 72:217-224, 1968.

Vitreous hemorrhage   (379.23)

DIAGNOSIS

Definition
Blood in the vitreous cavity.

Synonyms
None; usually abbreviated VH.

Symptoms
Sudden, painless loss of vision.
Sudden appearance of floaters and black spots: with or without flashing lights.

Signs
- The amount of blood in the vitreous cavity often determines the presenting visual acuity and the ability to examine the retina to determine the cause. The amount of blood, however, offers no help in determining the cause. Long-standing hemorrhage may take on a yellow appearance as the blood cells lose their hemoglobin.

Investigations
History of preceding symptoms.
Careful medical history: to rule out diabetes, hypertension, trauma, sickle cell disease, anti-coagulation therapy, and previous eye surgery.
Careful slit-lamp and dilated fundus examination of both eyes: even if the fundus is obscured by blood, often the fellow eye can provide clues on the possible cause.
B-scan ultrasound: to help rule out a retinal break or detachment if the retina cannot be visualized.

Complications
Secondary or "ghost cell" glaucoma: if the erythrocytes enter the anterior chamber, they can block the trabecular meshwork, causing a secondary elevation in intraocular pressure.

Pearls and Considerations
Causes loss of red reflex.

Referral Information
Usually needs to be referred to an ophthalmologist within 24 hr. If patient is known to have diabetes with a history of proliferative disease, may be referred within several days.

Differential diagnosis
Spontaneous posterior vitreous detachment (PVD).
Proliferative diabetic retinopathy.
Retinal break with or without detachment.
Retinal vein occlusion.
Macroaneurysm.
Age-related macular degeneration.
Sickle cell hemoglobinopathies.
Trauma.
Tumors and vascular anomalies.
Postoperative hemorrhage.

Cause
- Avulsion of a retinal blood vessel is the most common cause. Shearing effect on the ciliary body or damage to the iris can also cause blood to leak into the vitreous cavity.

Epidemiology
Most common causes [1]
PVD with a retinal tear (29%).
Proliferative diabetic retinopathy (20%).
Retinal vein occlusion (16%).
Vitreous detachment without a tear (12%).

Associated features
- Neovascularization of the iris may be seen in patients with diabetes and vascular occlusion. Drusen in the fellow eye may help with the diagnosis of age-related macular degeneration.

TREATMENT

Diet and Lifestyle
- Avoid heavy lifting.
- Sleep with head elevated on two pillows.
- Avoid contact sports and forms of exercise that would cause the hemorrhage to remain suspended in the vitreous cavity.

Pharmacologic Treatment
- Usually can continue use of prophylactic baby aspirin therapy without worsening vitreous hemorrhage.
- No pharmacologic treatment is recommended.

Nonpharmacologic Treatment
- Treat the underlying cause.

Pars plana vitrectomy: if the view remains cloudy for more than 2 mo, or much sooner if there is a high level of suspicion for a retinal tear or detachment.

Panretinal photocoagulation: for proliferative diabetic retinopathy, vascular occlusive disease, or sickle cell retinopathy.

Treatment aims
To treat underlying cause.
To restore visual acuity.
To prevent visual loss.
To avoid secondary complications (e.g., glaucoma).

Prognosis
Depends on the cause of the hemorrhage.

Follow-up and management
- Patients should be followed on a weekly basis. It is hoped the blood will clear, allowing a view of the fundus. If not, sequential B-scan ultrasound should be performed, looking for a retinal detachment.

Key reference
1. Lingren G, Sjodell L, Lindblom B: A prospective study of dense spontaneous vitreous hemorrhage, *Am J Ophthalmol* 119:458-465, 1995.

Appendix A: Techniques of ophthalmic medication administration

Eyedrops
1. Wash hands.
2. Instruct patient to lie down or to tilt head backward and look up.
3. Gently pull lower eyelid down until a pocket (pouch) is formed between eye and lower lid (conjunctival sac).
4. Hold dropper above pocket. Without touching tip of eyedropper to eyelid or conjunctival sac, place prescribed number of drops into the center pocket (placing drops directly onto eye may cause a sudden squeezing of eyelid, with subsequent loss of solution). Continue to hold the eyelid for a moment after the drops are applied (allows medication to distribute along entire conjunctival sac).
5. Instruct patient to close eyes gently so that medication will not be squeezed out of sac.
6. Apply gentle finger pressure to the lacrimal sac at the inner canthus (bridge of nose, inside corner of eye) for 1-2 min (promotes absorption, minimizes drainage into nose and throat, lessens risk of systemic absorption).
7. Remove excess solution around eye with a tissue.
8. Wash hands immediately to remove medication on hands. Never rinse eyedropper.

Eye Ointment
1. Wash hands.
2. Instruct patient to lie down or to tilt head backward and look up.
3. Gently pull lower eyelid down until a pocket (pouch) is formed between eye and lower lid (conjunctival sac).
4. Hold applicator tube above pocket. Without touching the applicator tip to eyelid or conjunctival sac, place prescribed amount of ointment (¼–½ inch) into the center pocket (placing ointment directly onto eye may cause discomfort).
5. Instruct patient to close eye for 1-2 min, rolling eyeball in all directions (increases contact area of drug to eye).
6. Inform patient of temporary blurring of vision. If possible, apply ointment just before bedtime.
7. Wash hands immediately to remove medication on hands. Never rinse tube applicator.

Miscellaneous Ophthalmic Agents

Uses

Miscellaneous ophthalmic agents are used to prevent and treat mild ophthalmic disorders, such as allergic conjunctivitis, keratitis, and dry eyes.

Action

Miscellaneous ophthalmic agents act in various ways. For example, *hydroxypropyl methylcellulose* stabilizes and thickens precorneal tear film, protecting and lubricating the eyes. *Azelastine, emedastine,* and *levocabastine* antagonize histamine (H₁) receptors, thus inhibiting histamine-stimulated responses in the conjunctiva, such as redness and itching. By stabilizing mast cells, *lodoxamide* prevents antigen-stimulated release of histamine, which inhibits type I hypersensitivity reactions. A broad-spectrum antiinfective, *sulfacetamide* interferes with the synthesis of folic acid that bacteria require for growth. *Vidarabine* blocks deoxyribonucleic acid (DNA) polymerase, blocking viral DNA synthesis.

Miscellaneous ophthalmic agents

Name	Indications	Dosages	Side effects
Azelastine (Optivar)	Relief of itching eyes caused by allergic conjunctivitis	1 drop 2 times/day	Transient eye burning or stinging, headache, bitter taste, eye pain, fatigue, flulike symptoms, pharyngitis, rhinitis, blurred vision
Emedastine (Emadine)	Treatment of signs and symptoms of allergic conjunctivitis	1-2 drops 2 times/day	Headache, bad taste, blurred vision, eye burning or stinging, dry eyes, tearing
Epinastine (Elestat)	Treatment of allergic conjunctivitis	1 drop 4 times/day	Headache, taste disturbance, drowsiness, blurred vision, eye burning or stinging, dry eyes, foreign body sensation, rhinitis
Hydroxypropyl methylcellulose (Artificial Tears, Isopto Tears, Tears Naturale)	Relief of eye dryness and irritation caused by insufficient tear production	1-2 drops 3-4 times/day	Eye irritation, blurred vision, eyelash stickiness
Ketotifen (Zaditor)	Temporary relief of itching eyes caused by allergic conjunctivitis	1 drop every 8-12 hr	Conjunctival infection, headache, rhinitis, eye burning or stinging, ocular discharge, eye pain
Levocabastine (Livostin)	Treatment of signs and symptoms of seasonal allergic conjunctivitis	1 drop 4 times/day	Transient eye stinging, burning, or discomfort; headache; dry eyes; eyelid edema
Lodoxamide (Alomide)	Treatment of vernal keratoconjunctivitis and keratitis	1 drop 4 times/day	Transient eye stinging or burning, instillation discomfort, itching eyes, blurred vision, dry eyes, tearing, headache
Olopatadine (Patanol)	Treatment of signs and symptoms of allergic conjunctivitis	1-2 drops 2 times/day	Headache, drowsiness, eye burning or stinging, foreign body sensation, pharyngitis, rhinitis, pruritus
Pemirolast (Alamast)	Prevention of itching eyes caused by allergic conjunctivitis	1-2 drops 3-4 times/day	Transient eye stinging or burning, instillation discomfort, itching eyes, blurred vision, tearing, headache
Sulfacetamide (Bleph 10)	Treatment of corneal ulcers, bacterial conjunctivitis, other superficial eye infections; prevention of infection after eye injury	1-3 drops every 2-3 hr; or 1.25- to 2.5-cm strip of ointment 4 times/day and at bedtime	Transient eye burning or stinging, headache, rash, itching eyes, eye swelling, photosensitivity
Vidarabine (Vira-A)	Treatment of keratitis or keratoconjunctivitis caused by herpes simplex virus, type 1 or 2	½ inch 5 times/day at 3-hr intervals; after reepithelialization, ½ inch 2 times/day for 7 days	Eye burning or irritation, itching eyes, tearing, eye pain, photophobia

Appendix B: Eye and topical agents

Topical Antiinflammatory Agents

Uses

Topical antiinflammatory agents relieve inflammation and pruritus caused by corticosteroid-responsive disorders, such as contact dermatitis, eczema, insect bite reactions, first- and second-degree localized burns, and sunburn.

Action

Topical antiinflammatory agents diffuse across cell membranes and form complexes with cytoplasm. These complexes stimulate the synthesis of inhibitory enzymes that are responsible for the antiinflammatory effects, which include inhibition of edema, erythema, pruritus, capillary dilation, and phagocyte activity. Topical corticosteroids can be classified based on potency, as follows:

- *Low-potency agents* provide modest antiinflammatory effects. These agents are safest for long-term application, facial and intertriginous application, use with occlusive dressings, and for infants and young children.
- *Medium-potency agents* are active against moderate inflammatory conditions, such as chronic eczematous dermatoses. These agents may be used for facial and intertriginous application for a limited time only.
- *High-potency agents* are effective in more severe inflammatory conditions, such as lichen simplex chronicus and psoriasis. These agents may be used for facial and intertriginous application for a short time only and can be used on skin thickened by chronic conditions.
- *Very-high-potency agents* offer an alternative to systemic therapy for local effects, such as with chronic lesions caused by psoriasis. Because they pose an increased risk of skin atrophy, these agents should be used only for short periods on small areas without occlusive dressings.

Topical corticosteroids

Name	Availability	Potency	Side effects
Alclometasone (Aclovate)	C, O: 0.05%	Low	Burning, stinging, irritation, itching, rash
Amcinonide (Cyclocort)	C, O, L: 0.1%	High	Same as above
Betamethasone dipropionate (Diprosone)	C, O, G, L: 0.05%	High	Same as above
Betamethasone valerate (Valisone)	C: 0.01%, 0.05%, 0.1%; O: 0.1%; L: 0.1%	High	Same as above
Clobetasol (Temovate)	C, O: 0.05%	High	Same as above
Desonide (Tridesilon)	C, O, L: 0.05%	Low	Same as above
Desoximetasone (Topicort)	C: 0.25%, 0.5%; O: 0.25%; G: 0.05%	High	Same as above
Dexamethasone (Decadron)	C: 0.1%	Medium	Same as above
Fluocinolone (Synalar)	C: 0.01%, 0.025%, 0.2%; O: 0.025%	High	Same as above
Fluocinonide (Lidex)	C, O, G: 0.05%	High	Same as above
Fluticasone (Cutivate)	C: 0.05%; O: 0.005%	Medium	Same as above
Halobetasol (Ultravate)	C, O: 0.05%	High	Same as above
Hydrocortisone (Cort-Dome, Hytone)	C, O: 0.5%, 1%, 2.5%	Medium	Same as above
Mometasone (Elocon)	C, O, L: 0.1%	Medium	Same as above
Prednicarbate (Dermatop)	C: 0.1%	—	Same as above
Triamcinolone (Aristocort, Kenalog)	C, O, L: 0.025%, 0.1%, 0.5%	Medium	Same as above

C, Cream; *G*, gel; *L*, lotion; *O*, ointment.

Miscellaneous Topical Agents

Uses

Miscellaneous topical agents are used to treat dermatologic disorders, such as acne, dermatitis, and infections. Some are also used to prevent certain dermatologic disorders and relieve localized pain.

Action

Miscellaneous topical agents act in various ways. Some *antiinfectives*, such as *docosanol, mupirocin*, and *penciclovir*, prevent viral or bacterial replication; *silver sulfadiazine* acts on bacterial cell walls, producing bactericidal effects. *Becaplermin* is a platelet-derived growth factor that stimulates new tissue growth to heal open wounds. *Capsaicin* depletes and prevents the accumulation of substance P (a mediator of pain impulses) from peripheral sensory neurons to the central nervous system, relieving pain. *Pimecrolimus* is an antiinflammatory agent that inhibits the release of cytokine, an enzyme that produces inflammatory reactions. *Tretinoin* decreases the cohesiveness of follicular epithelial cells and increases their turnover.

Appendix B: Eye and topical agents

Miscellaneous topical agents

Name	Indications	Dosages	Side effects
Azelaic acid (Azelex)	Treatment of mild to moderate acne vulgaris	Apply to affected area 2 times/day.	Pruritus, stinging, burning, tingling
Becaplermin (Regranex)	Treatment of lower-leg diabetic neuropathic ulcers extending into subcutaneous tissue or beyond	Apply once daily. After 12 hr, rinse ulcer and re-cover with saline gauze.	Local rash near ulcer
Capsaicin (Zostrix)	Treatment of neuralgia, osteoarthritis, and rheumatoid arthritis	Apply directly to affected area 3-4 times/day.	Burning, stinging, erythema at application site
Collagenase (Santyl)	Debridement of necrotic tissue in chronic dermal ulcers and severe burns	Apply once daily, or more frequently if dressing becomes soiled.	Transient erythema
Docosanol (Abreva)	Treatment of cold sores or fever blisters caused by herpes simplex virus, type 1 or 2	Apply to lesions 5 times/day at onset of symptoms and until lesions are healed, up to a maximum of 10 days.	Headache, skin irritation
Eflornithine (Vaniqua)	Reduction of unwanted facial and chin hair	Apply to affected area 2 times/day at least 8 hr apart.	Anemia, leukopenia, thrombocytopenia, dizziness, alopecia, vomiting, diarrhea, hearing impairment
Imiquimod (Aldara)	Treatment of external genital and perianal warts (condylomata acuminata)	Apply 3 times/wk before normal sleeping hours. Leave on skin for 6-10 hr, then remove. Continue for a maximum of 16 wk.	Local skin reactions, erythema, itching, burning, excoriation, flaking, fungal infection
Mupirocin (Bactroban)	*Topical:* Treatment of impetigo and infected traumatic skin lesions *Nasal:* Reduction of spread of methicillin-resistant *S. aureus*	*Topical:* Apply 3 times/day. *Nasal:* Apply 2 times/day for 5 days.	*Topical:* Pain, burning, stinging, itching *Nasal:* Headache, rhinitis, upper respiratory congestion, pharyngitis, altered taste
Penciclovir (Denavir)	Treatment of recurrent herpes labialis (cold sores)	Apply every 2 hr while awake for 4 days.	Headache, mild erythema, altered taste, rash
Pimecrolimus (Elidel)	Treatment of mild to moderate atopic dermatitis (eczema)	Apply 2 times/day.	Upper respiratory tract infection, nasopharyngitis, burning, pyrexia, cough, nasal congestion, abdominal pain, sore throat, headache
Povidone-iodine (Betadine)	External antiseptic action	Apply as needed.	Rash, pruritus, local edema
Sertaconazole (Ertaczo)	Treatment of superficial dermatophytic and candidal infections	Apply 2 times/day.	Headache, drowsiness, pruritus, erythema
Silver sulfadiazine (Silvadene)	Prevention and treatment of infection in second- and third-degree burns; protection against conversion from partial- to full-thickness wounds	Apply 1-2 times/day.	Burning feeling at application site, rash, itching, increased skin sensitivity to sunlight
Tretinoin (Retin-A)	Treatment of acne vulgaris	Apply once/day at bedtime.	Transient pigmentation changes, photosensitivity, local inflammatory reactions (peeling, dry skin, stinging, pruritus)

Metric System

Weight

kilogram = kg = 1000 grams
gram = g = 1 gram
milligram = mg = 0.001 gram
microgram = μg = 0.001 milligram

Volume

liter = L = 1000 milliliters
milliliter = mL = 0.001 liter

Household equivalents (approximate)

Utensil	Volume
1 teaspoonful	5 mL
1 tablespoonful	15 mL
1 teacupful	120 mL
1 tumbler glass	240 mL
1 pint	480 mL

Weight conversion: kilograms to pounds

Kilograms (kg)	Pounds (lb)
1	2.2
10	22
15	33
20	44
40	88
60	132
80	176

Appendix D: Abbreviations

ā	before
aa	of each
ab	antibody
abd	abdomen
ABGs	arterial blood gases
ac	before meals *(ante cibum)*
ACE	angiotensin-converting enzyme
ACEI	angiotensin-converting enzyme inhibitor
ACh	acetylcholine
ACT	activated clotting time
ACTH	adrenocorticotropic hormone
ad lib	as desired
ADH	antidiuretic hormone
ADP	adenosine diphosphate
ADR	adverse drug reaction
AIDS	acquired immunodeficiency syndrome
aka	also known as
ALT	alanine transaminase, serum
ama	against medical advice
amb	ambulation
amp	ampule
ANA	antinuclear antibody
ant	anterior
ANUG	acute necrotizing ulcerative gingivitis
AP	anteroposterior
APAP	acetaminophen
APB	atrial premature beats
aPTT	activated partial thromboplastin time
ARC	AIDS-related complex
AROM	active range of motion
ASA	acetylsalicylic acid (aspirin)
asap	as soon as possible
ASHD	arteriosclerotic heart disease
AST	aspartate transaminase, serum
AV	arteriovenous
A-V	atrioventricular
BAC	blood alcohol concentration
bid	twice a day *(bis in die)*
BM	bowel movement
BMR	basal metabolic rate
bol	bolus
BP	blood pressure
BPH	benign prostatic hypertrophy
bpm	beats per minute
BS	blood sugar
BUN	blood urea nitrogen

c̄	with
C	Celsius (centigrade)
C section	cesarean section (birth)
CA	cancer
Ca	calcium
CAD	coronary artery disease
cAMP	cyclic adenosine monophosphate
cap	capsule
cath	catheterization, catheterize
CBC	complete blood count
CCB	calcium channel blocker
CC	chief complaint
cc	cubic centimeter
cGMP	cyclic guanosine monophosphate
CHD	coronary heart disease
CHF	congestive heart failure
CK	creatine kinase
cm	centimeter
CML	chronic myeloid leukemia
CMV	cytomegalovirus
CNS	central nervous system
CO_2	carbon dioxide
CoA	coenzyme A
c/o	complains of
CO	cardiac output, carbon monoxide
COMT	catechol-O-methyltransferase
con rel	controlled release (dose form)
conc	concentration
COPD	chronic obstructive pulmonary disease
COX-2	cyclooxygenase 2
CPAP	continuous positive airway pressure
CPK	creatinine phosphokinase
CPR	cardiopulmonary resuscitation
CrCl	creatinine clearance
CRD	chronic respiratory disease
CRF	chronic renal failure
C&S	culture and sensitivity
CSF	cerebrospinal fluid
CTZ	chemoreceptor trigger zone
CV	cardiovascular
CVA	cerebrovascular accident (stroke)
CVP	central venous pressure
CysLt1	cysteinyl leukotriene receptor
D&C	dilation and curettage
del rel	delayed release (dose form)
DIC	disseminated intravascular coagulation

Appendix D: Abbreviations

DM	diabetes mellitus
DMARD	disease-modifying antirheumatic drug
DNA	deoxyribonucleic acid
DOB	date of birth
dr	dram
dsg	dressing
DVT	deep vein (venous) thrombosis
D_3W	5% dextrose (glucose) in distilled water
dx	diagnosis
EBV	Epstein-Barr virus
ECG, EKG	electrocardiogram
EEG	electroencephalogram
EENT	ear, eye, nose, throat
elix	elixir*
ENDO	endocrine system
EPO	erythropoietin
EPS	extrapyramidal symptoms
ESR	erythrocyte sedimentation rate
ext rel	extended release (dose form)
F	Fahrenheit
FBS	fasting blood sugar
FHT	fetal heart tone
FIO_2	inspired oxygen concentration
FSH	follicle-stimulating hormone
fx	fracture
g	gram
GABA	γ-aminobutyric acid
gal	gallon
GERD	gastroesophageal reflux disease
GGPT	γ-glutamyl transpeptidase
GHb	glycosylated hemoglobin
GI	gastrointestinal
G6PD	glucose-6-phosphate dehydrogenase
gr	grain
GR	glucocorticoid receptor
gtt	drops
GTT	glucose tolerance test
GU	genitourinary
Gyn	gynecology
HbA_{1c}	lab test for glycosylated hemoglobin
Hct	hematocrit
HCG	human chorionic gonadotropin
HDL	high-density lipoprotein
HEMA	hematologic system
Hgb	hemoglobin
HIV	human immunodeficiency virus

*Hydroalcoholic solution containing active drug(s).

H&H	hematocrit and hemoglobin
H&P	history and physical exam
5-HIAA	5-hydroxyindole acetic acid
HMG-CoA	3-hydroxy-3-methylglutaryl coenzyme A reductase
5-HT	5-hydroxytryptamine (serotonin)
H_2O	water
HPA	hypothalamic-pituitary-adrenocortical axis
HR	heart rate
HRT	hormone replacement therapy
hr	hour
hs	at bedtime (hora somni)
HSV	herpes simplex virus
HSV-2	herpes genitalis (herpes simplex virus type 2)
hypo	hypodermically
Hx	history
IBS	irritable bowel syndrome
ICP	intracranial pressure
ICU	intensive care unit
IDDM	insulin-dependent diabetes mellitus
I&D	incision and drainage
IgG	immunoglobulin G
IL-2	interleukin-2
IM	intramuscular
immed rel	immediate release (dose form)
inf	infusion
inh	inhalation
inj	injection
INR	international normalizing ratio
INTEG	relating to integumentary structures
IOP	intraocular pressure
IPPB	intermittent positive-pressure breathing
ITP	idiopathic thrombocytopenic purpura
IU	international units
IUD	intrauterine contraceptive device
IV	intravenous
IVP	intravenous piggyback
K	potassium
kg	kilogram
L or l	left
L	liter
lat	lateral
lb	pound
LDH	lactic dehydrogenase
LDL	low-density lipoprotein
LDL-C	low-density lipoprotein cholesterol
LE	lupus erythematosus

Appendix D: Abbreviations

LFT	liver function test
LH	luteinizing hormone
LHRH	luteinizing hormone–releasing hormone
liq	liquid
LLQ	left lower quadrant
LMP	last menstrual period
LOC	loss of consciousness
lot	lotion
loz	lozenge
LR	lactated Ringer's solution
LRI	lower respiratory infection
LVD	left ventricular dysfunction
m	meter
m^2	square meter
MAC	*Mycobacterium avium* complex
MAO	monoamine oxidase
max	maximum
META	metabolic
mEq	milliequivalent
mg	milligram
μg	microgram
MI	myocardial infarction
min	minute
mixt	mixture
mL	milliliter
mm	millimeter
mo	month
MPA	mycophenolic acid
MS	musculoskeletal
MVA	motor vehicle accident
Na	sodium
NC	nasal cannula
neg	negative
ng	nanogram
NIDDM	non–insulin-dependent diabetes mellitus
NKA	no known allergies
NMDA	*N*-methyl-D-aspartate
NMI	no middle initial
noc	nocturnal (night)
NPH	neutral protamine Hagedorn
NPO	nothing by mouth *(nil per os)*
NS	normal saline
NSAID	nonsteroidal antiinflammatory drug
NV	neurovascular
O_2	oxygen
OBS	organic brain syndrome

OC	oral contraceptive
OD	right eye *(oculus dexter)*
oint	ointment
OOB	out of bed
ophth	ophthalmic
OR	operating room
ORIF	open reduction, internal fixation
OS	left eye *(oculus sinister)*
OTC	over the counter
OU	each eye *(oculi unitas)*
oz	ounce
$\bar{p}$	after (post)
P	pulse
PABA	paraaminobenzoic acid
PAC	premature atrial contraction
$PaCO_2$	arterial carbon dioxide tension (partial pressure)
PaO_2	arterial oxygen tension (partial pressure)
PAT	paroxysmal atrial tachycardia
PBI	protein-bound iodine
PBP	penicillin-binding protein
pc	after meals *(post cibum)*
PCA	patient-controlled analgesia
PCN	penicillin
PE	physical examination
PG	prostaglandin
pH	hydrogen ion concentration
PMDD	premenstrual dysphoric disorder
PMS	premenstrual syndrome
PNS	peripheral nervous system
PO	by mouth *(per os)*
postop	postoperative(ly)
PP	postprandial
ppm	parts per million
preop	preoperative(ly)
prep	preparation
prn	as needed *(pro re nata)*
PSA	prostate-specific antigen
PT	prothrombin time
PTSD	posttraumatic stress disorder
PTT	partial thromboplastin time
PVC	premature ventricular contraction
PVD	peripheral vascular disease
q	every
qam	every morning
qd	every day
qh	every hour

Appendix D: Abbreviations

qid	four times a day
qod	every other day
qpm	every night
qt	quart
q2h	every 2 hours
q3h	every 3 hours
q4h	every 4 hours
q6h	every 6 hours
q12h	every 12 hours
qwk	every week
R	right
rap disintegr	rapidly disintegrating
RAR	retinoic acid receptor
RBC	red blood cell (or count)
RDA	recommended dietary allowance
rec	rectal
REM	rapid eye movement
RESP	respiratory system
rhPDGF-BB	recombinant human platelet-derived growth factor
RNA	ribonucleic acid
R/O	rule out
ROAD	reversible obstructive airway disease
ROM	range of motion
RTI	respiratory tract infection
Rx	therapy, treatment, or prescription
$\bar{s}$	without *(sine)*
SA	sinoatrial
SAN	sinoatrial node
SC	subcutaneous
sec	second
SERM	selective estrogen receptor modulator
SGOT	serum glutamic-oxaloacetic transaminase (now *AST*)
SGPT	serum glutamic-pyruvate transaminase (now *ALT*)
SIADH	syndrome of inappropriate antidiuretic hormone
sig	patient dosing instructions on prescription label
SL	sublingual
SLE	systemic lupus erythematosus
slow rel	slow release
SMBG	self-monitored blood glucose
SMZ	sulfamethoxazole
SOB	short of breath
sol	solution
ss	one half
SSRI	selective serotonin reuptake inhibitor
stat	at once
STD	sexually transmitted disease

surg	surgical
sus rel	sustained release (dose form)
supp	suppository
Sx	symptoms
syr	syrup*
T	temperature
$T_{1/2}$	drug half-life
T_3	triiodothyronine
T_4	thyroxine
tab	tablet
TB	tuberculosis
TBG	thyroxine-binding globulin
tbsp	tablespoon
TCA	tricyclic antidepressant
TD	transdermal
temp	temperature
TG	total triglycerides
TIA	transient ischemic attack
tid	three times daily *(ter in die)*
time rel	time release (dose form)
tinc	tincture, alcoholic solution of a drug
TMD	temporomandibular dysfunction
TMJ	temporomandibular joint
TMP	trimethoprim
TNF	tumor necrosis factor
top	topical
tPA	tissue plasminogen activator
TPN	total parenteral nutrition
TPR	temperature, pulse, respirations
TSH	thyroid-stimulating hormone
tsp	teaspoon
TT	thrombin time
Tx	treatment
U	unit
UA	urinalysis
ULDL	ultra-low-density lipoprotein
URI	upper respiratory infection
USP	United States Pharmacopeia
UTI	urinary tract infection
UV	ultraviolet
vag	vaginal
visc	viscous
VD	venereal disease
VHDL	very-high-density lipoprotein
VLDL	very-low-density lipoprotein
VO	verbal order

*Highly concentrated sucrose solution containing drug(s).

Appendix D: Abbreviations

vol	volume
VPB	ventricular premature beats
VS	vital signs
WBC	white blood cell (count)
WHO	World Health Organization
wk	week
WNL	within normal limits
wt	weight
yr	year
>	greater than
<	less than
≠	not equal
↑	increase
↓	decrease
2°	secondary

Common medications for treating open-angle glaucoma

Class	Generic name	Dosage	Side effects	Comments
Miotics	Pilocarpine	0.5%-6.0% drops, 2-4 times/day	Small pupil, blurred vision, dim vision, night blindness, headache, increased myopia, increased cataract, tearing, red eyes, increased ocular inflammation, retinal detachment, abdominal cramps, diarrhea, sweating, urinary retention	Systemic side effects more likely in smaller individuals; echothiophate is considerably more potent than pilocarpine or carbachol.
	Pilocarpine gel	4% drops, once/day		
	Carbachol	0.75%-3.00% drops, 2-3 times/day		
	Echothiophate	0.03%-0.25% drops, 1-2 times/day		
Prostaglandins	Latanoprost Bimatoprost Travoprost	0.005% drops, once/day	Increased iris pigmentation, burning, irritation, allergy, increased ocular inflammation, red eyes	Act by increasing uveoscleral outflow.
Combined α- and β-adrenergic agonists	Epinephrine Dipivefrin	1%-2%drops, 2 times/day 0.1% drops, 2 times/day	Red eyes, irritation, allergy, dilated pupil, blurred vision, pigment deposits in conjunctiva and tear ducts, increased blood pressure, rapid or irregular heartbeat, heart attack, headaches, anxiety, insomnia	Dipivefrin usually has fewer side effects than epinephrine, but less than 50% of patients have long-term tolerance for either drug.
Pure α$_2$-adrenergic agonists	Apraclonidine	0.5% drops, 2-3 times/day	Red eyes, irritation, allergy, dry eyes, dry mouth, decreased blood pressure	Brimonidine may have better long-term tolerance in patients than apraclonidine.
	Brimonidine	0.5% drops, 2-3 times/day		
Nonselective β-adrenergic blockers	Timolol	0.25%-0.5% drops, 1-2 times/day	Burning, allergy, corneal erosions, decreased corneal sensitivity, slow heartbeat, heart failure, low blood pressure, fainting, depression, loss of libido, fatigue, shortness of breath, asthma, decreased exercise tolerance, sudden death	Betaxolol (a selective β-blocker) has fewer side effects than the nonselective agents, but it is less effective in lowering intraocular pressure.
	Timolol gel	0.25%-0.5% drops, once/day		
	Levobunolol	0.25%-0.5% drops, 1-2 times/day		
	Metipranolol	0.3% drops, 2 times/day		
	Carteolol	1% drops, 2 times/day		
Selective β$_1$-adrenergic blockers	Betaxolol	0.5% drops, 2 times/day	See Nonselective β-adrenergic blockers.	
Carbonic anhydrase inhibitors	Betaxolol suspension	0.25% drops, 2 times/day		See Nonselective β-adrenergic blockers.
	Dorzolamide	2% drops, 2-3 times/day	Red eyes, irritation, allergy, tingling in fingers and toes, weakness, fatigue, depression, loss of appetite, weight loss, alteration of sense of taste, loss of libido, Stevens-Johnson syndrome, kidney stones, increased urination, acidosis, anemia, bone marrow suppression	Dorzolamide, the topical eyedrop, has less risk of side effects than the oral agents, acetazolamide or methazolamide; carbonic anhydrase inhibitors should not be in patients allergic to sulfa drugs.
	Acetazolamide	125- or 250-mg pills or 500-mg capsule, 1-4 times/day		
	Methazolamide	25- or 50-mg pills, 1-3 times/day		

Appendix F: Visual field defects   (368.4)

Definition

A visual field defect is a manifestation of a lesion somewhere in the visual pathway. Visual field defects are useful for localizing the abnormal area of the visual pathway but rarely are diagnostic of a specific disease entity. The table lists the types of visual field defects characteristic of lesions in various areas of the visual pathways, as well as some of the common diseases that may produce those defects.

Visual field defects, location, and common causative disease entities

Location of lesion	Visual field defect	Common disease entities
Transparent media	Generalized loss of sensitivity (368.45)	Corneal opacity, cataract, vitreous opacity or hemorrhage, miosis
Retina	Generalized loss of sensitivity (368.45)	Diabetic retinopathy, ocular ischemia, central retinal artery or vein occlusion, panretinal photocoagulation
	Localized scotoma (368.44)	Focal retinal lesions (e.g., tumors, inflammatory lesions, old scars, branch retinal vessel occlusions, macular degeneration, retinoschisis, retinal detachment)
	Ring scotoma, peripheral constriction (368.44)	Retinitis pigmentosa
Optic disc, peripapillary retina	Nerve fiber bundle defect: paracentral scotoma (368.41), sector or arcuate defect (368.43), altitudinal defect (368.43)	Glaucoma, arteritic and nonarteritic ischemic optic neuropathy, optic disc drusen, chronic papilledema, peripapillary choroiditis, hemiretinal vein or artery occlusion
Optic nerve	Nerve fiber bundle defect (see Optic disc, peripapillary retina), central and cecocentral scotoma (368.41)	Optic neuritis, toxic and nutritional optic neuropathies, traumatic optic neuropathy, orbital and optic nerve tumors, thyroid ophthalmopathy, orbital pseudotumor, orbital apex and sphenoid-ridge tumors
Optic chasm	Junctional scotoma, bitemporal hemianopic defects (368.47)	Pituitary tumors, craniopharyngioma, aneurysms, demyelinating disease, meningiomas
Optic tract, lateral geniculate body	Incongruous homonymous hemianopias (368.46)	Demyelinating disease, vascular occlusions, meningiomas, gliomas, aneurysms
Optic radiations	Homonymous quadrant and hemianopias (368.46)	Cerebral infarctions, intracranial tumors
Occipital cortex	Congruous homonymous scotomas or hemianopias, often with macular sparing (368.46)	Cerebral infarctions, intracranial tumors, closed-head trauma

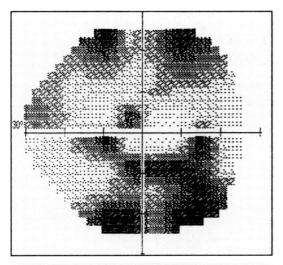

Figure 1 Glaucomatous visual field defect showing superior and inferior nerve fiber bundle types of defect.

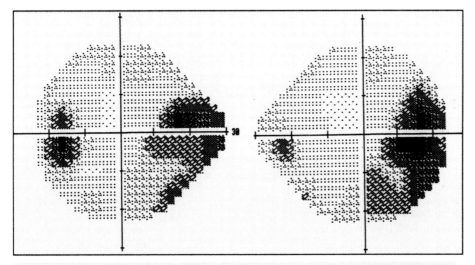

Figure 2 Left and right visual fields of a patient showing a left homonymous hemianopic visual field defect consistent with a lesion in the occipital lobe.

General references

Anderson DR: *Automated static perimetry*, St Louis, 1992, Mosby–Year Book.

Budenz DL: *Atlas of visual fields*, Philadelphia, 1997, Lippincott-Raven.

Harrington DO, Drake MV: *The visual fields text and atlas of clinical perimetry*, St Louis, 1990, Mosby.

Werner EB: Interpreting automated visual fields, *Ophthalmol Clin North Am* 8:229-257, 1995.

Appendix G: Nystagmus (379.50)

Cause

Nystagmus is an involuntary, rhythmic, biphasic oscillation of the eyes that results from a defect in tonus of the eye muscles from visual input disorders, labyrinthine disease, or disease of the central nervous system.

Natural History

The onset of *congenital nystagmus* usually is in the first few years of life and undergoes a metamorphosis in intensity and waveform. *Spasmus nutans* presents at 6 mo and lasts for 12 mo, usually resolving by 3 yr of age. *Acquired nystagmus* from a unilateral vestibular lesion recovers within 2 mo as vestibular tone is balanced again. *Central vestibular nystagmus* has a variable course depending on its cause.

Pathophysiology

Depends on type of nystagmus.

Nystagmus type	Description	Anatomic substrate
Congenital	Horizontal nystagmus with mixed waveform; remains horizontal in upgaze; intensity diminishes in a null zone and on convergence; worsens on fixation; inversion of optokinetic nystagmus response; latent component.	Unknown
Spasmus nutans	High-frequency, low-amplitude "quivering" of the eye in infants between 6 mo and 3 yr of age.	Unknown
Peripheral vestibular	Mixed horizontal and torsional waveform that intensifies when fixation is suppressed.	Inner ear
Rebound	When the eyes return to primary gaze after sustained eccentric gaze, there is a jerk nystagmus with fast phase in the opposite direction.	Cerebellum
Internuclear ophthalmoplegia	In eccentric horizontal gaze, an adducting deficit in one eye and a dissociated abducting nystagmus in the fellow eye.	Medial longitudinal fasciculus
Periodic alternating	Jerk nystagmus that reverses to the opposite direction every 90-120 sec.	Nodulus of cerebellum
Downbeat	Central vestibular jerk nystagmus with fast phase down.	Vestibulo-ocular projections in the cervicomedullary junction
Upbeat	Central vestibular jerk nystagmus with fast phase up.	Vestibulo-ocular projections in the medulla and cerebellum
Seesaw	One eye rises and extorts, whereas the other depresses and intorts.	Interstitial nucleus of Cajal
Convergence retraction	Opposed adducting saccades that retract and converge the eyes in attempted upgaze.	Dorsal midbrain
Superior oblique myokymia	Monocular, torsional-vertical, low-amplitude, high-frequency eye movement and high-amplitude, low-frequency eye movement.	Midbrain (fourth-nerve nucleus)
Ocular flutter	Intermittent bursts of horizontal saccades.	Selective cells in pons
Opsoclonus	Intermittent bursts of saccades in all directions.	Selective cells in pons
Oculopalatal myoclonus	Pendular, elliptical, vertical nystagmoid movement that moves synchronously with the palate.	Dentorubral-olivary pathway

General Information

The diagnosis of nystagmus is made on the basis of evaluating the position maintenance system.

Signs

- Nystagmus may present in one of three waveforms:

"Jerk" waveform: refers to slow phases (drifts) and quick phases (corrections). The slow phase reflects the underlying abnormality; however, the nystagmus is named by its "fast" phase.

Pendular waveform: describes a sinusoidal and rotational (circling movement) oscillation.

Rotary waveform: describes a circling movement.

- Nystagmus is also described by its *frequency* (low: <2 Hz; medium: 2-15 Hz; high: >15 Hz). *Amplitude* can be in millimeters or degrees (low: <1 mm or <7 degrees; medium: 1-3 mm or 7-21 degrees; high: >3 mm or >21 degrees). Intensity of the nystagmus is defined as amplitude times frequency.

Symptoms

The three most common symptoms are blurred vision, double vision, and *oscillopsia* (illusion that environment is moving). *Jerk nystagmus* creates the special effect that the world is moving in one direction. *Pendular nystagmus* creates the illusion that the world is rocking back and forth. A *superior oblique nystagmus* creates the illusion that the world is quivering.

Differential Diagnosis

Nystagmoid movements that mimic nystagmus include *saccadic intrusions* such as square wave jerks, macrosquare wave jerks, macrosaccadic oscillations, ocular flutter, opsoclonus, and superior oblique myokymia. These are classified as "saccadic oscillations" with and without "saccadic intervals."

Management

- *Yoked prisms* can be beneficial for congenital nystagmus. The prisms are coupled to place the eyes in the null zone, thereby reducing nystagmus intensity. This improves visual acuity and reduces head turn. Base-out prisms can damp the nystagmus by causing convergence. (Remember to add minus dioptric power to the lens prescription when this is done.) Yoked base-down prisms can be prescribed for patient with downbeat nystagmus.
- Baclofen can be effective in reducing the intensity of acquired periodic alternating nystagmus. Other medications used to treat central vestibular nystagmus include clonazepam, carbamazepine, and valproate.
- Only congenital jerk nystagmus is amenable to surgery (Kestenbaum procedure).

Examination Techniques

- A good way to detect and gauge nystagmus is with the direct ophthalmoscope. If the disc remains in the field of view, the nystagmus amplitude is approximately 4-5 degrees.
- Acquired nystagmus must be included in the differential in patients who complain of monocular diplopia.
- A patient with congenital nystagmus requires a trial frame to refract in the patient's null zone.

General references

Cogan DG: Internuclear ophthalmoplegia: typical and atypical, *Arch Ophthalmol* 84:583-589, 1970.

Davis DG, Smith JL: Periodic alternating nystagmus, *Am J Ophthalmol* 72:737-762, 1971.

Dell'Osso LF, Traccis S, Abel LA, et al: Contact lenses and congenital nystagmus, *Clin Vis Sci* 3:229-232, 1988.

Ellenberger C, Netsky MG: Anatomic basis and diagnostic value of opsoclonus, *Arch Ophthalmol* 83:307-310, 1970.

Leigh RJ, Zee DS: *The neurology of eye movements*, ed 2, Philadelphia, 1991, Davis.

Norton EWD, Cogan DG: Spasmus nutans: a clinical study of 20 cases followed two years or more since onset, *Arch Ophthalmol* 52:442-446, 1954.

Reinecke RD, Suqin G, Goldstein HP: Waveform evolution in infantile nystagmus: an electro-oculo-graphic study of 35 cases, *Binocul Vis* 3:191-202, 1988.

Page numbers followed by f indicate figures.

Index

Index

Index

Index

Episcleral veins, dilation, 141f
Episcleral venous pressure
    elevation, causes, 140
    measurement, 138
Episcleral venous pressure (elevation),
        glaucoma (association), 138-141
    diagnosis, 138, 140
    differential diagnosis, 138
    features, 138
    follow-up/management, 139
    prognosis, 139
    treatment, 139, 141
Episcleral venous pressure (elevation),
        orbital meningeal shunt (impact),
        141f
Episcleritis, 2, 150
Epithelial cells, presence, 115f
Epithelial disease, 195
Epithelioid cells, 265f, 323f
Erb-Goldflam disease, 232
ERG. See Echoretinography
Erythema. See Eyelid erythema
    extent, evaluation, 200
    presence. See Left upper medial canthus
Erythrocyte sedimentation rate (ESR), 24,
        190, 274
Erythromycin, 91, 251
Escherichia coli sepsis, 297
Esotropia, 8, 110-111
    diagnosis, 110
    differential diagnosis, 110
    epidemiology, 110
    follow-up/management, 111
    pathology, 110
    prognosis, 111
    treatment, 111
ESR. See Erythrocyte sedimentation rate;
        Westergren erythrocyte age-adjusted
        sedimentation rate
Essential/progressive iris atrophy
        (iridocorneal-endothelial syndrome),
        192-193
    classification, 192
    diagnosis, 192
    differential diagnosis, 192
    epidemiology, 192
    follow-up/management, 193
    pathology, 192
    prognosis, 193
    treatment, 193
Esthetic blemish, 8
Esthetic deformity, 220
Excision, 309
Exogenous bacterial endophthalmitis, 30
Exogenous endophthalmitis, 31
Exophthalmometry, 114
Exophthalmos, 176, 258. See also
        Noninfectious/nonendocrine
        exophthalmos; Ocular proptosis

orbit, cavernous hemangioma.
        See Right eye
Exorbitism, presence. See Graves' disease
Exotropia, 116-117
    creation, 239
    diagnosis, 116
    differential diagnosis, 116
    epidemiology, 116
    follow-up/management, 117
    prognosis, 117
    treatment, 117
Exposure keratitis, 260, 269
    impact, 267
External proton beam radiation, 207
External strabismus, 116
Extorsion, fundus camera (usage).
        See Left eye
Extracapsular cataract extraction (ECCE),
        38, 55
    endophthalmitis, postoperative
        development, 265f
Extramacular RPE, 72
Extraocular muscle (EOM), 108
    enlargement, 179f
    trapdoor entrapment, 224
Exudates, presence. See Neural retina
Eye agents, 330-333
Eyebrow arching, 36
Eyedrop use, history, 90
Eyelashes
    loss, 309f
    position, abnormality, 120
Eyelid conjunctivitis, follicular
        conjunctivitis (presence), 91f
Eyelid ectropion, 118-121
    classification, 118
    diagnosis, 118, 120
    differential diagnosis, 118
    follow-up/management, 119
    pathology, 118
    prognosis, 119
    treatment, 119, 121
Eyelid erythema, 125f
Eyelid hemorrhage, 122-123
    diagnosis, 122
    differential diagnosis, 122
    follow-up/management, 123
    immunology, 122
    prognosis, 123
    treatment, 123
Eyelid margins
    adjustment, 179
    blood vessels, prominence, 34
    inspissated oil gland, 34
    thickening, 118
Eyelid noninfectious dermatoses, 124-125
    classification, 124
    diagnosis, 124
    epidemiology, 124

follow-up/management, 125
immunology, 124
prognosis, 125
Eyelids
    discoloration, 122
    drooping, 102
    edema, 122
    fatigue, consistency. See Myasthenia
        gravis
    formation, destruction, 220
    growth/mass, presence, 306
    inflammation. See Chronic lid
        inflammation
    retraction, 176
        presence. See Graves' disease
    rubbing. See Cornea
    skin, redundancy, 102
    squamous cell carcinoma, 4
    sticking, symptom, 86, 90
    synkinesis, 221
Eyelid swelling, 34, 98, 126, 254
    cellulitis, acute ethmoiditis
        (impact), 257f
Eyes
    abduction movement, 244
    anterior chamber, blood (presence), 184
    constant wiping, 236
    crusting, 34
    enlargement, 152
    examination, 200, 238
    movement
        deficiency, 244
        limitation, 138. See also Bilateral eye
            movement
        pain, 252
    muscles, surgery, 11
    pain, 288
        symptom, 4, 52, 56
    rubbing, caution, 125
    skin excoriation, 236
    torsional righting, 96

F

FA. See Fluorescein angiography
Face, port-wine hemangioma, 136
Facial abnormalities, 116
Facial blemish, 266
Facial deformities, 266
Facial hemangioma, demonstration, 137f
Facial rash, 4
Farnsworth Munsell 100-hue test, 204
Farsightedness. See Hyperopia
Favism, 22
Fibrillar material, deposit, 166
Fibrosarcoma, 112
Fibrosis syndrome, 226-227
    diagnosis, 226
    differential diagnosis, 226
    epidemiology, 226

Index

Index

Index

Index

Index

Index